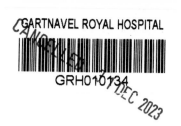

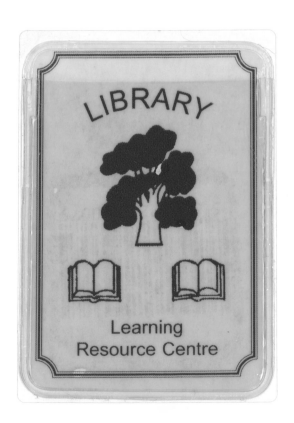

"Superb! The authors describe their evidence-based maintenance therapy for depression in great detail, while telling an engrossing (and well-referenced) story of how they developed their approach. Fascinating reading."
—*Ricardo F. Muñoz, PhD, Distinguished Professor of Clinical Psychology, Palo Alto University*

"A defining resource in the burgeoning arena of mindfulness-based therapies. The second edition incorporates new evidence from both clinical trials and neuroscientific studies of the mind, continuing the story of discovery of the mindfulness path out of chronic depression. Presented is up-to-date conceptual and clinical material that reflects the experience and wisdom of the authors, their colleagues, and the many individuals who have benefited from MBCT. As a graduate textbook for a course on either major depression or psychotherapeutic uses of meditation, this volume illustrates the theory and application of mindfulness-based approaches in an elegant and always readable manner."
—*Jean L. Kristeller, PhD, Department of Psychology, Indiana State University*

"Warmly written, accessible, and deeply insightful. This landmark book has played a key role in making mindfulness a central concern in clinical practice. The up-to-date second edition not only summarizes the extraordinary expansion of research evidence, but also is immensely practical and filled with clinical wisdom. Important, too, is its emphasis on compassion. A 'must' for all therapists interested in mindfulness."
—*Paul Gilbert, PhD, Head, Mental Health Research Unit, University of Derby, United Kingdom*

"A seminal book. Segal, Williams, and Teasdale have made a unique and enormous contribution to the field and have sparked a new generation of research in mindfulness-based approaches to emotional and physical conditions. This is a 'must read' book for anyone working in our field."
—Cognitive Behavioral Therapy Book Reviews *(on the first edition)*

"As a major plus, the book contains many practical tools useful to initiate an MBCT program, including client handouts. . . . The concepts discussed in this book are truly visionary."
—Psychiatry: Interpersonal & Biological Processes *(on the first edition)*

"Not your ordinary treatment manual for depression. . . . A skillful and practical integration of some key elements of a 2,500-year-old mind science with 21st-century cognitive psychology."
—Journal of Cognitive Psychotherapy *(on the first edition)*

"Readable and practical. An effective, brief group treatment for preventing depressive relapse is welcome news for patients, clinicians, and managed care companies alike."
— Psychiatric Services *(on the first edition)*

Mindfulness-Based Cognitive Therapy for Depression

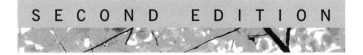

SECOND EDITION

Zindel V. Segal
J. Mark G. Williams
John D. Teasdale

Foreword by
Jon Kabat-Zinn

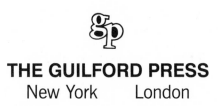

THE GUILFORD PRESS
New York   London

© 2013 The Guilford Press
A Division of Guilford Publications, Inc.
72 Spring Street, New York, NY 10012
www.guilford.com

Printed in the United States of America

This book is printed on acid-free paper.

Last digit is print number: 9   8   7   6   5   4   3   2

The authors have checked with sources believed to be reliable in their efforts to provide information that is complete and generally in accord with the standards of practice that are accepted at the time of publication. However, in view of the possibility of human error or changes in behavioral, mental health, or medical sciences, neither the authors, nor the editor and publisher, nor any other party who has been involved in the preparation or publication of this work warrants that the information contained herein is in every respect accurate or complete, and they are not responsible for any errors or omissions or the results obtained from the use of such information. Readers are encouraged to confirm the information contained in this book with other sources.

Library of Congress Cataloging-in-Publication Data

Segal, Zindel V., 1956–
  Mindfulness-based cognitive therapy for depression / Zindel V. Segal, J. Mark G. Williams, John D. Teasdale.—2nd ed.
      p. cm.
  Includes bibliographical references and index.
  ISBN 978-1-4625-0750-4 (hardcover)
  1. Depression, Mental—Treatment.   2. Mindfulness-based cognitive therapy.   I. Williams, J. Mark G.   II. Teasdale, John D.   III. Title.
  RC537.S44 2013
  616.85′270651—dc23
                                                                                2012018928

To Lisa, Ariel, Shira, and Solomon
—Z. V. Segal

To Phyllis, Rob, Jennie, and Annie
—J. M. G. Williams

To Jackie, Joe, and Ben
—J. D. Teasdale

About the Authors

Zindel V. Segal, PhD, is Distinguished Professor of Psychology in Mood Disorders at the University of Toronto—Scarborough. He is also the Director of Clinical Training in the Psychology Department's Graduate Program in Psychological Clinical Science. Dr. Segal's publications include *Interpersonal Process in Cognitive Therapy* (1990), *The Mindful Way through Depression* (2007), *Vulnerability to Depression* (2011), and *The Mindful Way Workbook* (2014). He is a founding Fellow of the Academy of Cognitive Therapy and advocates for the relevance of mindfulness-based clinical care in psychiatry and mental health.

J. Mark G. Williams, DPhil, is Professor of Clinical Psychology and Wellcome Principal Research Fellow at the University of Oxford. He also is Director of the Oxford Mindfulness Centre in the University of Oxford's Department of Psychiatry. Dr. Williams's publications include *The Psychological Treatment of Depression* (1992), *Cognitive Psychology and Emotional Disorders* (1997), *Suicide and Attempted Suicide* (2002), *The Mindful Way through Depression* (2007), *Mindfulness: Finding Peace in a Frantic World* (2011), and *The Mindful Way Workbook* (2014). He is a founding Fellow of the Academy of Cognitive Therapy and a Fellow of the Academy of Medical Sciences, the British Academy, and the Association for Psychological Science.

John D. Teasdale, PhD, held a Special Scientific Appointment with the United Kingdom Medical Research Council's Cognition and Brain Sciences Unit in Cambridge, England. His publications include *Affect, Cognition and Change* (1993), *The Mindful Way through Depression* (2007), and *The Mindful Way Workbook* (2014). Dr. Teasdale is a founding Fellow of the Academy of Cognitive Therapy and a Fellow of the British Academy and the Academy of Medical Sciences. He also is a recipient of the Distinguished Scientist Award from Division 12 (Society of Clinical Psychology) of the American Psychological Association. Since retiring, Dr. Teasdale has taught insight meditation internationally.

Foreword

I began the foreword to the first edition of this book with the words *"Mindfulness-Based Cognitive Therapy for Depression* is to my mind a seminal book." I can no longer say that. Ten years ago, it was seminal. Now, it is more appropriate and accurate to say that this new, revised, and updated edition is nothing short of transformational. As a professional book and as a treatment manual in particular, it sets a new standard of authenticity, fidelity, and relationality, not only in how it is structured, but, even more importantly, in how it is voiced—in other words, in its relationship with the reader as well as the subject.

This edition is in a class by itself, having exceeded in its first incarnation all expectations, although the underlying intention was, of course, there from the start: to make a profound difference for people at high risk for depressive relapse. Its appearance unleashed an avalanche of interest, clinical practice, and research throughout the world—indeed, it launched a whole new and highly sophisticated, evidence-based field within psychology and psychotherapy that did not exist 15 years ago. There is little doubt that the first edition, and the work of the authors upon which it was based, was a major contributor to the kinetics of the curve depicting the number of papers reporting on studies of mindfulness in the scientific and medical literature (Figure 1). At the time of this writing, this curve shows no signs of slowing down.

In reading this new version, appearing 10 years after the first edition, I was struck by two things. One was how much exquisite new material has been added, not just in the form of new chapters, but subtle revisions

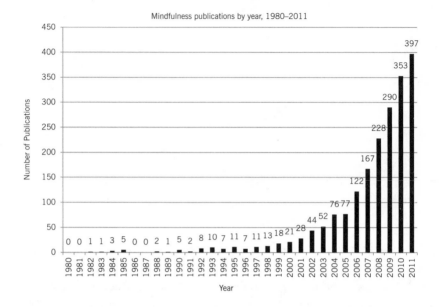

FIGURE 1. Results obtained from a search of the term "mindfulness" in the abstracts and keywords of the ISI Web of Knowledge database on March 19, 2012. The search was limited to publications with English language abstracts. Figure prepared by David Black, MPH, PhD, Cousins Center for Psychoneuroimmunology, Semel Institute for Neuroscience and Human Behavior, University of California, Los Angeles. Based on Williams and Kabat-Zinn (2011).

and restructuring of the text itself, refining, amplifying, and strengthening a number of key elements that 10 years of experience have made clear are critical to the effective delivery of mindfulness-based cognitive therapy (MBCT) in clinical settings, as well as to the understanding of the underlying and very clearly described theoretical framework upon which it rests. The other is that, in going back and forth between the first edition and this one to see exactly what was changed and in what ways, I was deeply moved all over again by how thorough, beautifully developed, and well argued the first edition was—in a tone at the same time invitational, logical, understated, and modest. I had forgotten. All that gold is still present. The authors have wisely kept vast swaths of the book as it was, since the basic rationale, structure, curriculum, and challenges of teaching MBCT have not changed. And into that material the authors have now seamlessly kneaded other essential ingredients that had intentionally been left to the side the first time, for reasons the authors themselves discuss. What we have now is this new and turbocharged version of MBCT, which we might call MBCT 2.0. While it is no different in essence from the first edition, it is now completely updated, more accessible, more complete, more supportive, and more explicit in what it takes to deliver such an intervention, which, after all, is the purpose of a treatment manual.

As in the first edition, the authors show themselves time and again to be master clinicians. This can be readily seen, for example, in their sensitivity and cautions about using self-compassion meditations with particularly vulnerable individuals. The authors are equally skillful mindfulness instructors. The new chapter on inquiry is a finely honed exegesis of that element of mindfulness-based interventions that many therapists find opaque or intimidating. It may still be intimidating, but we can no longer say it is opaque. They have parsed the unparsable, scripted the unscriptable, in a way that I have not seen done before, and they have done so with precision, sensitivity, and skill. I think all mindfulness-based instructors will be the beneficiaries of their gentle clarity and encouragement in this regard.

I for one have always been dubious about the possibility of "scripting" any aspect of a mindfulness-based intervention for those hoping to implement such a program, since our cardinal working principle is that the teaching has to come out of one's practice. Thus, to the bones of the curriculum need to be added the flesh and sinews of one's own experience with practice. In this edition, the authors have made it very clear that this is how they see it as well—in other words, that having one's own meditation practice as a deep, multidimensional, and textured resource for this curriculum is absolutely essential, not merely recommended. They are not saying that one cannot use elements of this work if one does not have one's own grounding in an ongoing practice of mindfulness. But they are explicitly saying that the work should only be called MBCT if indeed it is grounded in the instructor's own personal practice. They are both firm and compassionate on this point. Why? Because there is simply no other way to impart these practices to others and engage with them about their experiences with authenticity and depth without having inhabited them oneself over an extended period of time. Otherwise, as the authors themselves say, the intervention cannot possibly be "mindfulness based," and if it is not, then it cannot possibly be MBCT.

Here is a taste of the voicing:

> The ultimate aim of the MBCT program is to help individuals make a radical shift in their relationship to the thoughts, feelings, and body sensations that contribute to depressive relapse. The instructor's own basic understanding and orientation will be one of the most powerful influences affecting this process. Whether the instructor realizes it or not, this understanding colors the way each practice is presented, each interaction is handled. The cumulative effect of such coloring is that whatever the explicit message of the instructor's words, the more powerful influence, for good or ill, will be the nature of the instructor's basic, implicit views. (p. 64)

This is why it is so important for instructors (note they are not saying "therapists") to be aware of those basic, implicit views, and to refine and modulate their relationships to them through their own practice.

Elsewhere, they say: "The hallmark quality of an MBCT class, in fact, is that participants are treated more as guests than patients, with warm hospitality and respect for the courage that they show, even by turning up" (p. 137).

And again:

> Both the research data and our clinical experience suggest to us that only when people learn to take a different stance in relation to the "battleground" of their thoughts and feelings will they be able in the future to recognize difficult situations early and deal with them skillfully. Taking this different stance involves sampling a different mode of mind from that which we normally inhabit, *and which much therapy also inhabits*. It involves replacing the old mode of fixing and repairing problems with a new mode of allowing things to be just as they are, in order to see more clearly how best to respond. (p. 93, emphasis added)

This nonfixing and nondoing orientation may seem opaque to therapists at first blush, but inside its cultivation lies the potential for profound transformation and deep satisfaction on the part of both the patient and the therapist. Counterintuitive? Perhaps. Worth taking seriously? Without a doubt. This book effectively shows how the conditions for this *way of being in relationship to things* can unfold and be optimized.

New material in this edition, beyond the chapter on the inquiry process, includes mindful yoga; the day of mindfulness in the sixth week of the program; retitled chapters in some instances to refine the scope of particular sessions; a chapter devoted to, and a much stronger and more explicit emphasis throughout on, self-compassion, the embodiment of kindness, and their role in the curriculum; additional session handouts; and a tour-de-force look at the research to date in support of MBCT and how it might be exerting its effects on the tendency to relapse in major depression. It brings the biology of the "being mode" and the "doing mode" together with the effects of mindfulness training at the level of the body and at the level of the brain, underscoring the remarkable potential of paying attention and cultivating awareness in the systematic ways characteristic of mindfulness-based interventions.

To my mind, the introduction of mindfulness into psychological theory and into psychotherapy in the ways that MBCT is doing has the potential to enrich and transform the discipline itself and, ultimately, our understanding of the nature of the psyche and what we call the "self." Remarkably, recent brain studies by Zindel Segal's group (Farb et al., 2007) are elucidating different cortical networks that subtend two different modes of self-reference: one experiential, body based, and grounded in the present moment; the other thought based and grounded in a narrative of past and future, and, in some sense, potentially out of touch with the actuality of things. Mindfulness training has been shown to uncouple them, thus generating new possibilities for learning, growing, and healing. Such findings are essential evidence that the theoretical framework the authors put forward for understanding depressive rumination and the central role it plays in major depression, and the potential value of mindfulness in promoting a shift from a doing mode of mind to a being mode of mind, is very much on the right track.

In closing, I congratulate the authors on a remarkable job of offering to the world in a highly usable and friendly form a way of working with suffering and with the risks of depressive relapse that has rare efficacy and integrity. It also has potential applications far beyond depression. It will be interesting to see what another 10 years has in store for this still nascent field.

JON KABAT-ZINN, PhD

REFERENCES

Farb NA, Segal ZV, Mayberg H, Bean J, McKeon D, Fatima Z, Anderson AK. Attending to the present: Mindfulness meditation reveals distinct neural modes of self-reference. *Social Cognitive Affective Neuroscience* 2007; *2*: 313–322.

Williams JMG, Kabat-Zinn J. Mindfulness: Diverse perspectives on its meaning, origins, and multiple applications at the intersection of science and dharma [Special issue]. *Contemporary Buddhism* 2011; *12*(1): 1–18.

Acknowledgments

We are grateful to all those who, at different times and in different ways, have supported the further development and evaluation of mindfulness-based cognitive therapy (MBCT) and helped to sustain its vitality to a point where a second edition of this book is warranted. In addition to those named in the first edition, and although our thanks extend also to many whom we do not name, we would like to acknowledge the additional contribution of a number of people. From Toronto, we thank Susan Woods, Peter Bieling, Sona Dimidjian, Lucio Bizzini, Guido Bondolfi, Christophe Andre, Adam Anderson, Norman Farb, Graham Meadows, Patricia Rockman, and Stuart Eisendrath. From Oxford, we thank Catherine Crane, Danielle Duggan, Thorsten Barnhofer, Becca Crane, Sarah Silverton, Christina Surawy, Marie Johansson, Melanie Fennell, Antonia Sumbundu, and John Peacock. From Cambridge, we thank Christina Feldman, Willem Kuyken, Michael Chaskalson, Cieran Saunders (Ruchiraketu), Trish Bartley, and Alison Evans.

This book is not just an account of how we developed a treatment to prevent depressive relapse. It also chronicles our own step-by-step journey toward a very different paradigm for working with depression and its aftermath. In both areas, the staff of the Center for Mindfulness in Medicine, Health Care, and Society at the University of Massachusetts Medical School, especially Jon Kabat-Zinn, Saki Santorelli, Ferris Urbanowski, and Elana Rosenbaum, played a critical role, and further support over the years has been generously given by Melissa Blacker and Florence Meleo-Meyer.

We are also aware of how much our own thinking, as well as our teaching, has been influenced by other members of the mindfulness community. We continue to be extraordinarily fortunate to have the steadfast guidance, support, and wisdom of Jon Kabat-Zinn and Christina Feldman, both of whom have had a powerful influence on both what we taught and the style in which we taught. Other insight meditation teachers, especially Sharon Salzberg, Joseph Goldstein, Jack Kornfield, and Larry Rosenberg, have, through their written and spoken words, sharpened our understanding of the heart of mindfulness practice. Wherever we can trace a specific source for the way these teachers have influenced how we teach MBCT, we have acknowledged it, but we suspect that many of these influences may have become incorporated implicitly into our own approach, and we apologize if there is material we have failed to acknowledge.

Our efforts to continue this work past the point of our initial controlled analyses have been supported by grants from the National Institute of Mental Health (No. MH066992) and the Wellcome Trust (No. GR067797). Our personal support came from the Centre for Addiction and Mental Health, the University of Oxford, and the Medical Research Council of the United Kingdom.

We would also like to thank Jim Nageotte, Senior Editor at The Guilford Press, for his fine editorial guidance through the entire process. Also, Kevin Porter from A Musik Zone provided a steady hand and ear in producing the audio recordings.

Finally, our thanks and heartfelt appreciation go out to the courageous patients who took part in the MBCT groups. We are grateful to them for allowing us to reflect their experiences in this book. Working with them was, and continues to be, a vital part of our own learning and our inspiration. We are delighted that it was also of benefit to many of them.

Contents

PART III. EVALUATION AND DISSEMINATION

How to Use This Manual

The first edition of this manual included a number of forms and worksheets for readers to use as MBCT instructors and to distribute to participants. In this edition, you will once again find such forms; we gladly extend permission to individual book purchasers to make photocopies of these materials for their personal use with course participants. (Please see the particulars of this permission on the copyright page.)

For your convenience, we have also made the reproducible forms and worksheets available online (*www.guilford.com/MBCT_materials*), so individual book purchasers can download and print them as needed in a convenient 8½″ × 11″ size.

For this new edition, we have also created audio recordings of the mindfulness practice exercises in the book, which can be streamed directly from the Web or downloaded in MP3 format. Many participants find the recordings helpful, particularly when they are getting started practicing mindfulness. The audio tracks are available in two different locations: (1) on the instructor Web page, together with the reproducible forms and worksheets (*www.guilford.com/MBCT_materials*), and (2) on a Web page developed specifically for course participants (*www.guilford.com/MBCT_audio*). You can direct your course participants to *www.guilford.com/MBCT_audio* to access the recordings on their own. Alternately, you may wish to download the audio tracks yourself and burn them onto CDs or copy them to USB flash drives to distribute to participants at the first session.

Introduction

We would not have predicted that things would turn out like this. What you hold in your hands is the second edition of a book that was first published 10 years ago and was, in many ways, a fundamentally new departure for each of us. Little did we know that our attempts to understand recurrence processes in depression (and then to work out the practical implications of these understandings for prevention) would have the impact they have had. Looking back now, we can see that Jon Kabat-Zinn, in his Foreword to that edition, was more prescient. He said that the application of mindfulness in the domain of mental health would transform the field; that seeking to understand how these ancient wisdom practices could address the core processes maintaining vulnerability in depression, and to do so in the context of the latest psychological science, would be illuminating for all, allowing many who might otherwise take little notice to wake up to the huge transformative potential of cultivating moment by moment awareness.

In writing a second edition we faced several challenges. We needed to stay faithful to the intentions of the original but to be honest about any mistakes we had made. We wanted to explain better things that were unclear and have been misunderstood. We were keen to share new developments in both theory and practice, and to describe both aspects discarded in the light of experience and new elements included. A second edition has to say clearly what has changed, and what has remained the same.

In the first edition, we told the story of how, in 1992, we had started out to find a maintenance form of cognitive therapy, but found that both

1

laboratory and clinical findings, and our own experience, were pointing us in new directions. By 2002, after 10 years of research and a clinical trial, we offered in that edition our best insights into how we could understand ongoing risk of depression, and an eight-session program that might reduce that risk.

The reality is that by 2002, we had a reasonably firm foundation for some of the ideas that underpinned the program, but relatively little evidence for its effectiveness. After all, mindfulness as an approach to the treatment of depression was new to each of us. More than that, the problem we were seeking to tackle had emerged fairly recently within the field of depression. Only toward the late 1980s were clinicians coming to the stark realization that once a person has suffered depression on one occasion, it tends to recur. Previous treatments of depression had understandably focused on how to treat the acute episode, how to relieve the intense suffering of current depression. We wished to do something different: to help people stay well after an episode was over, to reduce ongoing risk. At the outset, we had not known how to do this. Far less did we think that an approach called insight (or "mindfulness") meditation might offer an answer.

This book retells and continues the story, starting with how we came to believe that this approach to depression was worth pursuing, based on the academic literature and our own research findings. The first step was to get a better theoretical understanding of recurrent depression; the second step was to implement these understandings. It was not plain sailing. The approach that later became known as mindfulness-based cognitive therapy (MBCT) was not our original intention, and even when we started down the road that took us to mindfulness, we did not call it MBCT.

In the first edition, we described in some detail the journey from the challenge of depression, through all our false starts to the provisional conclusion that mindfulness could be enormously empowering for many people who find themselves vulnerable to recurrence. We now need to go further, for there have been more studies revealing the nature of depression, more research evaluating the long-term effectiveness of antidepressants and other psychological treatments, more research on whether a mindfulness approach is effective, and for whom, and how, it works. In 2002 there were few studies using brain imaging; now there have been several key studies on what happens in the brain when people practice mindfulness.

Most striking of all has been the totally unexpected explosion of interest in using mindfulness for a large number of health and mental health conditions. In order to understand why this has happened, at least in the field of mental health in which we work, we need to go right back to the beginning of our collaboration. For at that time, we had not intended to go in this direction at all. So how on earth did we get from there to here?

Our story begins back in the summer of 1989. At that time Mark Williams and John Teasdale both worked at the Medical Research Council's Applied Psychology Unit (now called the Cognition and Brain Sciences Unit) in Cambridge, England, and Zindel Segal visited them in 1989, en route to the World Congress of Cognitive Therapy, which was meeting in Oxford that year. The three of us had a great deal in common, having each worked for some years on psychological models and treatment of depression. We were each to present papers at the Congress.

The discussion at that pre-Congress meeting in Cambridge was about the puzzles that recent research on cognition and emotion was throwing up and whether advances in this area could be applied to explain how negative thinking and feelings combine in depression with such debilitating results. Although we had each taken slightly different approaches, there was a good deal to share since we were examining the same problem, namely, how depression alters people's thinking in a way that first gets things stuck, then makes things worse.

Our conversations at that time were largely about the mechanisms that lie behind the changes in thinking and feeling that accompany depression. We were not focusing our attention on the treatment of depression because, by the late 1980s, there were already a number of psychological treatments whose effects were on par with those found for antidepressant medication. Further research on how to help people with current depression seemed unlikely, at that time, to add much to the field.

Instead, we focused our interest on why many people become depressed again once they have recovered from an episode of depression. The academic literature was uncertain. Some early studies seemed to suggest that if people continued to hold certain attitudes or core beliefs after recovery, then they would be the ones most likely to become depressed again. Examples include the beliefs "If I do not do as well as other people, it means I am an inferior human being" and "My value as a person depends greatly on what others think of me." Such attitudes or beliefs were thought to make depression more likely, largely because they link a person's sense of self-worth with events that, large or small, are often outside his or her control. A questionnaire called the Dysfunctional Attitude Scale had been developed to measure the degree to which people held such beliefs.

Increasingly, researchers were skeptical of the causal role of these attitudes in relapse. They pointed out that those patients who still held these sorts of beliefs at the end of treatment may not have fully recovered, so it was no wonder that they were more likely to relapse. Indeed, it remains true that the extent of residual symptoms following treatment is one of the best predictors of recurrence.

But there were other problems for this theory of why depression returns. Several studies were now showing that patients who had truly recovered, so that their depressed mood had returned to the average level of the general population, showed no evidence of this type of thinking style at all. Their core beliefs and attitude scores were normal despite the fact that these people, we knew, were very likely to become depressed again. In what way could these people be shown to be vulnerable? We continued to debate this question at the time, and we have more to say about it later. In any case, the Oxford Congress came and went, and, promising to keep in touch, we returned to our own academic homes.

Two years later, in 1991, there arose the opportunity to come together again to focus on the same issues. David Kupfer, who headed the Psychobiology of Depression Research Network of the John D. and Catherine T. MacArthur Foundation, asked Zindel Segal to develop a "maintenance" version of cognitive therapy for use with depressed patients to help them stay well once they had recovered from their acute episode. Maintenance therapy offers a way to continue treating recovered but at-risk patients. It is offered less frequently than regular therapy, but its aim is always the same: to support formerly depressed patients' use of skills to identify and address problems that, if ignored, could bring on depression. David Kupfer and Ellen Frank had just published a seminal study showing the value of such maintenance sessions for a type of structured treatment approach called interpersonal therapy (IPT). Could a maintenance version of cognitive therapy be similarly developed? Zindel, who was now Head of the

Cognitive Behaviour Therapy Unit at the Clarke Institute of Psychiatry (now the Centre for Addiction and Mental Health, Clarke Division), contacted Mark Williams (who had moved from Cambridge to the University of Bangor, Wales, and is now at the University of Oxford) and John Teasdale to discuss the possibility of working together on such a project.

Our first meeting was in Toronto, in April 1992. The notes from that meeting outline what such a maintenance cognitive therapy treatment would look like. It bears no resemblance to the approach we eventually developed. In the coming years, we would radically depart from the version of cognitive therapy in which each of us had been trained.

As this book explains, we first stepped away by adding an attentional training component to our cognitive therapy intervention. We found that this was not enough. We then discarded the "therapy" framework to work more fully within a mindfulness approach that emphasized holding thoughts and feelings in awareness rather than trying to change them. We finally moved toward an integration of core cognitive therapy principles with sustained mindfulness practice, and the 2002 book laid out this process in detail.

When the first edition was published, the impact of it on the therapy world astonished us. Early on in the process of developing MBCT, we had sometimes wondered how it would be received. We had anticipated that even if it proved helpful for some people, it would only ever occupy a small corner at the edge of therapeutic practice. It turns out that we had grossly misread the situation. For reasons that are still somewhat opaque, the mindfulness approach caught the mood of the times. In light of this growing acceptance, therapists were now starting to ask important questions about this new approach. For example, why choose MBCT, and what is it? Is it effective? How does it work? And who can teach it?

Why choose MBCT, and what is it? In 2002, this story was only just beginning to unfold. Ten years on, we need to see what has happened. So in this book we update the theory and research that motivates the use of a mindfulness approach for recurrent depression. We indicate what changes we have made to the program itself, what aspects we now realize were not clearly enough expressed, and what misunderstandings have resulted, and we'll try to be clearer. To this end, we reflect on what aspect of mindfulness is being cultivated by each aspect of the program, trying to answer some frequently asked questions.

Does it work? At the time of publishing the first edition, there was only a single trial to show that the intervention was effective at reducing risk of relapse. Although we had delayed writing the book until we knew the outcome of this trial, the data at this stage were very preliminary. Could they be replicated? Ten years on, we know the answer to that question. So we also review how this approach has fared in five new research trials that have evaluated it, two of which have compared MBCT and the most commonly used treatment to reduce relapse: continued antidepressant medication. The results are highly consistent: This approach is highly effective in reducing risk of relapse in those who have the longest and most recurrent history of depression.

Why does it work? At the time of the first edition, we had many guesses from our theoretical analysis and some laboratory work about what the range of possible critical mechanisms underlying the effectiveness of the intervention might be. But there had been little research examining what variables change during an 8-week program, or which of these changes are critical in preventing relapse and recurrence. The emerging answers are fascinating and add importantly to our knowledge.

And what does a clinician need to do to train and prepare to teach MBCT? In 2002, we were not so sure about this. Now, 10 years on, we have been involved in training several hundred prospective MBCT teachers all over the world. We give our current best thoughts on what background and experience seems best to prepare a teacher. Increasingly, we recognize the crucial importance of these factors—first, so that we do not harm those who come to us for help and second, so we can best ensure that patients are invited to participate in a program that will bring about profound and lasting freedom from suffering. We are now even clearer in our minds than we were in 2002, that when we use the term "mindfulness-based" we are not only referring to the fact that what is being taught in the class or clinic is "based in mindfulness," we are also saying that the "base" out of which skill as a teacher arises is his or her own daily mindfulness practice. To be clear, teachers who use this approach need skills as qualified and trusted professionals in their own field, but they also require the depth of practice and perspective that comes only from knowing, from the inside, what mindfulness practice is and what it is not. This means that *teachers* of mindfulness are *practitioners* of mindfulness in their own daily lives. Without a teacher having an ongoing mindfulness practice, whatever is being taught is not MBCT.

We begin by giving some background on depression itself. Looking back over the 20 years since we started this project, there remains no doubt that depression still poses one of the most pressing problems in the field of mental health. What did the situation look like in the late 1980s, and what new perspectives were emerging? We shall see that views of depression were changing, from depression as a single-episode problem to depression as a chronic, recurrent disorder. Health planners were beginning to wake up to the fact that depression was poised to be one of the major "diseases" of the 21st century, demanding new answers.

PART I
THE CHALLENGE
OF DEPRESSION

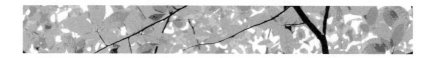

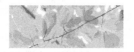 CHAPTER 1

Depression Casts a Long Shadow

Depression is a disorder of mood that affects a person's capacity to think clearly; undermines motivation to act; alters intimate bodily functioning, such as sleeping and eating; and leaves a person feeling stranded in the midst of searing mental pain and suffering he or she feels unable to do anything about. Each individual suffers alone, yet when we consider how many people suffer from depression, the figures are staggering. Based on data from both hospital and community studies, such mood disorders are among the most prevalent psychiatric conditions, a finding that is remarkably consistent all over the world. Recent epidemiological data from roughly 14,000 people, surveyed across six European countries, found that 17% of the population report some experience with depression in the past 6 months. When looked at more closely, serious major depression accounted for 6.9%, with minor depression accounting for 1.8%.[1] The remaining 8.3% of participants complained of experiencing depressive symptoms but did not view them as interfering greatly with either their work or social functioning. These numbers are closely comparable to rates reported in both Canadian[2] and U.S. samples.[3] At these levels, family physicians can expect to see at least one person with a significant depression during each day of clinical practice. When people are asked about their experiences with depression over longer periods of time, at any one time, 6.6% of the U.S. population have experienced clinical depression in the past year,[4] and between 18 and 22% of women and 7 and 11% of men will suffer a clinical depression during their lifetime.[5]

What is this depression? In its common usage the term suggests that one is "feeling down" or "blue," yet this characterization misses the

11

essential "syndromal" nature of the clinical disorder; that is, it consists of a combination of elements rather than a single feature. Clinical depression (sometimes also called "major depression") is a state in which persistent depressed mood or loss of interest occurs with other reliable physical and mental signs, such as difficulties sleeping, poor appetite, impaired concentration, and feelings of hopelessness and worthlessness. A diagnosis of depression is given only when a number of these elements are present at the same time, for at least 2 weeks, and are shown to interfere with a person's ability to perform his or her day-to-day activities.

Those who have been depressed know that there is no single face to the disorder, no single feature that tells the whole story. Some consequences of having depression are easier to recognize by the sufferer, including low mood and lack of concentration. Others may be harder to recognize because their main effects reduce the patient's ability to interact with loved ones and other family members, for example, lack of energy and preoccupation with negative themes and ideas. One of the most obvious tolls that depression exacts is increased risk for suicide. Suicide risk increases with each new episode, and there is a 15% chance that patients suffering from recurrent depression severe enough to require hospitalization will eventually die by suicide.[6] Depression is also rarely observed on its own. The most likely additional problem is anxiety.[7] The chances of a person with depression, for example, also suffering from panic disorder are 19 times greater than the odds of someone without depression experiencing panic.[8,9] Increased odds are also reported for simple phobia (nine times greater) and obsessive–compulsive disorder (11 times greater).

One of the most surprising and disturbing aspects to emerge from community-based surveys of depression and other mental illnesses is the low rate of mental health services use. There is a strange irony here. People with the most prevalent mental disorder are among the least likely to seek treatment. Of those seeking treatment, only 22% actually see a specialist for their problem and receive adequate treatment.[5] The failure to obtain care, especially in the case of depression for which effective treatments exist, has developed into an important public health issue. One response to this has been publicity to educate the public about the symptoms of depression and available treatment options. Depression screening days, now common in many hospitals, have helped to reduce the stigma associated with this disorder by portraying it as a legitimate medical/ psychological condition with well-documented clinical features.

Another change that has occurred in our understanding of depression over the past 20 years has been appreciation of the degree of disability associated with the disorder. In addition to the emotional pain and anguish suffered by those who are depressed, evidence suggests that the level of functional impairment is comparable to that found in major medical illnesses, including cancer and coronary artery disease. At the time we started this work, the work of Kenneth Wells and his colleagues had gone far in revealing many of the hidden costs and the nature of the social burden due to depression. For example, when we measure disability in terms of "days spent in bed," many people would be surprised to find that depressed patients spent more time in bed (1.4 days per month) than patients with lung disease (1.2 days per month), diabetes (1.15 days per month), or arthritis (0.75 days per month). Only patients with heart disease spent more time in bed (2.1 days per month).[10] As one might assume, the ripple effect of "bed days" on productivity at work is considerable. Workers suffering from depression have five times more work-loss days than do their healthy counterparts,[11] and depression is one of the most common causes of extended work absence in white-collar employees.[12]

The impact of these findings, as they entered the literature in the late 1980s and early 1990s, was that many people changed their views on the magnitude of the problem of depression. A World Health Organization projection for the year 2020 confirms these early warnings: Of all diseases, depression will impose the second-largest burden of ill health worldwide.[13] At the time we came together to consider the best treatment approach, depression was fast becoming the major challenge within the field of mental health.

EARLY OPTIMISM ABOUT THE TREATMENT OF DEPRESSION

With depression as the problem, where was the answer likely to be found? The truth was that by the end of the 1980s, there were a number of ways to combat depression. Antidepressant drugs, first discovered and used in the 1950s, had been refined to the point that a number of them had amassed decisive evidence for their efficacy. Most of these drugs targeted brain neurotransmitter function (the chemical messengers that allow neural impulses to cross from one nerve fiber to another at their junctions, or *synapses*). They worked by increasing the efficiency of the connections between brain cells and making greater quantities of neurotransmitters, such as norepinephrine or serotonin, available at the synapse.[14] Although how exactly this occurs remains in doubt, there is evidence to suggest that some drugs block the reuptake of neurotransmitters by other cells, whereas others actually stimulate nerve cells to release more neurotransmitter. By the end of the 1980s, antidepressants had become, and still remain, the frontline treatment for clinical depression.[15] However, there are alarming indications that for mild to moderate depression, they are not any more effective than an inert placebo,[16] and that even if they are effective, for some people (for reasons we don't yet understand) they begin to lose their power after 1 or 2 years of continuous treatment.[17]

By the late 1980s, psychological treatments of depression were also starting to come into their own. There were at least four broad approaches to the problem, all of which were structured and time-limited. Each had some degree of empirical support. Behavioral approaches emphasized the need to increase depressed persons' participation in reinforcing or pleasure-giving activities,[18] while social skills training corrected behavioral deficits that increased depressed persons' social isolation and rejection.[19] Cognitive therapy[20] brought together a number of behavioral and cognitive techniques, with the joint aim of changing the way a person's thoughts, images, and interpretation of events contribute to the onset and maintenance of the emotional and behavioral disturbances associated with depression. Finally, IPT[21] stressed that learning to resolve interpersonal disputes and changing roles would alleviate depression. Cognitive and interpersonal therapies came to be seen as "gold standards" in psychological treatment, largely because support for these interventions reflected three important features that are still rare in psychological treatment research: The therapies were tested in multiple studies in different centers; they used clinical patients who met standard diagnostic criteria for depression; and when evaluated against antidepressant medication, their efficacy was judged to be equivalent.[22]

With all these treatments for depression available, surely the problem had been solved. Unfortunately, as treatments for current depression demonstrated their efficacy, research showed that a major contributor to prevalence rates across the world was the *return* of new episodes of depression in people who had already experienced one episode. The scope of the problem had changed.

DEPRESSION AS A CHRONIC, RELAPSING CONDITION

Why had this aspect of depression not been noticed before? First, because much of the data on which our understanding of depression was based came from studies conducted in the earlier part of the 20th century. At that time, the first onset of serious clinical depression tended to be late middle age, so the opportunity to see longer patterns of recurrence did not exist. Decade by decade, as the second part of the century unfolded, a different pattern emerged, with the first onset of depression being seen earlier and earlier, until the average age of onset had fallen to the mid-20s, with many people experiencing their first episode during adolescence. The tragic effect of earlier onset is that there is now a whole lifetime to observe what happens after a single episode of depression—and the newer research studies started to tell a different and disturbing story.

Second, we had not realized how recurrent depression could be because there had been no studies in which patients who recovered from the disorder had been followed and evaluated at regular intervals. Only with this type of information can there be a complete understanding of how depression waxes and wanes over the life cycle, and how its natural course develops. Such studies allow us to calculate the likelihood of *spontaneous remission* (in which a person gets better without treatment) and to evaluate the relative costs of using treatments that carry significant risks or side effects against the costs of leaving depression untreated. There was little in the way of hard data on these issues until the mid-1980s. Now, newer studies identified patients once they were no longer depressed, then followed them over 1- to 2-year intervals.

One of the first such studies, conducted by Martin Keller and colleagues in 1983,[23] followed 141 patients diagnosed with major depressive disorder for 13 months and reported that 43 (33%) had relapsed after having been well for at least 8 weeks. Clearly, patients in recovery faced a major challenge in maintaining their health and the gains of treatment. All the research since that time has told a similar story: that at least 50% of patients who recover from an initial episode of depression will have at least one subsequent depressive episode,[24] and those patients with a history of two or more past episodes will have a 70–80% likelihood of recurrence in their lives.[6] Up to this point, mental health professionals distinguished between "acute" conditions (short-term) and "chronic" conditions (long-term, lasting over 2 years), noting that some depressions might *appear* acute, but many depressed people who recover remain "chronic" in the sense of increased, long-term vulnerability. In a widely quoted review, Judd concluded that "unipolar depression is a chronic, lifelong illness, the risk for repeated episodes exceeds 80%, patients will experience an average of 4 lifetime major depressive episodes of 20 weeks' duration each" (p. 990).[25] Findings such as these have helped to shape the current consensus that relapse and recurrence following successful treatment of depression are common, debilitating outcomes (see Figure 1.1[26]).

From the perspective of the early part of the 21st century, it is easy to forget that this emphasis on recurrence was quite new at the time. Up to the late 1960s and early 1970s, the focus had been on developing more effective treatments for acute depression. Relatively little attention was paid to a patient's ongoing risk. This new research signaled the need to take into account the risk of relapse that remained during recovery, when making decisions about the type of treatment to offer.

Keller's data suggested a large difference in prognosis between patients with no history of depression and those with at least three previous depressive episodes. These two groups relapsed at significantly different rates—22% for "first timers" versus 67% for patients with a history of three or more episodes. Patients recovering from their first episode of depression were shown to be at a critical juncture in the developmental course of their disorder. They "have a substantial probability of prompt

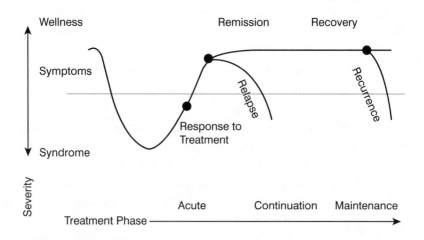

FIGURE 1.1. Depression as a chronic relapsing condition.

relapse, and should they relapse, they have approximately a 20% chance of remaining chronically depressed" (p. 3303).[23] As later data from a 5-year follow-up of patients with chronic and nonchronic affective disorder suggested,[27] those who relapse very soon after recovery are the ones whose depression becomes a long-lasting condition.

Distinguishing among patients on the basis of the number of past episodes continues to be one of the most reliable predictors of future depression, bearing out Keller's earlier observations. While the threshold in Keller's study was set at three past episodes, now the more common cutoff is two episodes. It is important to note that the principle of separating these two groups on the basis of their risk for relapse is still endorsed. In fact, the *Diagnostic and Statistical Manual of Mental Disorders* (DSM-IV-TR) of the American Psychiatric Association[28] qualifies the diagnosis of major depressive disorder with the term "recurrent" for those patients with a history of at least two depressive episodes.

HOW COULD DEPRESSIVE RELAPSE AND RECURRENCE BE PREVENTED?

With a clearer view of the burdens that depression imposes on its sufferers came a corresponding urgency to develop treatments that might help. Because major depression was now seen to be a recurrent disorder, it seemed imperative to look at ways of expanding the types of care offered to patients. The evidence seemed to suggest that if one relied on medication, there was a need for a longer-term approach.

Although the conclusion was not wholly welcome to those uncomfortable with long-term administration of medication, the evidence implied that a clinician should continue to prescribe antidepressants after depressed patients had recovered from the episode for which they sought help in the first place. What sort of study could be used to test the necessity of such continuation treatment?

The answer is a study in which all patients receive the same medication until they have recovered, and are then randomly allocated either to a condition in which the active drug is swapped for a placebo (an inert pill) or one in which they continue to receive the active drug. (Patients agree beforehand to participate in such a study but do not know the group to which they are assigned.) That is what Glen and his colleagues did in a seminal study in the 1980s. All patients were allocated to receive drug or placebo once they had got better on the active drug. The results were clear: Some 50% of the patients who were switched to the placebo became depressed again, compared to only 20% of the patients treated with active medication.[29]

One feature of this result was particularly important. Glen and colleagues found that depression came back much more quickly than would be expected if it were a new episode. This suggested that patients were experiencing not a new episode (a "recurrence"), but the worsening of a previously controlled episode that had not yet run its course (a "relapse"). The more general implication of this result was that although individuals suffering an episode of depression might feel better after taking antidepressant medication, if they stopped the medication before the episode had run its course, they risked rapid relapse.

By the late 1980s, many clinicians endorsed the view that it was best to prevent future episodes of depression by prescribing antidepressant medication *prophylactically* (i.e., to prevent the occurrence of a future episode, and not just to treat the existing episode). Clinicians started to distinguish between *acute, continuation*, and *maintenance* use of antidepressant medication to refer to treatment at the different stages of the depression (see Figure 1.1). So prescribing antidepressants with the aim of relieving current symptoms during an episode was called *acute treatment*. Prescribing antidepressants for 6 months beyond the period of recovery from the episode of depression was called continuation treatment, and extending antidepressants for as long as 3 to 5 years following recovery was referred to as *maintenance treatment*. The American Psychiatric Association's current practice guidelines for depression are based on this framework.[30,31]

But note a very important assumption behind these guidelines: that antidepressant drugs do not provide a long-term cure. Their effects do not outlast their use. To put it another way, antidepressants have their effects by suppressing symptoms; they do not target the supposed causes of the episode itself.[32,33] Nevertheless, given that the risk for early recurrence increases with each episode experienced, and that the interval between recurrences tends to shorten over time,[34] it remained important to prevent the return of symptoms in any way possible. For many, the message of this and similar, later studies was clear: To prevent future depression, continue the same treatments that worked in alleviating the acute episode of depression.

PSYCHOTHERAPY AS A MAINTENANCE TREATMENT

The gains achieved through extending pharmacological treatment of depression beyond initial recovery were, by the late 1980s, well documented and extremely important. Yet effective alternatives to the continued use of antidepressant medication in the recovery phase were still required. At any given time, such long-term drug treatment is not suitable for a considerable number of people. For example, pregnant women and women who wish to breast-feed their babies are discouraged from taking such medication, as are those undergoing major surgery. Others cannot tolerate the side effects of antidepressants, and still others decline to take the medication. In a study of 155 depressed outpatients, 28% stopped taking antidepressants during the first month of treatment, and 44% had stopped taking their medication by the third month.[35] In general, the proportion of patients that does not take the prescribed antidepressant medication is estimated in the 30–40% range.[36] An online survey of 1,400 patients in the United States, conducted by the National Depressive and Manic–Depressive Association, found that only one-third of patients receiving maintenance antidepressant therapy were satisfied with the quality of their treatment.[37]

Could psychotherapy help? After all, there was evidence that negative life events often precede the return of episodes of depression. Such events often involve losses, arguments, rejections, and disappointments. Surely, then, psychotherapy could play an important role in helping patients manage the interpersonal consequences of these events, thus reducing the risk of recurrence. This was the rationale behind the groundbreaking study of maintenance IPT conducted by Ellen Frank and her colleagues.[38]

What was new about this study was that patients were first treated for their episode of depression with a combination of interpersonal therapy and the antidepressant, imipramine, then continued to receive therapy for 3 years, even though they had already recovered. For patients, the experimental part of the study started once they had recovered from their episode of depression. Results from the Frank and colleagues study showed that maintenance IPT significantly extended how long they stayed well. For patients who received maintenance IPT, the average survival time until the next episode was greater than 1 year. By contrast, patients receiving only placebo during the maintenance phase had a depression-free period of only 21 weeks.

These findings spoke directly to central concerns in the field. They demonstrated for the first time that psychotherapy, like antidepressant medication, could reduce the chances that depression would return. Interestingly, patients receiving medication actually stayed well longer than those receiving only maintenance IPT. However, patients on maintenance IPT still did much better than patients receiving only placebo. These findings opened the door to using psychotherapy as a preventive measure and challenged the field to develop theoretical models to clarify which skills depressed patients ought to be taught to prevent relapse.

The finding that IPT could be used in a maintenance format to keep people well was very important, and it was not long before clinicians started to wonder whether other forms of psychotherapy might also be used in this way. The problem was that, at the time, many psychotherapy researchers had put their energies into developing better and more effective treatments for acute depression, and had not considered developing "maintenance" versions of their therapies. If this field was to progress, others would need to do what Frank and her colleagues had done, and begin to examine how best to offer psychological treatments to keep people well once they had recovered.

The possibility of developing a maintenance version of cognitive therapy to parallel the maintenance version of IPT provoked the interest of members of the John D. and Catherine T. MacArthur Foundation's Psychobiology of Depression and Affective Disorders Research Network. The network director, David Kupfer, invited Zindel Segal to explore how to produce such a maintenance treatment. Kupfer was also to play an important role later in the development of our ideas, when he allowed us to stray from our initial brief and to follow our growing feeling that such a maintenance form of cognitive therapy was too narrow an approach. But we are running ahead of our story. We were asked to develop a maintenance version of cognitive therapy, and that is where we started.

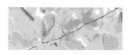 CHAPTER 2

Why Do People Who Have Recovered from Depression Relapse?

DEVELOPING A MAINTENANCE VERSION OF COGNITIVE THERAPY

In April 1992, the three of us met to discuss the possibilities of developing a maintenance version of cognitive therapy. We were optimistic about being able to adapt current cognitive therapy for depression in a way that could be applied to patients in recovery. We believed that such a treatment would draw on skills patients had learned during the acute phase of treatment. In order to understand why this therapy was a good place to start, it may be helpful to provide a brief background.

Cognitive therapy was pioneered by Aaron T. Beck in the 1960s and 1970s, as a structured, time-limited approach to depression. Beck had noticed how often the themes of loss, failure, worthlessness, and rejection were featured in the thinking of his depressed patients. Until this time, most clinicians had assumed that this negative thinking was merely a surface feature of depression, caused by an underlying biological disturbance or psychodynamic conflict. According to these prevailing views, if the underlying problem were treated, then the thoughts would get better.

Beck realized that the causal sequence could work equally well the other way around. Negative thinking could itself *cause* depression. In addition, even if such thinking had not been the first cause of an episode, it could certainly *maintain* the episode once it had started. For example, if a person believes 100% that "I've got no friends" or "Nobody likes or respects me," then he or she will be less likely to phone a friend for support or to accept invitations, and as a result will become more isolated. This sequence of events will make the person's recovery from low mood even more difficult. Thoughts and feelings could interact with each other in a damaging, vicious spiral.

Beck's therapy took these thoughts seriously. He encouraged his patients to "catch" whatever thoughts were going through their minds when their mood shifted. They would write the thoughts down and bring them to therapy sessions, where they could be evaluated in the light of evidence for and against them. Home practice was scheduled, during which patients would gather more evidence and gradually extend their activities to restore a sense of mastery and pleasure in their daily lives. Difficult situations for patients were cognitively rehearsed during the therapy session, and alternative options to tackling them generated and discussed. Patients were taught to be vigilant for long-term beliefs, attitudes, and assumptions they might hold, and to look out for situations where these might trigger depressed mood.

It is interesting now to reflect on why cognitive therapy became so successful. Partly it was because Beck used evidence from both the clinic and the experimental laboratory to substantiate his ideas, drawing in a wide range of clinicians and scientists. He also incorporated many behavioral techniques that shared features with the widely used behavior therapies for anxiety-based problems. But success was equally due to Beck's insistence on carefully assessing both processes and outcomes with valid and reliable measures, on applying the therapy to an important clinical problem that structured psychotherapies had neglected, and on evaluating the treatment against the standard existing treatment (antidepressant medication). Any one of these factors might have made cognitive therapy prominent in the field, but with all of them combined, the case for using this approach with depressed patients was overwhelming, and by the time we were meeting, cognitive therapy had become a (if not *the*) major psychotherapeutic alternative to medication.

If we were to plan a maintenance form of cognitive therapy, it would clearly make most sense for patients to use many of the same techniques to prevent future depression: activity scheduling, rating mastery and pleasure, thought monitoring and challenging, cognitive rehearsal, generating alternative options, and noticing and dealing with dysfunctional attitudes. A maintenance treatment might consist of monthly meetings in which these skills were renewed, deepened, and practiced. It would also make sense for the therapy to inform and train patients to notice early indicators of relapse or recurrence.

At this point, the question of what such a manual for maintenance cognitive therapy would contain seemed relatively uncontroversial. There seemed to be an emerging consensus that the cognitive therapy approach to prevention of depressive relapse/recurrence should primarily depend on continuing to use those cognitive techniques that were helpful in treating the acute episode.

However, it was not long before our discussions led us to ask whether we should consider alternative approaches. First, we had become aware of the sheer enormity of the problem of depression (see Chapter 1), compared with the scarce resources of psychotherapy. The number of trained cognitive therapists was clearly not going to meet the demand, so to ask such therapists to add maintenance therapy to their already busy caseloads was only likely to prevent them from seeing newly referred patients. There needed to be a more cost-efficient solution than to continue to rely on one-to-one psychotherapy. The second problem with believing that maintenance cognitive therapy would be the answer to relapse was that, by 1992, it was becoming clear that treating acute depression with "standard" cognitive therapy already prevented relapse in many patients.

THE LONG-LASTING EFFECTS OF COGNITIVE THERAPY

Up to that point, four studies had compared cognitive therapy with antidepressants for the treatment of acute depression, and examined how patients fared over the next 12 to 24 months after initial recovery.[39–42] All four trials had found that cognitive therapy prevented relapse, findings subsequently further confirmed by Hollon and colleagues in 2005.[32] Patients whose medication was discontinued upon their recovery had, as expected, fairly high rates of relapse/recurrence (varying between 50 and 78%), as shown in Figure 2.1.[43]

However, Figure 2.1 also shows that the proportion of patients who relapsed or needed further treatment was substantially reduced if cognitive therapy alone was used to treat the depression. In this case, rates of

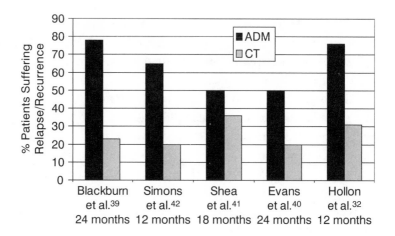

FIGURE 2.1. Comparison of relapse rates for depressed patients receiving either cognitive therapy (CT) or antidepressant medication (ADM).

recurrence were reduced to 20–36%. These studies appeared to provide relatively compelling evidence that cognitive therapy, even if used only in the acute phase, could reduce the risk of future relapse. Taken together with the evidence that maintenance IPT could reduce rates of relapse/recurrence, there could be little doubt that psychological treatments could play a major role in dealing with the increased burden of depression faced by individuals and society. Yet evidence from studies of cognitive therapy, like the relapse rates shown in Figure 2.1, had two important implications for the chances of producing a maintenance version, the first negative, the second more positive.

First, if cognitive therapy were shown reliably to reduce rates of relapse following recovery to the level of 20–36%, then why develop a maintenance version at all? Of course, it is always possible to do better, and perhaps with some fine-tuning, relapse rates could drop even lower, perhaps to 10–15%. As we saw it, however, this was more a question of modifying the existing components of the cognitive therapy package, perhaps by adding interventions to address residual symptoms, than actually designing an intervention for depressed patients in recovery.

But, second, the data clearly implied that the practice of cognitive therapy had taught people something that, once learned, protected them against future depression. This implication was potentially of enormous significance. Recall that up to this point, both pharmacological and psychological approaches had assumed that once a person had recovered, the best way of dealing with the risk of relapse was to extend whatever treatment he or she had *already* received. The words "continuation" and "maintenance" carry with them this assumption. But why should the options be so confined? Why not use one approach to deal with acute depression and another to keep people well once they have recovered?

For the first time, we began to see that this way of looking at the problem gave rise to new possibilities for sequencing treatment. If we could understand how cognitive therapy had its protective effect, we might then devise a way of teaching that "something" to people who had recovered from their depression. This could be done even if people had not had cognitive therapy when they were depressed. In particular, patients could take antidepressant medication during acute depression (and since this remained the most common treatment for depression, it seemed a sensible option), then use a maintenance version of cognitive therapy to stay well. Patients not able to take maintenance medication would be protected after recovery by learning the same principles and practices that cognitive therapy teaches to acutely depressed patients.

There were other benefits to this approach. Patients would not have to continue to take antidepressant medication indefinitely. Furthermore, such a maintenance version of cognitive therapy delivered in a group format could have tremendous advantages in cost-efficiency. It would also allow greater numbers of patients to be helped compared to standard individual cognitive therapy.

What would such a treatment look like, could it be developed, and how effective would it be? Answers to these questions would depend very much on our ability to answer two basic questions. First, what are the important psychological mechanisms involved in depressive relapse? Second, how are these modified during the course of acute cognitive therapy? Only after answering both questions could we begin to think about offering patients who had never had cognitive therapy the same type of protection. As we see later, several pointers in the research literature indicated how the first question might be answered. However, the second question remained unanswered: At that time, we simply did not know how cognitive therapy's effects reduced risk of relapse. We needed to go back to basics.

COGNITIVE VULNERABILITY TO RELAPSE
AND RECURRENCE

As we have seen, one of the major contributions of the cognitive model of emotional disorders during the 1970s and 1980s was its assertion that the way we think about ourselves, the world, and the future can have a major effect on our emotions and behavior.[44] So far, the model as we have described it only applies to the *onset* of an episode and how long it *persists* once it has established itself. Negative thinking can cause and maintain depression. But what of ongoing *vulnerability*, the risk of becoming depressed again once the person has recovered from an episode? With respect to such vulnerability, Beck proposed that early in life, vulnerable individuals acquire certain assumptions or attitudes that persist into adulthood and become traits that endure throughout their lives.[45] When someone sees the world from such a point of view, his or her risk of suffering depression increases because when a negative event occurs, it is seen through the lens of the underlying belief, bringing about feelings of sadness that may be out of proportion to the event itself. In the Introduction, we mentioned briefly the questionnaire that Weissman and Beck[46] constructed as a way to measure these dysfunctional attitudes: the Dysfunctional Attitude Scale. It is now time to detail how this measure of vulnerability progressed from yielding disappointing results to intriguing and important new insights into the nature of depressive relapse.

ARE PERSISTING DYSFUNCTIONAL ATTITUDES
THE CAUSE OF RELAPSE?

Items on the Dysfunctional Attitude Scale describe attitudes or assumptions that reflect, as it were, a personal contract for maintaining self-worth. As long as the conditions of the contract are met, the person is fine. If, for example, someone believes that "to be happy, I must succeed in everything I do," then his or her mood is fine so long as he or she does not fail at anything. If he or she fails an exam at college or is turned down for a promotion, the conclusion is likely "I cannot be happy" or "I cannot live with this failure." It is not hard to see how these dysfunctional attitudes were seen as enduring traits that rendered some people vulnerable to clinical depression.

What, then, did the clinical cognitive model predict about previously depressed patients' scores on the Dysfunctional Attitude Scale? Since we knew that these patients were undoubtedly vulnerable to future depression, and certainly at higher risk than people who had never been depressed, the prediction was clear. Formerly depressed patients, even if not depressed now, should have higher scores on the Dysfunctional Attitude Scale than those who had never been depressed. It was relatively easy to set up studies in which previously depressed and never-depressed participants' levels of dysfunctional attitudes were compared. Rick Ingram and colleagues reviewed over 40 such studies done around that time and, with very few exceptions, their conclusions were clear. Although Dysfunctional Attitude Scale scores were elevated in patients during an episode of depression, the scores of recovered patients, tested in normal mood, were not distinguishable from the scores of never-depressed people.[47] There have been few occasions in clinical psychology research on which such a strong prediction has been rejected in such a clear-cut way. Persistent dysfunctional attitudes and assumptions were not the cause of relapse.

SAD MOODS CAN REAWAKEN NEGATIVE THOUGHT PATTERNS: A BASIS FOR UNDERSTANDING VULNERABILITY

If there was no good evidence for the existence of dysfunctional attitudes as persistent traits, how was vulnerability to depression to be explained cognitively? At this point, it was necessary to step back from the research on dysfunctional attitudes to consider briefly another, parallel strand of research. This other research program, begun by, among others, John Teasdale and colleagues, was concerned not with understanding the effect of thinking on mood, but with examining the other side of the vicious circle: the effect that mood has on thinking. They used experimental induction of sad moods in which participants read sad statements or listened to sad music for 5–10 minutes. The effects of the mood inductions were short-lived and reversible, but provided a valuable window on the types of changes in thinking brought on by mild depression.

Several studies found that if nondepressed people were experimentally induced into mild depressed moods, then they showed negative biases in memory. They were less likely (and took longer) to recall pleasant events in their lives, and more likely to recall negative events. Previous researchers had observed such biases in clinical depression but had been inconclusive about how such biases were caused.[48,49] Depressed people might recall more negative memories simply because they had experienced more such events, or because they evaluated their whole lives as negative. The experimental work showed that the biasing effects of depression on memory were not simply the result of more negative events in depressed persons' lives. Such negative events undoubtedly occur, but, to add to the misery, people who are depressed must also cope with a mood-induced bias that focuses more on negativity in their lives and less on any positive aspects.

This suggested a different way of looking at vulnerability. Perhaps the important difference between individuals who had recovered from depression and those who had never been depressed was not in how they thought about things when their moods were fine, but in what came to mind when they were feeling sad. Could the answer to what makes people vulnerable to future depression lie in the patterns of negative thinking previously associated with experiences of depression? We already knew some of the central symptoms of depression: guilt; remorse; and negative, self-critical thinking. During an episode of depression, people experience both depressed mood and negative thinking. What if, during an episode, the brain forms an association between one and the other? In the future, the occurrence of just one element (mood) would bring about the other (change in thinking patterns). For people who have been depressed in the past, even normal, day-to-day sadness might have serious consequences.

Teasdale[49] put forward such a "differential activation hypothesis," the idea being that sad moods were likely to reactivate thinking styles associated with previous sad moods. These styles would differ from one individual to another, depending on individuals' past experiences. Teasdale suggested that differential accessibility could help us understand depressive relapse. Whereas most people might be able to ignore the occasional sad mood, in previously depressed persons a slight lowering of mood might bring about a large and potentially devastating change in thought patterns. These thought patterns would most often involve global, negative self-judgments such as "I am worthless" and "I am stupid."

Experiments were carried out to test these ideas. In these studies, people who were no longer depressed, but who had been depressed in the past, were examined with and without mood induction. The question was: How would formerly depressed people react to experimental induction of a sad mood, and how would such a mood impact their thinking compared to that of people who had never been depressed? The results from a number of such studies (reviewed by Segal & Ingram[50]) suggested that even when the sadness brought about by the experiment was similar in previously depressed and never-depressed persons, the mood had a more telling impact for those with a history of depression. People who had been depressed before showed an exaggerated cognitive bias.

The negative thinking reactivated in recovered patients would act to maintain and intensify the moods in a series of vicious cycles. In this way, in persons with a history of major depression, states of mild sadness would be more likely to progress to more intense and persistent states, increasing the risk of future onset of major depressive episodes. This very simple but powerful idea succeeded in turning attention away from measuring the levels of dysfunctional or biased thinking in nondepressed mood, and focused instead on how easily mood could reactivate this thinking.

SAD MOODS REACTIVATE VULNERABLE ATTITUDES AND BELIEFS

At the end of the 1980s, the work of Jeanne Miranda and Jacqueline Persons added new and important evidence. In several studies, they looked at the effects of mood, not on measures of memory, as Teasdale had done, but on the very same measure of dysfunctional attitudes that had yielded the earlier disappointing results. They found that when never-depressed individuals reported feeling sad, their belief in such attitudes changed relatively little. By contrast, when formerly depressed patients reported feeling sad, they were more likely to endorse dysfunctional attitudes than when their moods were fine. For example, when sad, such persons were more likely to believe that to be happy, they must succeed in everything they did.[51,52]

These findings pointed to the same conclusion that Teasdale had reached: Just a small increase in sadness, for those who had been depressed before, could lead to a reinstatement of the thinking patterns they had experienced when depressed. To use a computer analogy, the "depressive thinking" program had not really been wiped from the hard disk during recovery; small shifts in mood could reinstall it, as if it had never been absent.

Our thinking at the outset of the MacArthur project was that the degree to which people showed mood-activated reinstatement of negative thinking patterns most likely predicted relapse and recurrence in depression. Two subsequent studies have confirmed this hypothesis. Zindel Segal and his colleagues[53,54] induced a temporary sad mood in depressed patients who had just completed treatment (either antidepressants or cognitive therapy) at the Centre for Addiction and Mental Health in Toronto. Their aim was to determine the effect of the treatments on dysfunctional beliefs: particularly, whether the treatments effected changes in the beliefs in response to increases in sad mood. Segal and colleagues also wanted to see how well mood-related changes on the Dysfunctional Attitude Scale predicted patients' subsequent relapse.

The results from both studies showed that those patients with the greatest increase in dysfunctional beliefs following the "mood challenge" were more likely to suffer a relapse over the subsequent 30 months.[53,54] Furthermore, those patients who had undergone cognitive therapy showed less reactivity: Their dysfunctional attitudes shifted less in response to the mood challenge. This was further confirmation of our rapidly forming view that such "cognitive reactivity," the tendency to react to small changes in mood with large changes in negative thinking, was the issue that had to be addressed in order to prevent depression. Furthermore, data from other sources suggested that cognitive reactivity might have a cumulative effect, with each episode of depression increasing the likelihood of yet another episode.

PATHWAYS TO RELAPSE
ARE MORE EASILY ACTIVATED OVER TIME

In 1992, Robert Post,[34] an eminent biological psychiatrist, published a paper in which he suggested that rather than remaining constant, the relationship between psychological stress and depressive relapse changes over time. He reviewed a large amount of data suggesting the need to revise our view of the link between stressful events and the onset of depression. Previous discussion of the impact of events on depression largely had been limited to whether negative life events are sufficient to cause the onset of depression, or whether they need to occur in combination (or interaction) with other vulnerability factors. The data reviewed by Post suggested a more complex picture. *Early* episodes of depression were, indeed, often preceded by significant negative events. However, as more episodes of depression were experienced, stressful events played a progressively less important role. Kendler and colleagues[55] tested Post's conjecture by calculating *odds ratios*, a statistic that indicates the relative odds of depression arising in the presence of a life event compared to the absence of a life event. They showed that although the risk of further depression increases each time a person experiences an episode, the contribution of life events to that risk declines with successive episodes. Post has argued that each new episode contributes to small changes in the neurobiological threshold at which depression can be triggered, and that, with time, this threshold is lowered to the point that episodes seem to occur spontaneously, as if independent of circumstances in the person's life. Although the Kendler and colleagues data suggest that even after 40 previous episodes, the odds of becoming depressed are still higher in the presence of a stressful event, the overall pattern is one in which the onset of a new episode is more easily triggered. Although these studies were conducted within a neurobiological understanding of depression, the emerging ideas were very consistent with our view that repeated episodes of depression could make the psychological processes involved in the onset of a new episode more autonomous.[56]

THE RUMINATIVE MIND

Let us take stock for a moment. We have seen that persistence of "dysfunctional" ways of looking at the world cannot explain why some people remain vulnerable to future depression. When depressed people recover, their view of the world appears, on the face of it, to be restored to normal. In any event, it resembles the view of someone who has never been depressed. But despite this apparent normality, depression leaves its mark. What remains, once depression is over, is a tendency to react to small changes in mood with large changes in negative thinking.

Note that we have focused up to now on the way mood can bring to mind certain types of thoughts, memories, beliefs, and so on. We have, as it were, focused on the *contents* of consciousness. But there was also increasing evidence that people who are vulnerable to depression differ from other people in the *way* they try and deal with depressed mood itself.

Susan Nolen-Hoeksema, in a number of important studies during the 1990s, had shown that there are marked differences in people's reactions to depressive moods and situations. Some people respond to low mood by acting in ways that focus attention on themselves, while others do things that take their minds away from themselves. Nolen-Hoeksema refers to the first way of reacting as the "ruminative response style," and assesses people's tendency to react in this way with her Response Styles Questionnaire. By contrast, others are less likely to ruminate, and many engage in activities that allow them to distract themselves from such feelings. People who tend to use such distraction techniques are more likely to experience more short-lived depressed moods.

A dramatic early illustration of the importance of the ruminative response style came from a study by Nolen-Hoeksema and Morrow.[57] This study took advantage of the fact that they had assessed people on their measure of ruminative response style shortly before the 1989 Loma Prieta earthquake in California. They found that people who reported (before the earthquake occurred) a tendency to respond to depression by ruminating had the highest depression scores following the earthquake. Subsequent research studies have reported similar results: Attempting to think ourselves out of depression, especially once the thinking has taken on a brooding, repetitive nature, actually results in more prolonged depression, the exact opposite outcome from that which was intended.

One of the problems of research that finds an association between a cognitive trait, such as ruminative response style on one hand, and depression on the other, is that we can never be sure that the depression is not being caused by a third factor (e.g., another personality trait, such as neuroticism) that simply correlates with ruminative tendencies. There is a way out of this difficulty, however. It is possible to mimic the effects of different cognitive styles in the laboratory, and to examine their impact on mood. In this case, Nolen-Hoeksema and her colleagues carried out experiments in which nondepressed college students were given a mood induction procedure, then randomly allocated to one of two conditions. In the first condition, they were given instructions to think about themselves, and why they were the way they were (the "rumination" condition). In the second condition, they were instructed to think about things unrelated to themselves (the "distraction" condition). Results showed that the mood induction produced more persistent and intense sadness in the rumination group.

This sort of experiment can also address other important aspects of rumination. For example, why does rumination persist if it does so much damage? When asked why they chose to ruminate about their feelings in this way, many people said that they believe it would give them a better understanding of their emotions, and that this would help them solve their problems.[58] Using an experimental approach, Lyubomirsky and Nolen-Hoeksema found that the opposite was true.[59] They asked people either to ruminate about, or to distract themselves from, their sad mood, and then assessed subjects' ability to solve problems by using the means–ends problem-solving task. This widely used task gives participants the beginning of a story about a problematic situation (e.g., a relationship breakup) together with a "happy ending." Participants complete the story to say how the problem was solved. The results of this study revealed a dramatic contrast between belief and reality. Participants who ruminated about their mood *believed* they were beginning to understand themselves and their problems better, but actually they showed a reduction, rather than an improvement, in their ability to solve problems. They seemed trapped by a sense that they were on the verge of solving their problem, so that when they found that they were actually *further away* from the very solution they were looking for, they took this as a message to redouble their efforts to ruminate.

With Nolen-Hoeksema's findings, and the work comparing depression-induced negative thinking in recovered depressed and never-depressed people, we now had two important approaches to what makes people psychologically vulnerable to depression: first, the relatively easy accessibility of negative material (thoughts, memories, attitudes) when mood is low and, second, the way some people handle such negative moods and material by ruminating about them. Which approach should be chosen, or might both play a role? In the end, it turned out that these were not alternatives. In reality, they were two aspects of an entire "package" of changes brought about by depression. Let us take a particular example to illustrate this.

Imagine the following situation: Mary has just returned from work, tired and looking forward to a relaxing evening of television. A message on the answering machine indicates her partner will be late coming home. She feels disappointed, angry, and upset. She brings to mind other occasions earlier in the month, when the same thing happened. A thought about possible unfaithfulness comes to mind. She dismisses the thought, but it returns with greater vividness as she imagines that she heard some laughter in the background on the taped message. She feels nauseated. But it does not end there. With increasing speed, her mind conjures up images of the possible future: separating, seeing lawyers, getting divorced, buying another place, living in poverty. She can feel herself getting more upset as anger turns to depression and she recalls episodes in the past when she was rejected and alone. She "knows" that all their mutual friends probably would not want to know *her* anymore. Tears well up in Mary's eyes and she is left wondering what she can do. Sitting at the kitchen table, she says to herself, "Why does this always happen to me?" Mary tries to work out why it is that she always reacts this way. Note the avalanche of feelings, thoughts, and body sensations here. But note also that it is not just the negative material that causes Mary to be upset, nor is it simply the *way* she deals with it. Rather, it is as if a whole mode of mind, a configuration or pattern of negative mood–thoughts–images–body sensations, has been "wheeled into place" in response to this situation. This mode of mind includes *both* the easily accessible negative material *and* the tendency to deal with it by ruminating. But it also includes feedback loops involving the effects of emotion on the body. This only makes it harder for Mary. She may well need to take skillful action to address her concerns about her partner, but the track down which her rumination has taken her makes it *less* likely that such skillful actions will come to mind.

Like Mary, people who are vulnerable to depression spend a good deal of their time ruminating about why they feel the way they do, and trying to understand their problems and personal inadequacies. They believe that thinking about things in this way should help them find ways to reduce their distress, but the method they use to achieve that aim is tragically counterproductive. In fact, in this state of mind, repeatedly "thinking about" negative aspects of the self, or of problematic situations, serves to perpetuate rather than to resolve depression.

We wrote up these "best guesses" about the causes of vulnerability to depression in a paper in 1995.[60] What we believed was happening to cognitively vulnerable people was as follows: At times of lowering mood,

old habitual patterns of cognitive processing switch in relatively automatically. This has two important effects. First, thinking runs repeatedly
around fairly well-worn "mental grooves," without finding an effective
way forward out of depression. Second, this thinking itself intensifies
depressed mood, which in turn leads to further thoughts. In this way,
through self-perpetuating vicious cycles, otherwise mild and transient
mood can escalate into more severe and disabling depressed states. We
have more to say in Chapter 4 about this model and its effect on our
understanding of how we might take a radically different approach to
reducing the risk of relapse. As we see it, *the task of relapse prevention is
to help patients disengage from these ruminative and self-perpetuating modes
of mind when they feel sad, or at other times of potential relapse.* With this
model of vulnerability in our minds, we return to the question of how
cognitive therapy achieves its effects.

HOW DOES COGNITIVE THERAPY REDUCE RELAPSE AND RECURRENCE IN DEPRESSION?

Although, by the late 1980s, there had been studies showing that cognitive therapy reduces risk of relapse, nobody knew how it had this effect.
As we have seen, the original clinical model underlying cognitive therapy
for depression suggested that vulnerability to depression is related to the
persistence of certain underlying dysfunctional attitudes or assumptions.
From this perspective, reduction in risk of relapse following cognitive
therapy would be seen as the result of specific effects of cognitive therapy in reducing those dysfunctional attitudes. This hypothesis received
little empirical support.[61] In studies in which cognitive therapy produced
significantly better long-term outcomes than pharmacotherapy, the two
treatments often did not differ on posttreatment measures of dysfunctional thinking (Dysfunctional Attitude Scale).[62] This extremely important finding reinforces the view that the *level* of such attitudes, when
people are not depressed, is not the point at issue.

What then were the cognitive processes through which cognitive
therapy reduced relapse and recurrence in depression? At the time that we
considered this central question, it was generally assumed that cognitive
therapy, which primarily targets changing belief in depressive thoughts

and dysfunctional attitudes, had its effects through changes in the *content* of depressive thinking. Our more detailed theoretical analysis suggested a different possibility.[60] Although the explicit emphasis in cognitive therapy was on changing thought content, we realized that it was equally possible that when successful, this treatment led implicitly to changes in patients' *relationships* to their negative thoughts and feelings. Specifically, as a result of repeatedly identifying negative thoughts as they arose, and standing back from them to evaluate the accuracy of their content, patients often made a more general shift in their *perspective* on negative thoughts and feelings. Rather than regarding thoughts as necessarily true or as an aspect of the self, patients switched to a perspective within which negative thoughts and feelings could be seen as passing events in the mind that were neither necessarily valid reflections of reality nor central aspects of the self. The importance of such "distancing" or "decentering" had previously been recognized in discussions of cognitive therapy,[20] but usually as a means to the end of changing thought content, rather than as an end in itself.

Others, however, had suggested a more central role for decentering. Rick Ingram and Steve Hollon suggested that "cognitive therapy relies heavily on helping individuals switch to a controlled mode of processing that is metacognitive in nature and focuses on depression-related cognition . . . typically referred to as 'distancing' . . . the long-term effectiveness of cognitive therapy may lie in teaching patients to initiate this process in the face of future stress" (p. 272).[63]

This alternative perspective on how cognitive therapy might produce its effects represented a fundamental shift in our understanding. Previously, we, and others, had seen decentering as one of a number of things going on in cognitive therapy. Our analysis suggested that it was central. As we conceived it, then, decentering meant seeing thoughts in a sufficiently wider perspective, to be able to see them as simply "thoughts" rather than necessarily reflecting reality. This fundamental aspect of cognitive therapy protected people against future depression. If such decentering did not take place, patients would be left arguing with themselves about whether their thoughts were true or not, marshaling evidence for or against a negative thought, and at risk of simply getting caught up in the thought pattern.

The shift gave us the freedom to consider alternative approaches to relapse prevention. The task was to find ways to teach people to decenter from their negative thoughts, preferably in a way that would take up the cognitive "space" in a mind otherwise filled with ruminative thoughts. (We have not said much about this aspect of the model, for it takes us too far afield. Suffice it to say that most models of mind assume that conscious, aware forms of information processing take up space in a "limited capacity channel." This implies that if the limited channel can be filled with nonruminative material, the person, for that period, will simply be unable to ruminate. See Teasdale and colleagues[60] for more details of this aspect of our thinking.)

Could we get at these processes directly? That is, could we find a way to bring about a shift in a person's relationship to his or her negative thoughts and feelings, in a way that would have no elements explicitly directed at changing thought content?

As we considered these questions, John Teasdale was reminded of possibilities he had considered almost a decade earlier, at a time when he was working at Oxford in the University Department of Psychiatry. He already had an interest in meditation. Knowing this, a colleague had invited him to a talk by the U.S.-born Buddhist monk Ajahn Sumedho. During the talk, John was struck by the parallels between the core ideas of the Buddhist analysis of suffering, as described by Sumedho, and the basic assumptions of cognitive therapy. Both approaches stressed that it was not experience itself that made us unhappy, but our *relationship* to experience (in the Buddhist analysis) or our *interpretation* of experience (in the Beckian analysis). It was also clear that a central aspect of Buddhist mindfulness meditation involved learning *to relate to thoughts as thoughts* (i.e., as mental events rather than "the truth" or "me"). In this way, individuals could free themselves from the effects of unhelpful thought patterns that might otherwise control their actions or create unhappy states of mind.

Inspired by this talk, John began to wonder whether it might be possible to help depressed patients by teaching them to see their negative thoughts *as* thoughts, that is, to decenter from them. Colleagues greeted these ideas with sympathetic interest but raised the critical, but awkward, question, "How?" And this was where things got stuck. Because, at that time, there seemed to be no obvious way that the subtleties of Buddhist insight meditation could be offered to patients in a form that might be part of a brief, structured, psychological treatment.

And so, although John continued to explore the use of other forms of meditation with depressed patients (e.g., Teasdale[64]), the idea of using meditation to help patients decenter from their negative thoughts was put on the shelf. It might have stayed there a long time, but, fortunately, luck intervened, in the visit of one of our colleagues, Marsha Linehan.

Marsha had spent part of her 1991 sabbatical leave with John Teasdale and Mark Williams at the Medical Research Council's Applied Psychology Unit in Cambridge. She had used the concept of decentering in her development of dialectical behavior therapy.[65] She had worked many years developing this psychological treatment for people who presented clinicians with some of their most challenging problems: those with a diagnosis of borderline personality disorder. In the treatment manual she developed, numerous exercises trained patients to pay attention to their experience in ways that allowed them to observe events as they were occurring. She had introduced a training procedure called "mindfulness" in the service of helping her patients protect themselves from their more powerful thoughts and emotions, by showing them how to step back from them and relate to them less literally.

While in Cambridge, as well as telling us about her own work, Marsha had mentioned the name of Jon Kabat-Zinn. He, it appeared, had developed a brief, structured program to teach mindfulness in a health care setting with patients suffering from chronic pain. Now, over a year after that sabbatical conversation, as we looked for ways to train recovered depressed patients to decenter from depressive thinking, the memory of that conversation, and of the thoughts prompted by Ajahn Sumedho's talk, came to mind: Could Jon Kabat-Zinn's program now offer us the way forward that John had looked for but been unable to find back in 1984? We decided to look more closely at the work of Kabat-Zinn.

MINDFULNESS

Jon Kabat-Zinn described mindfulness in this way: "Mindfulness means paying attention in a particular way: on purpose, in the present moment, and nonjudgmentally" (p. 4).[66] This was remarkable in its directness and simplicity. How was mindfulness used in practice? Kabat-Zinn's Stress Reduction Clinic at the University of Massachusetts (UMass) Medical Center had several unique features. In it, he taught participants the ancient practice of mindfulness meditation, adapted from its use as a spiritual practice to extend its availability and relevance to patients suffering from a variety of chronic physical illnesses. His aim was to equip patients with ways of responding to the stress in their lives that allowed them to step out of those mental reactions that often worsened the stress and interfered with effective problem solving.

We did not know much about Kabat-Zinn's work. We happened to be meeting in Toronto at the time we were considering whether it might be relevant. We knew he had written a book about his stress reduction program, *Full Catastrophe Living*, so the three of us took a break, walked to the Cavendish bookstore close to the Clarke, bought three copies, and spent the next few hours engrossed in it.

The accounts of what his patients were getting out of the program bore a striking similarity to what we were beginning to see as the central change process in cognitive therapy. It became rapidly clear how the mindfulness Kabat-Zinn was teaching fostered a decentered relationship to mental contents by training people to take a wider perspective, in order to observe their thinking as it was occurring. For example, there is a story in the book[67] about a patient who had just recovered from a heart attack. He found himself washing his car in his driveway at 10 o'clock at night, using floodlights for illumination! All of a sudden, he had the realization that he didn't have to be doing this. The idea that he must wash his car was just a thought. It was just that he never stopped to question what he thought needed doing. The way Kabat-Zinn expressed this could not have summed up more accurately what we had in mind when we were trying to understand how cognitive therapy had its decentering effects:

> It is remarkable how liberating it feels to be able to see that your thoughts are just thoughts and that they are not "you" or "reality."
> . . . The simple act of recognizing your thoughts as thoughts can free you from the distorted reality they often create and allow for more clear-sightedness and a greater sense of manageability in your life. (pp. 69–70)[67]

This most significant element struck a chord with us at that time.

There were a number of other reasons to believe that this approach might be relevant. First, the mindfulness practice Kabat-Zinn taught to his patients involved exercises in awareness. According to our understanding of the factors that allow the thought–affect cycles to self-perpetuate, any exercise in purposeful awareness would have the advantage of "taking up capacity" in the limited information-processing channel. This would starve the vicious ruminative cycles of the resources needed to maintain them.

Second, such practice at becoming aware of thoughts, feelings, and body sensations might meet the need we had identified to help patients recognize at an early stage the times they were most likely to slide into depression. Mindfulness exercises might provide an early warning system of an impending avalanche, so that it could be stopped before the rocks started to slide.

Third, we could not ignore a further aspect of the mindfulness-based stress reduction (MBSR) program at UMass: classes of 30 or more people at a time. Here was an approach that promised to meet the larger need of an increasing number of patients suffering from depression. And all this took place in a context where no attempt was made to deal with the particular content of any individual's thoughts.

Here was another way to reach the same end of decentering that we considered critical to the relapse prevention effects of cognitive therapy. MBSR, a fully developed and highly cost-efficient treatment program with increasing empirical support, could be made available to many patients. Could we use this as a template in developing our own approach with recovered depressed patients? While these skills had not been shown to be applicable to problems in clinically depressed patients, there was encouraging evidence for their efficacy in related disorders that often went along with depression (e.g., chronic pain,[68] generalized anxiety disorder[69]). There was also evidence that some form of mindfulness practice was maintained on a regular basis by a majority of patients up to 3 years after the initial training had been completed.[70]

In summary, mindfulness appeared to offer a number of possibilities for approaching relapse prevention. We saw it as providing alternative methods for teaching decentering skills, training patients to recognize when their mood was deteriorating, and using techniques that would take up limited resources in channels of information processing that normally sustained ruminative thought–affect cycles.

MAKING CONTACT WITH THE STRESS REDUCTION CLINIC AT UMASS MEDICAL CENTER

So why, then, did we not rush to Worcester, Massachusetts, and embrace these ideas? We discussed the possibility of contacting Kabat-Zinn, but we could not easily agree on whether this was a good idea. There were reasons to be cautious. For one thing, such an exploration of mindfulness and awareness training would take us away from our brief to design a maintenance form of cognitive therapy. Furthermore, only one of us had experience with meditation practice, on the basis of which he believed it might hold promise for patients who had been depressed. Indeed, John Teasdale had moved from Oxford to Cambridge in 1985 with an explicit plan to investigate the possible benefits of meditation in dealing with depressed mind states.

But we also had to recognize a more skeptical view. What evidence was there that mindfulness meditation was any more effective than relaxation training? Hadn't one of the earliest studies examining psychological treatment, that by McLean and Hakstian in 1979, shown the unequivocal superiority of cognitive-behavioral therapy over relaxation in treating depression?[71] And if we were attracted because of its affinity with cognitive therapy principles and practice, why not stay with cognitive therapy? Finally, we must admit that we were unsure how such a move might affect our scientific colleagues. Meditation seemed too close to a form of religious practice, and though each of us had a different "take" on religion, we all felt that such personal issues were best left outside the laboratory and the clinic.

So, although there were many reasons for exploring mindfulness further, we had many reservations. We agreed in the end that we would at least explore further the mindfulness approach. We would contact Kabat-Zinn and pilot-test some of the mindfulness exercises with one or two patients. At this stage, it was not clear which way the project would go. Differences of opinion can be seen in the different tone of two letters. The first was sent by Zindel Segal to John Teasdale; the second, by

John Teasdale to Jon Kabat-Zinn. Only when we went through our own archives to prepare this book did we notice the curious juxtaposition of attitudes, sent, by a strange coincidence, on the very same day.

Zindel Segal's letter betrays an uneasy tone:

> *. . . I have had the opportunity to try out the "just pay attention to your breathing" technique with a patient who is 6 months post depression. Her reaction was generally receptive and she agreed to keep a log for a month and practice "observing her attention wander and return to her thoughts." My reaction, on the other hand, is that I was teaching her to meditate!!!, and this made me feel somewhat uncomfortable. It will be interesting to compare notes in January . . .*

John Teasdale's letter to Jon Kabat-Zinn was very different. It refers to his long-lasting interest in this subject and is explicit in its enthusiasm about exploring new territory:

> *. . . given the apparent importance of streams of negative thoughts in the maintenance of clinical depression, I have become increasingly interested in the possible use of meditation-related procedures . . .*

And:

> *I have been very impressed by your ability to extract the essence of Buddhist mindfulness meditation and to translate it into a format that is accessible and clearly very effective in helping the average U.S. citizen. For both personal and professional reasons, I would very much like to explore the applicability of your work to treatment of depression.*

Our collective mix of enthusiasm and curiosity on one hand, and diffidence and alarm on the other, might not be atypical of the reactions of other behaviorally and cognitively trained therapists. Despite a good degree of skepticism and differences among us, it was clear from reading and listening to the tapes used in the program that MBSR included at least some elements that might be very helpful to the maintenance version of cognitive therapy we still expected to develop. We wanted to see firsthand what actual skills patients were learning in MBSR, whatever the philosophy behind their delivery.

We now had a theoretical model that emphasized the importance of changing patients' relationships to their negative thoughts and feelings. We had moved away from thinking that the key ingredient in cognitive therapy (the reason why it had such long-lasting effects) was that it changed a person's degree of belief in his or her thoughts and attitudes. Instead, we believed that the key was whether people could learn to take a decentered perspective on their patterns of thinking. If this were true, then there was no need to change the content of people's thoughts, but only how they related to this content. We had recognized that in the MBSR program there appeared to be an emphasis on decentering from which we might learn. We visited Jon Kabat-Zinn in October 1993 to sit in on some mindfulness classes.

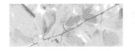 CHAPTER 3

Developing Mindfulness-Based Cognitive Therapy

Jon Kabat-Zinn set up the Stress Reduction Clinic (offering MBSR) at the University of Massachusetts Medical Center in Worcester in 1979. By the time we were in contact with him, he and his colleagues had helped more than 10,000 people with a range of conditions, including heart disease, cancer, AIDS, chronic pain, stress-related gastrointestinal problems, headaches, high blood pressure, sleep disorders, anxiety, and panic. By 1993, the clinic had already evaluated the efficacy of its approach with patients suffering from anxiety disorders[69] and chronic pain.[68] The evidence showed that most participants experienced not only long-lasting physical and psychological symptom reduction but also deep positive changes in attitude; behavior; and perception of self, others, and the world.

What did the Stress Reduction Clinic at UMass actually do? The program consisted of eight weekly 2½-hour sessions, at which instructors met with around 30 patients. The program, then and now, involves a great deal of commitment. For example, the between-session daily practices (lasting up to 1 hour a day) are an essential element of the program. People are told that it may be stressful to take the stress reduction program!

The primary work of the program is intensive training in mindfulness meditation. The aim is to increase patients' awareness of present, moment-to-moment experience. They receive extensive practice in learning to bring their attention back to the present, using a focus on the breath as an "anchor," whenever they notice that their attention has been diverted to streams of thought, worries, or general lack of awareness, and then build on this attentional training to bring openhearted awareness and clarity of seeing to their experience, including those aspects of experience that they fear most.

FIRST IMPRESSIONS

On our first visit to the Stress Reduction Clinic, we were invited to sit in on Session 1 of the MBSR program led by Jon Kabat-Zinn. The classes were held in a large, carpeted conference room. The first thing we noticed was that the composition of the group was different from what we were accustomed to, in that many patients appeared to be dealing with very difficult medical conditions. On the other hand, the majority of the class did not have severe mental health problems: These participants seemed happy to be in the class, and relatively willing to share their experiences. Although we knew that the clinic originally had been set up to deal with severe and chronic physical illness and disability, it remained unclear whether the experience would be relevant to relapse in depression as we had thought. This was especially so since depression, like other mental health problems, brings with it a certain "heaviness"—an almost palpable sense of ongoing trauma and impending crisis. Added to this is the feeling of shame and self-disgust that recurrent mental health problems can bring, different in many respects from that which comes with physical problems that feel less "shameful" to the person.

The theme of the first MBSR class focused on becoming more aware of the tendency we all have to be on automatic pilot much of the time; how we do ordinary things (e.g., eating) in everyday life without really being aware of what we are doing. Later on, the instructor led the class through an exercise that involved bringing awareness to different parts of the body in turn (the "body scan"). The instruction was simply to pay attention, moment by moment, to sensations in each part of the body, rather than trying to alter them in any way.

Although the content of the session was different, nothing appeared inconsistent with our own understanding of the basic processes underlying cognitive therapy's effects. In fact, the emphasis on being more aware of things, of stepping out of automatic pilot, was central to our view that people who have been depressed need to learn to be more aware of the early warning signals indicating times when their mood might deteriorate. Here were some practices that might help them do just that.

The program builds on the initial experience with the body scan, introducing (in later sessions) meditation on the breath, the body, sights, and sounds. More attention is paid to body sensations than is common in most psychological treatments for depression, using mindful movement to explore in some detail different patterns of body sensations and reactions to them. But in addition, participants are taught, whatever their chosen focus of attention at any moment, to allow, as best they can, thoughts, feelings, and sensations to come and go in the mind. The instruction is to notice how the mind often tends to become attached to an experience judged to be positive, and avoids or escapes an experience judged to be negative. In addition to noting this in daily practice, at one point in the course, participants are given home practice in which they keep a diary of pleasant and (a week later) unpleasant events. They are asked to pay special attention to thoughts, feelings, and body sensations associated with each event they record.

After the first class, the curriculum for subsequent sessions always prioritizes meditation practice (i.e., the instructor leads the class in a practice such as a body scan, or a sitting meditation with focus on the breath). The remainder of each session mixes dialogue, further practice, poetry, story, and awareness exercises, all in the service of helping participants become more aware of the "here and now" (for details, see Kabat-Zinn's *Full Catastrophe Living*[67]). The basic message of the program is that we all (whether patients or clinicians) frequently find ourselves swept away by the currents of thought and feeling related to the past, present, or future. We often lose the vividness of the present moment by "being somewhere else." When we are able to be in the present moment, we become more awake in our lives, more aware of each moment, and more aware of the choices open to us.

Although some of the vocabulary used in the stress reduction program was not what we would normally use in cognitive therapy, it appeared to us from our first visit, together with our reading about the program and listening to its recorded guided meditations, that we could relatively easily combine the two approaches without having to make too many changes in the way we worked with patients. We were particularly attracted to the fact that patients in the program learn generic skills of attentional control. Because these skills are generic, learning does not depend on the presence of negative thoughts and feelings. They can be practiced on a wide range of experiences in everyday life. This looked as if it would suit our purposes very well, for we wanted a procedure that could be used when patients were not currently feeling depressed. At this point, patients would be looking for something to increase positive well-being and perhaps reduce the risk of future depression, rather than something to reduce current symptoms of depression.

For our purposes, there seemed to be another advantage of the MBSR program over traditional therapy. Since we wanted a program for people between episodes, it had to be suitable at a point when people were not actually seeking treatment. The stress reduction techniques of MBSR, such as focusing on breathing or mindful movement based on yoga, are those that many people choose to do in their spare time as a way to promote health and well-being. This boded well for a prophylactic approach.

Furthermore, participants in MBSR are asked to practice mindfulness skills on a daily basis as part of their home practice, and the evidence suggested that they continue to do this long after they have completed the MBSR program (up to 3 years[70]). This seems to be a valuable way to keep new learning active, so it is very relevant to depressed patients in recovery, whose task is to remain prepared for an event that might not happen until months, or even years, later. If patients ran into difficulties, the daily practice ensured that the skills could be recalled and implemented more easily. In addition, it seemed to us that practice in increased awareness of momentary experience made it more likely that patients would detect, at the earliest possible stage, any signs of incipient relapse. Patients would therefore be more likely to take appropriate action at a point when interventions have the greatest chance of success. We began to see how we might design a program that, in combining MBSR and cognitive therapy into a new form of cognitive therapy, would help recovered depressed patients stay well.

REASONS TO BE CAUTIOUS: THE PERSONAL PRACTICE OF MINDFULNESS AND FULFILLING PROMISES

In that first visit, the instructors at UMass sounded a note of caution. If we were serious about incorporating mindfulness in our approach, then, as prospective instructors, we would have to have our own mindfulness meditation practice. Frankly, we were not at all sure about this. After all, we did not intend to teach MBSR, but to incorporate some of its techniques into our maintenance form of cognitive therapy. We were interested mainly in the theoretical and practical convergence we could see between mindfulness and cognitive approaches and the need to notice warning signs earlier; the need to decenter from negative thoughts; and the need to deploy attention in ways that would starve the self-perpetuating, relapse-related thought–affect cycles of cognitive resources. None of this seemed to require us to develop a mindfulness meditation practice. So we simply "took note" of their opinion on the issue: We could think about that later.

We had seen enough on our first visit to confirm our view that MBSR might be a convenient vehicle to teach many of the principles and practices of decentering, and to bring about a reduction in risk of relapse. Of course, we had only witnessed Session 1, but given that at that time we had a pretty definite view of what changes had to be brought about in formerly depressed patients, we could easily imagine that the remainder of the sessions (if we had time to sit in on them) would also confirm our view.

As it was, we decided to incorporate mindfulness into a "regular" cognitive therapy format—a format that would incorporate the problem-solving approach with which we were familiar. This seemed a good compromise. It allowed us to avoid having to adopt wholesale the values and practices associated with meditation. And there was much in the MBSR program we could use.

However, there was a second reason to be cautious. Combining cognitive therapy with another, different approach (no matter how similar) was not what we had been funded to do. Incorporating any MBSR techniques might be construed as changing cognitive therapy too much to qualify as simply a maintenance version of the therapy. Furthermore, we felt that we needed an approach that could be taught to patients who had never had cognitive therapy at the acute stage of their depression. What we were suggesting represented a move away from a standard maintenance therapy (i.e., a therapy that extended the acute phase of treatment into the maintenance phase), toward an approach that might have wider applicability, but this was not what we had promised to develop for the MacArthur Foundation.

It was unclear how best to proceed, and in the end, we decided to face the issue head on and contact David Kupfer to discuss the dilemma and find out what the MacArthur Foundation might think of this new plan. His decision was to be an important turning point in the project. He encouraged us to develop whatever treatment we thought most effective. In his mind, one of the operational definitions of success was that we should be able to be manualize whatever form of preventive treatment we developed, and that it be judged theoretically and empirically credible enough to evaluate once the MacArthur project was over. Such manualization has become a critical aspect of clinical trials methodology.[72] Without it, an approach cannot be reliably taught by other clinicians, which is essential if it is to be available more widely to patients who need it. Over the next few weeks and months, we drew up a preliminary manual of a treatment that combined some MBSR and cognitive therapy strategies.

ATTENTIONAL CONTROL TRAINING

In order better to reflect the central role played by attentional training in our preventive intervention, we decided to call our version of cognitive therapy "attentional control training." The aim of attentional control training was to combine mindfulness and cognitive approaches to enable patients to increase their awareness. This would have three positive consequences. First, awareness would enable patients to notice when they were about to undergo dangerous mood swings. Second, awareness itself would take up those scarce processing resources that might have been supporting rumination, thereby weakening it. Third, patients could then decenter or exit from the more automatic, depression-linked patterns of thought that these moods habitually brought to mind. At that point, techniques from cognitive therapy could allow patients to deal with the negative thoughts that any sad moods might reactivate.

This sounded great in theory, but we needed to check out these ideas. Would the treatment be useful to our patients, and would the rationale be compelling to our academic colleagues? In relation to the first issue, we decided that we would each run our own pilot group. In relation to the second, we would send our draft treatment manual to the MacArthur Research Network for comments.

For our pilot classes, we used the 8-week group structure developed at the UMass Stress Reduction Clinic as the basis of attentional control training and modified it to deal with themes of preventing depressive relapse (though shortening the length of each session to 2 hours). We taught mindfulness by having the class listen to a 20-minute audiotape of mindfulness instructions by Kabat-Zinn that we had shortened for the purpose. We asked participants to listen to the tape once a day as home practice. The pilot groups also watched an episode of the television program *Healing from Within* (one of the Bill Moyers series *Healing and the Mind*, produced by the Public Broadcasting Service), which featured the 8-week MBSR program at the Stress Reduction Clinic.

The feedback we received from the 8-week pilot program was very revealing. Some of the patients in each group appeared to do well. It was as if they learned the skills and used them effectively to deal with problems in their lives. Other patients, however, experienced considerable difficulty in applying the skills of attentional control and observation to their emotional upheaval. To be honest, this outcome may have reflected a number of silent assumptions on our part. Reflecting now on how we ran those groups, it was as if we believed that this approach would be OK for mildly negative thoughts and feelings, but not for more severe and persistent ones. In our pilot classes, any suggestions we made to participants to increase awareness of difficult issues were politely refused. We withdrew the suggestions quickly, for we had little confidence that we could deal with such difficulties using this approach.

Our intention was that participants gradually acquire the skills of decentering, so they might subsequently use them when at risk of their thoughts and feelings spiraling out of control. But participants' experiences and behavior did not fit our carefully constructed plans. They may have recovered from depression, but they wanted to bring to the discussion the many ups and downs in their lives. The problem was that patients were looking for help in dealing with these unwanted emotions early in the program, before they had time to learn the skills of decentering and thought answering that we saw as crucial.

So how were we to respond to this situation? Recall that our main intent behind attentional control training was to teach patients skills for decentering, which would allow them to step out of the "automatic pilot" state of mind or mode, in order to nip in the bud the escalation of self-sustaining patterns of depressive thought. But what do you do when patients have emotional ups and down that cannot be dealt with by decentering from thoughts alone? What do you do when patients have tried to decenter and the negative feelings are still there? We had assumed that we would naturally move into a cognitive therapy mode for dealing with these concerns.

However, with a group of 10 or more patients, there never seemed to be enough time for the instructor to deal with everyone's problems. To handle these problems with the same thoroughness as individual cognitive therapy would normally involve identifying negative thoughts feeding unwanted emotions, considering evidence for and against such thoughts, reviewing alternative possibilities, setting behavioral experiments, and so on. Although some therapists had developed cognitive therapy in a group format, we wanted to teach other skills, too, and along with standard cognitive strategies, there was simply not enough time to do both adequately. The skills in attentional control, which were crucial to the decentering we wanted to teach participants, seemed not to be deliverable in the format we had envisioned.

Something was not quite right, but what was it? The theoretical perspective we had brought to the problem of relapse seemed coherent. Equally, the changes we had made in aspects of MBSR as we incorporated them into attentional control training seemed harmless enough. For example, we had chosen to use 20-minute audiotapes because we were not completely confident that patients would listen to longer tapes. At UMass the tapes are 40–45 minutes long. But it did not seem very plausible that these kinds of procedural changes could explain all our difficulties. It seemed that something more fundamental was amiss.

These difficulties in implementing the attentional control training program were not our only problem. We had sent a draft version of the manual to Kupfer for his comments in the winter of 1994. He sent it out for review. To our chagrin, the review of our work was skeptical of its contribution. The concerns raised were that we focused too much on mindfulness training, leaving out the valuable cognitive therapy–based components that patients really needed. The review concluded that while the "emphasis on discrete exercises and homework-based practice would provide effective learning experiences, it is still unclear how the mindfulness techniques contribute to controlling the risk of future depressive disorder." The very thing we thought was innovative failed to impress the reviewer as being relevant at all.

At this point, we were at a crossroads. We had worked hard to bring in new ideas to define the challenges faced by depressed patients in recovery and the types of interventions that would address them more directly. In spite of this, however, we had clearly not convinced this reviewer that anything new was necessary. He or she saw in our proposals only a weakening of accepted cognitive-behavioral principles and practice. In retrospect, the reviewer was right. In our first draft manual, there were possibly too few cognitive and behavioral techniques. If the patients were not going to be taught cognitive therapy skills, then there was the danger that they would be left in no-man's-land, between a therapy that had proven effectiveness in reducing relapse and a new set of principles and practices that, for depression, were dangerously unproven. We had to make a decision: Either go back to the original plan to draw up a maintenance version of cognitive therapy to be used by patients when they were well, or make much clearer the potential of the clinical implementation of the mindfulness-based approach.

WHAT WERE THE INSTRUCTORS IN MINDFULNESS-BASED STRESS REDUCTION ACTUALLY DOING?

We arrived at the Stress Reduction Clinic at UMass Medical Center for the second time in the spring of 1995, with fewer certainties. But there was another important difference. On our first visit, we had seen the first session of one class and had only talked (and read) about the remainder of the program. On this second visit, we had the chance to sit in on three different classes midway through the program, a time when participants were working with difficult physical and emotional issues. We now saw differences between attentional control training and the MBSR mindfulness approach that we had not seen before. In particular, we saw how experienced mindfulness teachers like Saki Santorelli, Ferris Urbanowski, and Elana Rosenbaum worked with participants' painful emotions. They did not try to fix or give solutions to problems raised. When patients said they felt sad or afraid, or that they had judgmental or hopeless thoughts, they were taught a radically different approach, one that encouraged them to "allow" difficult thoughts and feelings simply to be there to bring to them a kindly awareness, to adopt toward these thoughts and feelings a more "welcoming" than a "need to solve" stance. For us, this was more than a problem of fine-tuning attentional control training. In order to proceed any further, it was vital that we understand the nature of this difference. Without it, our attempts to integrate cognitive therapy and MBSR meaningfully would likely stop there.

Instead of translating into cognitive therapy what we saw in MBSR, we decided to look again at all aspects of MBSR, rather than just at those parts that fit our preexisting theory. We thought again about the fact that all the MBSR instructors were themselves practicing mindfulness meditation, and that they seemed able to embody the same gentle approach to patients' difficulties that the patients themselves were being encouraged to take. The stance of the instructor was itself "invitational." In addition, there was always the assumption of "continuity" between the experiences of the instructor and those of participants. If class members described becoming aware of how they had been criticizing themselves, for example, the experience of dealing with self-critical thoughts was something the instructor had in common with others in the class. The assumption here was simple: that minds tend to operate in similar ways, and there is no basis for discriminating between the minds of those seeking help and those offering it.

OUR OWN MINDFULNESS PRACTICE?

As we contemplated this change, we became aware of an issue that we could not put off any longer: our own mindfulness practice. Recall that when we first visited the Stress Reduction Clinic and started our pilot work, we had seen MBSR as mostly a vehicle for teaching participants attentional control as a skills training exercise. We felt that the technique could be adequately conveyed using the audiotapes of Kabat-Zinn's meditation instructions both in class and for home practice. This view ran counter to the spirit of the message we were getting from the staff at the Stress Reduction Clinic.

The staff at the Stress Reduction Clinic had consistently emphasized the importance of instructors having their own meditation practice, and within minutes of first meeting us, they asked about our personal commitment to the practice of mindfulness. We had now seen for our-selves the remarkable way they were able to embody a different relation-ship to the most intense distress and emotion in their patients. And we had seen the MBSR instructors going further in their work with nega-tive affect than we had been able to do in the group context by staying within our therapist roles. We now saw more clearly how these two things were connected: *that this ability to relate differently to negative affect came from having their own ongoing mindfulness practice, so that they might teach mindfulness out of their experience of it.* A vital part of what the MBSR instructor conveyed was his or her own embodiment of mindfulness in interactions with the class.

This ultimately persuaded us of the wisdom of the advice we had not wholly heeded on our first visit. Participants in the MBSR program learn about mindfulness in two ways: through their own practice, and when the instructor him- or herself is able to embody it in the way issues are dealt with in the class. This was different from our earlier concep-tion of mindfulness as a technique in which patients could be trained by a therapist who might or might not have been mindful him- or herself. If the therapists themselves are not mindful as they teach, the extent to which class members can learn mindfulness will be limited. Just as in rock climbing, those who are learning need to feel that the instructor has both the skill and experience to deal with the difficult situations that arise. In the same way, mindfulness training involves the instructor participating alongside the patient, not giving instructions, as it were, from the bottom of the rock face. The challenge to us as clinicians, and as scientists, was to participate in mindfulness, to experience it from the inside. We com-mitted ourselves to developing a regular mindfulness meditation practice.

Committing to doing something is one thing; doing it is quite another. We experienced many struggles in doing this "simple" thing that we had asked our patients to do. Finding time in a busy schedule, or perhaps getting up 45 minutes earlier than usual, was difficult. There was, we discovered, a wonderful array of excuses on a particular day to take a break from the discipline of daily practice. Then, there was the issue of how much of this we could disclose to professional colleagues (a minor issue, as it turned out; it constantly surprises us how many of our colleagues also do some practice like this and have not told anyone). We remembered what we had heard mindfulness instructors say to their patients: that taking the stress reduction classes is stressful. Now we knew what they meant. Apart from anything else, we found that our respect for our patients rose enormously, perhaps even more for those who struggle and struggle yet still turn up each week for the class.

As time passed, we were able to incorporate the experience with the mindfulness practice into our further reading and into discussions with each other, and with the teachers at the Stress Reduction Clinic in our subsequent visits. Our difficulties in implementing attentional control training had taught us something very important. It had helped us to realize that the approach we had been developing to reduce relapse in depressed patients required revision, and we now felt we could look again to see what these revisions should be. Our perspective about what patients needed to learn in class and in home practice had changed radically. We found ourselves more confident that patients already had within themselves the resources they needed to move forward in the way they handled their problems. The issue turned on how best to empower them to do so, and this would require us to change both our theory and our practice.

IMPLICATIONS FOR OUR APPROACH: THE NATURE OF DECENTERING

We could now see that our theoretical analysis had taken us only part of the way. We had stressed the importance of the change in relationship to thoughts that cognitive therapy brought about when it protected a person against relapse. This is what we had meant by decentering. But we could now see that our understanding of "decentering" was at once too specific, yet not specific enough.

In the first place, our understanding was too specific because it referred mainly to thoughts. This was quite understandable given that our starting point had been an attempt to understand the role of decentering in thought change in cognitive therapy. But the MBSR program was teaching people to explore how they might have a different relationship not only to thoughts but *also* to feelings, body sensations, and impulses to act, that is, to the whole mind–body state.

In the second place, our understanding of decentering was not specific enough. "Decentering" is an ambiguous term: It can be done in a number of ways, and with a number of different attitudes. For example, decentering can be seen as a "stepping away from." But this might mean ignoring a problem and hoping it will go away. Or it might mean trying to dissociate from thoughts or feelings to suppress, repress, or otherwise avoid them. The mode of mind one brings to decentering is critical. The stance of the mindfulness approach is one of *welcoming* and *allowing*. It is invitational and compassionate. It encourages "opening" to the difficult and adopting an attitude of gentleness to all experience.

Broadening the scope of decentering beyond the realm of thinking brings all experience within this attitude of allowing and welcoming. So long as we focused only on thoughts, we offered participants a restricted view of the means to deal with negative feelings and sensations. Broadening the scope might allow participants to learn how they might deal directly with feelings, thoughts, impulses, and body sensations, rather than (as we had planned in attentional control training) dealing with negative feelings by identifying and changing related patterns of negative thought. Extending the application of decentering to feelings, impulses, and body sensations allowed more "ways in" to difficult experiences. Even when negative thinking was the predominant feature, this alternative approach allowed participants to handle such negative thoughts by bringing, as it were, a "friendly awareness" to the parts of the body affected by the thought–affect–behavior cycle. The difficulty of describing these processes in words further emphasizes the importance of understanding them "from the inside," from the perspective of ongoing mindfulness practice.

FROM THERAPIST TO INSTRUCTOR: TEACHING PEOPLE A NEW WAY OF RELATING TO EXPERIENCE

Looking back now, given where we were coming from, it is understandable that we would see mindfulness as a technique that could fit straightforwardly into a cognitive therapy framework. In our own training, we had been taught that when faced with a difficult clinical problem, we should collaborate with the patient on how best to solve it by seeing what thoughts, interpretations, and assumptions might be causing or exacerbating the problem. We anticipated taking the same approach in developing attentional control training, bolting mindfulness techniques onto this basic therapy framework. However, it became clear from our later visits to the Stress Reduction Clinic that unless we changed the basic structure of our treatment, we would continually revert to dealing with the most difficult problems by searching for more elaborate ways to fix them. Instead, it now appeared to us that the overarching structure of our treatment program needed to change from a mode in which we were therapists to a mode in which we were instructors. What was the difference? As therapists, coming as we did from the cognitive-behavioral tradition, we felt a responsibility to help patients solve their problems, "untie the knots" of their thinking and feeling, and reduce their distress, staying with a problem until it was resolved. By contrast, we saw that the MBSR instructors left responsibility clearly with the patients themselves, and saw their primary role as empowering patients to relate mindfully to their experience on a moment-by-moment basis.

Instructors in MBSR encouraged participants to let go of the idea that problems might, with enough effort, be "fixed." If fixing worked, then fine. But the mindfulness approach was explicit about the danger that such attempts at fixing might merely reinforce people's attitude that their problems were the "enemy," and that once they were eliminated, everything would be fine. The problem is that this approach may encourage further attempts to solve problems by ruminating on them, and these attempts often keep people trapped in the state from which they are trying to escape. This is something that family therapists have emphasized for years[73]; it is central to Linehan's concept of self-invalidation,[74] and there is good experimental support for the notion.[75]

Of course, it is understandable that someone who is in distress will want to avoid further suffering. The MBSR approach, however, was that a skillful response would involve, first, recognizing how quickly we react by jumping in and trying to solve the problem. It emphasized letting go of the attempts at problem solving and, instead, purposely standing back to see what it feels like to see the problem through the lens of nonreactivity, and to bring a kindly awareness to the difficulty.

This approach ran completely counter to the commonly held, but mistaken, view of meditation as a way to clear the mind or escape or shut out unwanted thoughts and feelings. The MBSR instructors did not help participants shut off or get rid of their negative experiences. Instead, they encouraged patients to discern from their own experience how fighting against unwanted thoughts, feelings, impulses, and body sensations sometimes created more tension and inner turmoil. With time, some of the tension itself could be reduced. Instead of continuously "feeding" the tension by participating in what their thoughts or feelings demanded, participants stayed close to this mental struggle by finding a calm place from which to observe and explore it.[67]

We could see more clearly why MBSR used body-focused awareness exercises, including a body scan exercise that involved focusing awareness on each part of the body in turn, as well as stretches, mindful walking, and yoga. These were not simply added extras, but a central way in which a person might learn to relate differently to his or her experience. The MBSR approach allows participants to see how negative thoughts and feelings are often expressed through the body. These sensations, too, could be held in awareness and observed, not pushed away. Awareness of the effect of negative thoughts and feelings *in the body* gave participants another place to stand, another perspective from which to view the situation. For us, this learning to work with difficulties through the body was to become a central message. This approach offered an alternative to avoidance of difficult or painful thoughts, feelings, or body sensations. Instead, it suggested a measured and reliable way of "turning toward" and "looking into" these experiences. It also suggested that breathing or a neutral focus in the body could be used as a base or center from which to steady oneself if the work of looking at one's experience became overwhelming. Both of these ideas seemed to have the effect of "leveling the playing field," so that *any* experience, regardless of its perceived valence or importance, was seen as worthy of the person's attention.

Based on what we had seen, we concluded that class members were not just being exposed to a set of skills or techniques to be used at the first sign of stress. They were actually learning *a more general mode of mind that was especially helpful in relating to difficult experiences*. Participants' regular meditation was teaching them to understand the nature of their thoughts, simply as thoughts, and to observe the relationship they had to them. More than that, their meditation also cultivated a new attitude toward all experience, including feelings, body sensations, and impulses to act.

MINDFULNESS-BASED COGNITIVE THERAPY

In summary, our deeper understanding of what was actually going on in the MBSR program was directly relevant to the difficulties we had experienced in our initial attempt to use attentional control training. We had first come to MBSR through our belief that decentering and developing a different relationship to negative thinking was the key to cognitive therapy's ability to prevent relapse. We found that decentering was also important in the MBSR program. We then tried to use decentering to "nip in the bud" low-level negative thoughts and feelings. However, for more intense feelings, we had reverted to a conventional cognitive therapy approach, only to find there was just not enough time in the attentional control training group context to use this approach effectively. We saw how the MBSR instructor's "decentered" stance, to even the most intense negative experiences, utilized decentering more widely and deeply than we did. We finally realized why Kabat-Zinn had called his book *Full Catastrophe Living.*[67] Rather than helping people avoid the catastrophes in their lives, he and his colleagues were teaching them how to embrace them and to live in the midst of them. This new perspective provided us with the springboard we needed to move forward.

Having a springboard is one thing; having the resources to allow you to use it is another. Throughout the period of development we have described, we had been drafting and redrafting applications to two funding bodies, both of which finally approved applications that enabled a multicenter research project to go ahead. One grant was from the United Kingdom's National Health Service's Wales Office of Research and Development for Health and Social Care, and the other was from the National Institute of Mental Health in Washington, D.C. These funding bodies allowed us to build on the work we had done for the MacArthur Foundation, to finalize the manual, and to evaluate our prophylactic intervention. The submissions that they approved reflected their interest in the link between the mindfulness intervention and our theoretical model that pointed to the reactivation at times of lowered mood, of patterns of persistent thought–affect–body cycles similar to the patterns that had occurred during a person's previous depressions. We were clearly saying that for depressive relapse, this was the risk factor that needed to be altered.

We could now write the final draft of the treatment manual, out of our new understanding of how best to capture the decentering that we believed had been a critical factor in cognitive therapy. We would do so in the context of a mindfulness approach that used awareness of all experience as grist for the mill in preventing future depression. We now had an eight-session program that was closely modeled on MBSR yet contained some important differences. Those differences were to be found in the elements of cognitive therapy and theory—easily missed but critically important—that address the specific vulnerabilities and exacerbating factors that make depression recurrent, and create so much agony for sufferers and their families.

We were finally in a position to submit our model to a scientific test, in the form of a first randomized clinical trial. The results of this trial, together with later trials, are reported in Chapter 19. In brief, participants in the 8-week program were much less likely to become depressed again in the 12 months following their participation. Furthermore, we were surprised to find that the more "chronic" participants benefited more from the program than those with a shorter history of depression. Results showed that those who had suffered more episodes of depression in the past, and therefore had the greatest risk of relapse or recurrence, were helped more by the program than those who had experienced fewer episodes and were thus at less risk.

Following the completion of the trial, we became less sure that the title "attentional control training" conveyed the essence of the approach. We had incorporated cognitive therapy principles and practice into a mindfulness framework. It had become mindfulness-based cognitive therapy.

PART II

MINDFULNESS-BASED COGNITIVE THERAPY

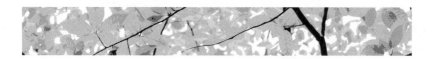

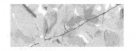 CHAPTER 4

Doing and Being

Before starting out on a journey into new territory, it is important to have as clear a map of the terrain as possible. In earlier chapters, we have described the ups and downs of the project, and how our early theoretical model was shaped and reshaped by the research and clinical findings, and by our experience in exploring the mindfulness approach. We have shown how the earlier maps we had drawn needed to be changed. Having redrawn these maps several times, there is a danger that the situation remains rather unclear, that we have left a map so filled with scribbles and amendments that it might be difficult to see which road is going where. Nowhere yet have we described the overall model on which we settled, the map that would guide our use of the mindfulness approach in preventing depression. In this chapter, therefore, we lay out, as best we can, our understanding of the psychological factors involved in the risk of relapse, and what it is that MBCT has to do if it is to help people with their vulnerabilities.

There is an additional, important reason for being very clear about what overall model is guiding treatment. Chapters 7–18 describe the program, session by session. You will see that it includes a range of practices, techniques, and exercises. But we believe the effectiveness of the whole is more than the sum of these parts. Our experience with mindfulness training and, before that, cognitive therapy has convinced us that the techniques that a therapist or instructor uses are, by themselves, not enough. Rather, it is the way that those procedures are woven together with other aspects of the total treatment context that determines just how much change will occur in those taking part in the program. The most enduring changes in patients in the MBCT program seem to come when instructors embody in their teaching an accurate and effective understanding of the processes of depressive relapse and the ways in which mindfulness impacts them. The teaching of specific skills and techniques, then, provides a vehicle to communicate shifts at a deep level of understanding, as well, of course, as an opportunity to acquire a new "bag of tools" for dealing with particular problematic situations.

What, exactly, does this mean? This is not an easy question to answer. The key idea is that patients make radical changes in the underlying views, or mental models, that shape their relationship to negative thoughts and feelings. Such shifts in view reflect the accumulated effects of repeated learning experiences, framed in a particular way, rather than the effects of general discussion of ideas or the blind application of techniques. We hope that in the following chapters, as we describe the program session by session, you will get some sense of how it weaves experiential and conceptual input together to create those shifts, and that the accumulating effects will lead to changes in your own mental models. However, reading about others' experiences is not the same as having those experiences oneself. So we offer here some conceptual scaffolding that may aid the integration of the material in the following chapters into changes in underlying views in the mind. In doing so, we inevitably repeat some of what we have discussed in Chapters 1–3. The aim here is to draw from that material an integrated model that underlies the MBCT program.

The ultimate aim of the MBCT program is to help individuals make a radical shift in their relationship to the thoughts, feelings, and body sensations that contribute to depressive relapse. The instructor's own basic understanding and orientation will be one of the most powerful influences affecting this process. Whether the instructor realizes it or not, this understanding colors the way each practice is presented, each interaction is handled. The cumulative effect of such coloring is that whatever the explicit message of the instructor's words, the more powerful influence, for good or ill, will be the nature of the instructor's basic, implicit views. So let us, as best we can, describe the understanding that, we believe, underpins effective use of MBCT.

UNDERSTANDING RELAPSE: A WORKING MODEL

Relapse involves the reactivation, at times of lowering mood, of patterns of negative thinking similar to the thought patterns that were active during previous episodes of depression. These patterns pivot around a particular "view" or "model" of depressive experience. Within this view, the self is felt to be inadequate, worthless, and blameworthy, and negative thoughts are seen as accurate reflections of reality. Reactivation of these patterns of thinking is automatic. It comes about by itself rather than as the result of a deliberate decision. Indeed, the reappearance of these old patterns of thought is often the last thing for which anyone would wish. The patterns themselves also seem automatic, in the sense that the mind runs around some very well-worn mental grooves, or ruts, as old mental habits switch in and run off. Again, the thinking here is more a matter of the mind "doing its own thing" than of conscious decision and choice.

Although we speak of patterns of negative thinking, relapse actually involves the reactivation of a whole package of characteristic thoughts, feelings, and physical sensations. These different aspects of experience interact through feedback loops to create and re-create, moment to moment, an ongoing state of mind. If left unchecked, this state of mind can spiral down to a more severe and persistent state of depression and bring on relapse.

From this analysis, we can see that the central task of MBCT is to give patients the understanding and skills that will enable them to recognize and free themselves from these states of mind—to empower them to step out of the habitual, automatic patterns of mind and body that are reactivated by depressed mood and make them vulnerable to further episodes of depression.

THE RUMINATIVE MIND

If relapse involves the reactivation of states of mind based on old mental habits, the question naturally arises: Why does the mind keep these habits when they seem to be so unhelpful? The answer seems to be that these states of mind are seen as ways to achieve some highly desired goals.

Ironically, one of these goals is to prevent or reduce these very same states of mind. But, tragically, as we have seen, the strategies used to achieve that goal are quite counterproductive. They have exactly the opposite effect to that intended. Take, for example, the situation in which we are upset for days after a store clerk has been rude or an acquaintance has taken 2 days to return a phone call. We remain upset not so much because of the original situation, but because our minds go round and round some well-established grooves trying to work out why we got so upset in the first place. Worrying away at the problem in this way, far from helping us out of the hole of unhappiness into which we find ourselves sinking, means that we dig ourselves deeper into the very hole from which we are trying to escape.

There is a tragic mismatch between the strategies built into these well-rehearsed patterns of thinking and what is actually required to change such self-perpetuating states of mind. The old mental habits deceive us into attempting to "think" our way out of our problems. This involves ruminatively dwelling on current emotional states, past negative events, and all the problems that will be created if things don't change. At the heart of this rumination is a "discrepancy monitor": a process that continually monitors and evaluates the self and the current situation against a model or standard—an idea of what is desired, required, expected, or feared. Once this discrepancy monitor is switched on, it will find mismatches between how things are and how we think they should be. That is its job. Registering these mismatches motivates further attempts to reduce these discrepancies. But, crucially, dwelling on how things are not as we want them to be can, naturally enough, create further negative mood. In this way, our attempts to solve the "problem" of feeling sad by endlessly thinking about it can keep us locked into the state of mind from which we are doing our best to escape.

If we have previously experienced just how awful major depression can be, it is natural that we would be deeply invested in avoiding further depression, and that we would persist in trying to get rid of depression, even when these efforts have failed over and over again. In reality, a more skillful response would be to abandon those attempts and disengage from the state of mind that is creating the risk of relapse.

How can we do this? How can we help patients in MBCT learn to relate more skillfully to the states of mind that arise as they become depressed when, at the time that they take the program, they have recovered and are relatively free of depression? Is there some way in which we can use aspects of everyday experience as the basis for learning? To answer these questions, we need first to say something about how the mind works more generally.

MODES OF MIND

The activities of the mind are related to patterns of brain activity. Different mental activities, such as reading a book, painting a picture, or talking to a loved one, each involve different patterns of interaction between networks of nerve cells in the brain. The networks involved in one activity are often different from those involved in another activity. Networks can also be linked together in different patterns. If we looked into the brain, we would see shifting patterns in the activity of networks and in their connections with each other as the mind moves from one task to another. For a while, one pattern predominates, then a shift occurs, so brain networks that previously interacted in one pattern now do so in a different configuration. Over time, we would see the different activities of the mind reflected in continually shifting and evolving patterns of interaction between brain networks.

If we looked long enough, we would see that a limited number of core patterns of brain activity and interaction seem to crop up as recurring features in a wide variety of different mental activities. These core patterns reflect some basic "modes of mind."

We can think of these modes of mind as loosely analogous to the gears of a car. Just as each gear has a particular use (starting, accelerating, cruising, etc.), so each mode of mind has its own particular characteristics and functions. Over the course of a day, as the mind switches from one kind of activity to another, the underlying mode of mind changes—a little like the way that in a car, driven through a busy city, will undergo a continuous series of changes from one gear to another. And in much the same way a car can only be in one gear at a time, when the mind is in certain modes, it will not be in other modes at the same time.

The fact that a limited number of fundamental modes of mind underpin a wide variety of mental activities has important implications. It opens a way for us to use aspects of everyday experience to teach patients new ways to relate to the kind of mind states that support rumination and lead to relapse. We can think of mindfulness training as a way to teach individuals how to become more aware of their mode of mind ("mental gear") at any moment, and the skills to disengage from unhelpful modes of mind and to engage more helpful modes. We might describe this as learning to shift mental gears. In practice, this task often comes down to recognizing two main modes in which the mind operates, and learning the skills to move from one to the other. These two modes are known as "doing" and "being."

The "Driven–Doing" Mode

The ruminative state of mind is actually a variant of a much more general mode of mind that has been called the "doing" mode. The job of this mode of mind is to get things done—to achieve particular goals that the mind has set. These goals could relate to the external world—to make a meal, build a house, or travel to the moon—or to the internal world of self—to feel happy, not make mistakes, never be depressed again, or be a good person. The basic strategy to achieve such goals involves the discrepancy monitor we have already mentioned. First we create an idea of how we want things to be, or how we think they should be. Next, we compare that with our idea of how things are right now. If there is a difference between how things are and how we want them to be, then we generate thoughts and actions to try to close the gap. We monitor progress to see whether the gap is increasing or decreasing, and adjust our actions accordingly. We know we have reached our goal when our idea of how things are coincides with our idea of how we want them to be.

There is nothing inherently wrong with this doing mode. In fact, quite the reverse: This approach has worked brilliantly as a general strategy for solving problems and achieving goals in the *impersonal, external* world—whether those goals be as humble as buying all the items on our weekly shopping list or as lofty as building a pyramid. It is natural, then, that we should turn to this same doing mode when things are not as we would like them to be in our *personal, internal* worlds—our feelings and thoughts, or the kind of person we see ourselves to be. And this is where things can go terribly wrong.

But before we go on to describe how, it is important to forestall any possible misunderstanding. We are in no way suggesting that the doing mode *necessarily* causes problems—it does not. It is only when the doing mode "volunteers for a job it can't do"[76] (p. 40) that problems arise. In many, many, areas of our lives, the doing mode volunteers for a job it *can* do, and our lives are the better for it. To make the distinction clearer, we call problematic applications of this mode *driven–doing*, as opposed to the more general *doing*. This issue is so important that we will return to it later.

If action can be taken straightaway to reduce a discrepancy, and such action is successful, there is no problem. But what if we cannot find any effective actions, and our attempts to think up possible solutions get nowhere? With an external problem we might simply give up and get on with some other aspect of our lives. *But once the self becomes involved, it is much more difficult simply to let go of the goals we have set.* For example, if we are upset because a long-standing relationship has just ended, there will be many potential discrepancies between current reality and how we wish things to be. We may wish for restoration of the relationship, or for the start of another relationship. Most likely, we also wish we were not so upset. There may be solutions we could find. But what if we begin to feel that we are bound to end up alone, concluding that there is in us some basic failure as a person that caused the relationship to fail? This conclusion suggests no ready solution, and the discrepancy remains. And yet *we cannot let go* because we have such a central need not to be this kind of person—what could be more important to us than our own sense of identity?

The result of all this is that the mind continues to process information in doing mode, going round and round, dwelling on the discrepancy and rehearsing possible ways to reduce it. And our continued dwelling on the way we are not as we would like to be just makes us feel worse, taking us even further from our desired goal. This, in turn only serves to confirm our view that we are not the kind of person we feel we need to be in order to be happy.

The mind will continue to focus in this way until the discrepancy is reduced or some more immediately urgent task takes the focus of the mind elsewhere, only to return to the unresolved discrepancy once one has dealt with the other task. When the doing mode is working on internal,

BOX 4.1

The Doing Mode of Mind Can Be Really Helpful—but Often Isn't

We can make clearer the distinction between helpful and unhelpful applications of doing mode by considering a simple task—driving across town to take part in a meeting.

In the helpful version, the goal set is simply "be in the conference room of the Marshall Building by 2:00 P.M.." Doing mode then devises a sequence of subgoals and actions to achieve that goal and puts them into action. If the action plan runs into problems, such as an unanticipated traffic jam because of an accident, then doing mode searches for alternative actions (find another route) and if none is available, accepts the inevitability of arriving late. We make our apologies, briefly consider ways we might avoid similar problems in the future, and that is that—no need to dwell further.

In the driven–doing version, the self becomes entangled in the goal: "Be punctual at this meeting, as a conscientious person should be, so that others will respect you and value your contribution." (As this is a habitual pattern of goal setting, we may not necessarily be consciously aware of what we have "added extra.") When we get stuck in a traffic jam with this goal in mind, we add a further layer of "story" to our anticipation of arriving late: "I should have foreseen this. What will people think of me? We'll never get the contract now." We become anxious and agitated; we arrive at the meeting looking hot and bothered, with our minds more focused on our worries and concerns about others' judgments of us than on presenting a convincing argument. The meeting goes badly, we don't get the contract, and we come away dwelling on what a failure we are as persons. This is not something that we can accept as easily as the simple fact "I arrived late," and we spend hours ruminating on its implications, and what it means for our lives and future more generally.

self-related goals like this, we can more accurately call it the "driven–doing" mode.

If we look closely, we will see the driven–doing mode, so central to the ruminative thought patterns of recurrently depressed patients, in action in very many areas of our lives. Whenever there is a sense of "have to," "must," "should," "ought," or "need to," we can suspect the presence of this mode.

How else might we recognize the driven–doing mode subjectively? Its most common feature is a recurring sense of unsatisfactoriness, reflecting the fact that the mind is focused on processing mismatches between how we need things to be and how they actually are. Driven–doing mode also involves a sense of continuously monitoring and checking up on progress toward reducing the gap between these two states ("How well am I doing?"). Why? Because where no immediate action can be taken to reduce discrepancies, the only thing the mind can do is continue to work on its ideas about how things are and how they should be, in the hope of finding a way to reduce the gap between them. This it will do over and over again.

In this situation, because the "currency" with which the mind is working consists of thoughts about current situations, desired situations, explanations for the discrepancies between them, and possible ways to reduce those discrepancies, these thoughts and concepts will be experienced mentally as "real" rather than simply as events in the mind. Equally, the mind will not be fully tuned in to the full actuality of present experience. It will be so preoccupied with analyzing the past or anticipating the future that the present is given a low priority. In this case, we are aware of the present only in a very narrow sense: The only interest in it is to monitor success or failure at meeting goals. The broader sense of the present, in what might be called its "full multidimensional splendor," is missed.

Driven–doing underlies the ruminative thought patterns that engender relapse. It also underlies many of our reactions to more everyday emotional experiences—we habitually turn to this mode to free ourselves from many kinds of unwanted emotion. It follows that we can use such everyday emotional experiences, and other reflections of the general driven–doing mode of mind, as training opportunities to learn skills that enable us to recognize and disengage from this mode. We return shortly to a discussion of how we might do this. For the moment, let us consider an alternative mode of mind, "being."

THE "BEING" MODE

The full richness of the mode of "being" is not easily conveyed in words—its flavor is best appreciated directly, experientially. In many ways, it is the opposite of the driven–doing mode. The driven–doing mode is goal-oriented, motivated to reduce the gap between how things are and how we think we need them to be; our attention is narrowly focused on these dis-crepancies between actual and desired states. By contrast, the being mode is not devoted to achieving particular goals. In this mode, there is no need to emphasize discrepancy-based processing or constantly to monitor and evaluate ("How am I doing in meeting my goals?"). Instead, the focus of the being mode is "accepting" and "allowing" what is, without any imme-diate pressure to change it.

"Allowing" arises naturally when there is no goal or standard to be reached, and no need to evaluate experience in order to reduce discrepan-cies between actual and desired states. This also means that attention is no longer focused narrowly on only those aspects of the present that are directly related to goal achievement; in being mode, the experience of the moment can be processed in its full depth, width, and richness.

Doing and being differ in their time focus. In doing, we often need to work out the likely future consequences of different actions, anticipate what might happen if we reach our goal, or look back to memories of times when we have dealt with similar situations to get ideas for how to proceed now. As a result, in doing mode, the mind often travels for-ward to the future or back to the past, and the experience is one of not actually being "here" in the present much of the time. By contrast, in being mode, the mind has "nothing to do, nowhere to go" and can focus fully on moment-by-moment experience, allowing us to be fully present and aware of whatever is here, right now. Doing mode involves thinking about the present, the future, and the past, relating to each through a veil of concepts. Being mode, on the other hand, is characterized by direct, immediate, intimate experience of the present.

The being mode involves a shift in our relation to thoughts and feelings. In doing mode, conceptual thinking is a core vehicle through which the mind seeks to achieve the goals to which this mode of mind is dedicated. This means, as we have seen, that thoughts are seen as a valid and accurate reflection of reality and are closely linked to action. In doing mode, the relationship to feelings is primarily one of evaluating them as "good things" to hang on to or "bad things" to get rid of. Making feelings into goal-related objects in this way effectively crystallizes the view that they have an independent and enduring reality.

By contrast, in being mode, the relation to thoughts and feelings is much the same as that to sounds or other aspects of moment-by-moment experience. Thoughts and feelings are seen as simply passing events in the mind that arise, become objects of awareness, and then pass away. We can recognize here the "decentered" perspective to which we attached such importance in our analysis of the way that cognitive therapy has its effects. In the being mode, feelings do not so immediately trigger old habits of action in the mind or body directed at hanging on to pleasant feelings or getting rid of unpleasant feelings. There is a greater ability to tolerate uncomfortable emotional states. In the same way, thoughts such as "do this, do that" do not necessarily automatically link to related actions, but we can relate to them simply as events in the mind.

In being mode, there is a sense of freedom and freshness as experience unfolds in new ways. We can be responsive to the richness and complexity of the unique patterns that each moment presents. In doing mode, by contrast, this wonderful multidimensional complexity of experience is boiled down to a narrow, one-dimensional focus: What does this have to say about my progress in reaching my goals? Discrepancies between actual and goal states then trigger fairly well-worn, general-purpose habits of mind that may have worked well enough in other situations. But, as we have seen, when, in the driven–doing mode, the goal is to be rid of certain emotional states, these habits can backfire and lead to perpetuation rather than cessation of unwanted mind states.

Clearly, doing and being are fundamentally different modes of mind. Before drawing out the implications of this difference for MBCT, it is important that we be very clear on one point: *Being mode is not a special state in which all activity has to stop.* Doing and being are both modes of mind that can accompany any activity or lack of activity. Recall that we gave a particular name to the type of doing mode that causes problems— "driven–doing"—and this point may become clearer. For example, it is possible for one to try to meditate with so much focus on being someone who gets into a deeply relaxed state that if anything interrupts it, one feels angry and frustrated. That would be meditating in a driven–doing mode rather than a being mode because the meditation is "driven" by the need to become a relaxed person. Or take another example: It is your turn to do the dishes and there is no way out of it. No one is going to rescue you from this chore. If you do the dishes with the aim of finishing them as quickly as possible to get on to the next activity and are then interrupted, there will be frustration, since your goal has been thwarted. But if you accept that the dishes have to be done and approach the activity in being mode, then the activity exists for its own sake in its own time. An interruption is simply treated as something that presents a choice about what to do at that moment rather than as a source of frustration.

THE CORE SKILL

The core skill that the MBCT program aims to teach is the ability, at times of potential relapse, to recognize and disengage from mind states characterized by self-perpetuating patterns of ruminative, negative thought. Such patterns, if left unchecked, are likely to produce a downward spiraling of mood and, eventually, the onset of relapse. In MBCT, participants learn how to disengage from one mode of mind and enter another, incompatible, mode of mind that will allow them to process depression-related information in ways that are less likely to provoke relapse. This involves moving from a focus on content to a focus on process—away from cognitive therapy's emphasis on changing the content of negative thinking, toward attending to the way all experience is processed.

The basic tool to effect this change of mental modes, or shift of mental gears, is the intentional use of attention and awareness in particular ways. By choosing what we are going to attend to, and how we are going to attend to it, we place our hand on the lever that enables us to change mental gears.

How do participants in the program learn to do this when, in recovery, the mind states that provoke relapse do not occur very often and are therefore not available for learning? As we have already noted, relapse-related mind states are actually particular examples of the much more general driven–doing mode of mind. In our culture, this mode of mind is extremely prevalent, and participants almost certainly engage it as their "default" mode of mind in many situations. This means that this mode occurs again and again during the program and may become especially apparent during the exercises, practices, and interactions that take place in the sessions themselves and in the home practice. In the sessions, this mode of mind arises under not only participants' own noses but also the nose of the instructor. In this way, with sufficient skill on the part of the instructor, much of the content of the program, both planned and unplanned, can be used as opportunities to recognize and disengage from driven–doing mode. It is, of course, even more helpful if participants have opportunities to do this work in relation to unpleasant emotional states in general, and to depression in particular. For this reason, the instructor has a very real basis for welcoming the occurrence of such states as "grist for the mill" and as ideal opportunities for teaching the core skills at the heart of the program.

When can participants find opportunities to cultivate being mode? In principle, this mode of mind can be practiced in all situations. In practice, the tendency to enter doing mode is so pervasive (especially when one is learning a new skill such as how to "be"!) that very simple learning situations have to be set up, and the instructor has to embody being mode more or less constantly in those situations in order to facilitate entry into this mode of mind.

The driven–doing mode has a strong tendency to keep itself going and to reassert itself once the mind has switched to another mode of processing. It is particularly important, therefore, that the mode to which the mind switches after disengaging from driven–doing be incompatible and inconsistent with that mode, in the same way that it is not possible to be in forward and reverse gears in a car at one and the same time. Being mode is an ideal candidate for such an initial, alternative mode into which to switch. Once that initial switch has been made, it may be appropriate for patients to learn how to enter, intentionally, some other mode, for example, one that will facilitate skillful, planned action to alleviate any persisting depressed mood.

In the end, we need to balance being and doing in our lives. Whether it is because the culture we live in exalts doing, or because driven–doing is often propelled by automatic, well-worn routines, it can easily crowd out other ways of being with one's experience. We can learn to switch out of automatic pilot by bringing our awareness to the present moment. When we do this, we start to see that we have a choice, and this is often the first step in taking care of ourselves differently in the face of sad moods.

MINDFULNESS AS A CORE SKILL

Mindfulness has been described as "the awareness that emerges through paying attention on purpose, in the present moment, and non-judgmentally to things as they are."[76] [(p. 47)] As such, mindfulness fits remarkably well the requirements that our analysis has identified as a core skill to be learned in a relapse prevention program. Awareness of the patterns of thought, feelings, and body sensations that characterize relapse-related mind states (and the driven–doing mode of mind more generally) is an essential first step in recognizing the need for corrective action. Intentionally (on purpose) changing the focus and style of attention is the "mental gear lever" by which processing can be switched from one cognitive mode to another. And the nonjudgmental, present-moment focus of mindfulness indicates that it is indeed very closely related to the being mode of mind. In other words, mindfulness provides both the means to change mental gears when disengaging from dysfunctional, "doing-related" mind states, and an alternative mental gear, or incompatible mode of mind, into which to switch.

THE STRUCTURE OF THE MINDFULNESS-BASED COGNITIVE THERAPY PROGRAM

In the following chapters, we describe in detail, session by session, the MBCT program. Immersed in the detail of each session, it is easy to lose sight of the overall aim and structure of the program. It may therefore be helpful to remember that the aim of early sessions is to teach participants to recognize driven–doing mode in its many manifestations and to begin the cultivation of being mode by intensive, formal mindfulness practice. You will see this theme repeated quite a lot as the sessions unfold. Such repetition is there to remind participants again and again of the core themes, for practice provides many opportunities to recognize that being mode is no longer present, to disengage from the prevailing mode, and to return to mindful being. As mindfulness skills develop, training focuses more specifically on recognizing when, in everyday life, negative emotions and reactions trigger driven–doing, and on learning how to disengage from that mode, enter being mode, and how, if necessary, to "turn toward" and explore difficult and uncomfortable emotions. Subsequently, the simple skill of disengagement from emotion-related modes of mind is supplemented by additional coping strategies that provide patients with a range of options for responding more skillfully to negative emotion. Finally, the skills taught are integrated around the ultimate aim of the program: staying well and preventing future relapse.

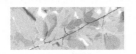

CHAPTER 5

The Eight-Session Program
How and Why

Our aim in the chapters that follow is to give a detailed sense of MBCT, session by session. Those who are primarily interested in getting the flavor of MBCT may, after reading this introduction, proceed straight to Chapter 7, where we begin to describe Session 1. This chapter is intended for those who contemplate the possibility of actually teaching MBCT. Here, we focus in some detail on the "how and why" of running sessions within this approach. Some may find it helpful to return to this section after reading the description of the eight-session program. Others may find this chapter a useful opportunity to ground their perception of MBCT in concrete detail, before going on to the more narrative description that follows.

For those interested in pursuing this approach further, we have provided more practical details both in this introduction and by including the handouts that we gave, section by section, to participants after each session (including details of the home practice following each session). We have included a short chapter (Chapter 21) with websites and other resources that we hope will be helpful to MBCT instructors and their patients.

YOUR OWN PRACTICE

The starting point for those wishing to teach MBCT for recurrent depression is to have had accredited training in counseling or psychotherapy, or as a mental health professional with experience in mood disorders.

In addition, training in behavioral or cognitive therapy or an equivalent evidence-based approach to depression, as well as experience in running groups, is needed. Although we do not insist that someone have full training in cognitive *therapy*, it is essential to have an understanding of depression vulnerability from the perspective of cognitive *theory*—through such understanding our treatments have progressed over the years. Recognizing the patterns of thoughts and feelings that create vulnerability both refines the actual teaching of mindfulness and enhances its relevance to class participants.

With these competencies in place, it is then essential that instructors have firsthand, ongoing experience of mindfulness practice. Why is this so? First, it is inevitable that some patients will experience difficulties with the practice that the instructor will not be able to approach with "intellectual" knowledge alone. A swimming analogy may help to illustrate the point. A swimming instructor is not someone who knows the physics of how solids behave in liquids, but he or she knows how to swim. It is an issue not just of credibility and competence but of the teacher's ability to embody "from the inside" the attitudes he or she invites participants to cultivate and adopt. When we started this work, we believed that it was unreasonable to expect all instructors to have experienced such mindfulness practice, or even to have practiced before. We have changed our minds about this.

Our own conclusion, after seeing for ourselves the difference between using MBCT with and without personal experience of using mindfulness practice, is that instructors should not embark on teaching this material before they have extensive personal experience with its use, as well as "sitting in" on an MBCT course as a participant. These necessary requirements are not in themselves sufficient, and complete training guidelines can be found in Chapter 21. We therefore recommend as a minimum that prospective instructors have a daily formal mindfulness practice in their own lives for at least a year before they embark on teaching it to clients. Without such experience, the approach cannot be called mindfulness-based cognitive therapy; in fact, it is not mindfulness-based anything at all, since "mindfulness-based" actually *means* teaching from the basis of your own mindfulness practice.

For those new to the mindfulness approach, we give some pointers for how to go about learning more in Chapter 21. And if you find that the mindfulness approach is not for you, remember that there are many very effective ways to treat depression, so you have many alternative approaches to explore—and you will surely help many people through your clinical skill and wisdom.

WORKING WITH RECOVERED DEPRESSED PATIENTS

There are a number of constraints in working with people who have had such serious episodes of depression. First, because they may have overcome their episodes of depression with the help of antidepressants, they may have a "biological" model of their illness. Such a model is perfectly understandable given their experience, and any psychosocial approach needs to take account of it. With this in mind, we suggest taking time during initial assessment interviews (see later) to discuss how both biological and psychosocial factors may play a role in the onset, maintenance, and recurrence of depression.

A second constraint in working with recovered patients is that in remission, symptoms of depression are, by definition, "low level." Previous psychological treatments developed for depression assume that clients experience relatively "loud" phenomena—persistent low mood, negative thoughts and images, severe biases in memory and judgment, inability to experience pleasure and inactivity, and suicidal thoughts and impulses. An important aim of the mindfulness-based approach is therefore to teach clients to be more aware of even small changes in their mood. Since the symptoms are not "loud," clients are taught to listen for the whisper.

A third constraint is that recurrence, when it comes, may not occur until, on average, a year has passed. Teaching clients *about* such recurrence by simply extending their *knowledge* of how to prevent relapse is unlikely to affect an event that is so far in the future. The aim must therefore be to teach *procedures and skills*. MBCT emphasizes daily practice during the active phase of the program, in the expectation that participants will learn skills they cannot easily forget, precisely because they have learned a new way of being in their lives. As part of the research trials described in Chapter 19, between two and four follow-up meetings are offered to participants in the year following the 8-week program. Such a pattern of follow-up meetings may not be suitable in all settings, but some type of continuing contact is always valuable—an opportunity for participants to reconnect with the formal practice in a class setting.

PLANNING AND PREPARATION FOR SESSIONS

Each session contains a large amount of work to be done: the relevant handouts to distribute; audio tracks to be copied; the inevitable setting-up of the room before each session, perhaps writing key issues on the black- or whiteboard; and positioning the chairs. In other words, each session needs *planning*. But we found (often to our disadvantage, when we had not left sufficient time for it) that each session also needed *preparation*; that is, we needed to prepare ourselves. When looking at the videotapes of our sessions after the research was over, we could easily identify the times when we had just rushed in from another meeting versus those when we had prepared ourselves by taking the time for things to settle. With this in mind, we recommend that you prepare yourself for each session, so that you not only approach each class with practical arrangements running smoothly but also embody the balance of openness and "groundedness" that participants are invited to experience for themselves. But there is another factor: a sense of preparation that comes from your ongoing mindfulness practice. This allows you some degree of flexibility of approach in the classes: to stay in the moment and, if necessary, let go of the plan you have made, drawing on other components of the MBCT program to respond to what is most cogent in the participants' experience.

Such talk of careful preparation may give an impression that the aim is to "succeed." Our final word should therefore be one of caution. At the outset, doing this work may create more stress! Just finding the time for yourself to practice each day may demand many lifestyle changes. Both instructors and participants may understandably expect some immediate gain from such sacrifice. But the more such expectation of change is uppermost in your mind, the more elusive it may become. As best you can, therefore, suspend judgment and invite participants to do the same. Emphasize the empirical approach. To borrow from the first formal practice used in the program, "Don't try too hard—whatever comes up, accept it, for that is what you are feeling right now."

OVERVIEW OF MINDFULNESS-BASED COGNITIVE THERAPY

The Initial Assessment Interview

This initial assessment interview, which lasts around 1 hour, conducted with each prospective participant, is based on the initial material sent to participants before they attend (see Handouts 6.1 and 6.2 in Chapter 6). This material explains some aspects of depression and the program, and can be used as a starting point for dialogue between instructor and participant. The aim of the initial interview is as follows:

1. To learn about the factors that, for each participant, have been associated with the onset and maintenance of depression.
2. To explain something of the background of MBCT and explore with each participant how it might help him or her.
3. To emphasize that MBCT will involve some hard work, and a need for patience and persistence in that work over the course of the 8 weeks.
4. To determine whether the person is likely to benefit at this time. In general, instructors will not take participants into the program (a) if they are actively suicidal *and* have no other form of counseling support (they are enrolled in the classes if they have other such support); (b) if they are currently abusing drugs or alcohol; or (c) if the prospective participant or the teacher feels that this is the wrong approach or the wrong time given his or her circumstances (e.g., in the midst of a major life crisis).

The Classes

In this book, we give an outline *theme and curriculum* for each of the eight classes at or near the beginning of each session, and the *participant handouts* are reproduced at the end of each session.

Class size depends on the facilities available, but MBCT—especially since it is used for people who are highly vulnerable to serious mood problems—requires relatively small classes. We have classes of around 12 in our research, but we note that a class that is too small can be problematic

TABLE 5.1. Recorded Mindfulness Practices

Session		Track
1	Raisin Exercise	2
	Body Scan	3
2	10-Minute Sitting Meditation—Mindfulness of the Breath	4
3	Stretch and Breath Meditation	6
	Mindful Movement—Formal Practice	5
	3-Minute Breathing Space—Regular Version	8
4	Sitting Meditation	11
	Mindful Walking	7
	3-Minute Breathing Space—Responsive Version	9
5	Working with Difficulty Meditation	12
6	10-Minute Sitting Meditation	4
	20-Minute Sitting Meditation	10
	Bells at 5 Minutes, 10 Minutes, 15 Minutes, 20 Minutes, and 30 Minutes	13

because the instructor can too easily revert to a "therapy" rather than a "class" mode.

The instructor also needs to consider how to provide participants with the recorded mindfulness meditations to enable home practice between sessions (see Table 5.1). One option is for instructors to burn CDs or load USB flash drives with the downloadable MP3 files available at *www.guilford.com/MBCT_materials* and distribute these at the first session. A second option would be to distribute the address of the Web page developed specifically for course participants (*www.guilford.com/MBCT_audio*), from which they can stream or download the recordings directly.

Core Aims

The overarching aim is to help people who have suffered from depression in the past to learn skills to help prevent depression coming back:

- By becoming more aware of body sensations, feelings, and thoughts, from moment to moment.
- By developing a different way of relating to sensations, thoughts, and feelings—specifically, mindful acceptance and acknowledgment of unwanted feelings and thoughts rather than habitual, automatic, preprogrammed routines that tend to perpetuate difficulties.
- By being able to choose the most skillful response to any unpleasant thoughts, feelings, or situations that they meet.

The Structure

MBCT prioritizes learning how to pay attention on purpose, in each moment and nonjudgmentally. Learning the basics of mindfulness is the focus of Sessions 1–4. First, participants become aware of how little attention is usually paid to daily life. They are taught to become aware of how quickly the mind shifts from one topic to another. Second, having noticed that the mind is wandering, they learn how to bring it back to a single focus. This is taught, first, with reference to parts of the body and to breathing. Third, the participants learn to become aware of how this mind wandering can allow negative thoughts and feelings to escalate, without their being aware that this is happening.

Only when a person has become aware of these aspects is he or she likely to use MBCT to be vigilant for mood shifts, then move on to handle them. Handling mood shifts involves the second phase of MBCT and is dealt with in *Sessions 5–8*. Whenever a negative thought or feeling arises, the instructions emphasize allowing it simply to be here, exploring it as it is, before taking steps to respond skillfully by using specific strategies. How is this done? Participants learn how to become fully aware of the thought or feeling, then, having acknowledged it, to move their attention to their breathing for a minute or two before expanding attention to the body as a whole. We call this the *breathing space*. Introduced first in Session 3, it becomes the common thread through the rest of the program, gradually allowing participants to weave what is being learned from the formal practices into everyday life. The use of the breathing space develops in Sessions 3 to 7 as participants deepen their practice. At first, participants learn to take a 3-minute breathing space three times each day. From Session 4, they add to this by seeing how the breathing space may be used at times of difficulty, when it may turn out to be sufficient to handle difficulties in the moment, to free participants from the unpleasant thoughts or feelings. Gradually we invite participants to see the breathing space more explicitly as the essential first step in dealing with difficulties, after which they may choose how best to respond.

First, they may choose simply to "reenter"—to return to the flow of their lives with a more grounded and spacious presence, in better shape to relate to whatever life has to offer. Or following Session 5, they may choose to deal with the difficulty by noting the part of the body it affects, and bringing awareness to that part of the body, using the breath to open and soften to the sensation rather than tighten and brace around it. Or (following Session 6) they may deal with difficulties by seeing more clearly how negative thoughts arise with mood and are then taken to be true; how adhesive these thoughts are, and how they may be seen and held in awareness as "mental events." Or (following Session 7) they may choose to deal with a difficulty by taking action specifically chosen for its ability in the past to bring some pleasure or sense of mastery. Because of the large variety of contexts in which the breathing space is used, it is important to emphasize its *flexibility*. It will not always be possible for participants to close their eyes and take exactly 3 minutes, but pausing (1) to acknowledge what is going on, (2) to gather themselves by going to the breath, before (3) expanding the focus of attention to sense the wider perspective of the here and now comprises a three-step "mini-meditation" that is an important first step.

Finally, participants are encouraged to become more aware of their own unique warning signs of impending depression, and to develop specific action plans for when this might occur. We came to believe that MBCT should combine both the generic themes of mindfulness approaches in general and help in dealing with the specific problems that depression poses. But all the time, in the background, was the overall theme of changing the relationship with what was most difficult.

Differences In Participants' Approaches to the Classes

Participants' different past experiences account for their very different ways of approaching the classes. Some know a great deal of what the classes will be about; many know nothing and are very scared of what they may be asked to talk about or do. We take time at the start of the first class not only to emphasize confidentiality but also to say that, after they have introduced themselves to the group, participants need feel no pressure at all to say anything during the classes. We also talk at that point about the skill of really *listening* to what another person is saying. Quite often, while someone else is talking, many of us are working out how we can best help him or her, or determining what we are going to say next. Learning to pay attention means really learning to be attentive to what others are saying, while they are saying it. Those who choose to say little in a class may nevertheless contribute much to the class by their very presence, as well as by using their gift of listening.

Guiding Practice

We found that the way we led the formal practice set the scene for the rest of each class. Some of the ways we helped ourselves to embody staying fully present during the guidance follow:

• Using the present participle when describing actions we would like participants to take. For example, " . . . noticing whether your mind has wandered . . . " or " . . . bringing your attention back to the breath" (rather than "Notice whether . . . " or "Bring your attention back . . . "). (*Note.* In languages where the " . . . ing" form is not available, it will be important to find ways to guide the practices without it feeling as if "orders" are being given.)

• Starting the meditation by asking people to spend a few moments being aware of their posture. It is recommended that the back be erect, with the base of the spine gently curved inward, but not stiff. If someone is sitting on a chair, then it is important to sit partly forward in the seat, so that the back does not need to be supported by the chair frame, and to use cushions if necessary, so that the hips are raised above the level of the knees. Of course, if the person has a bad back or back pain, then some type of support for the back may be necessary. Encourage participants to check the alignment of the back, neck, and head. Intentionally creating a posture that embodies dignity, stability, and alertness allows us to bring these qualities to the sitting itself.

• Delivering instructions for the meditation in a matter-of-fact way. Note that this is not a relaxation exercise, so there is no need to adopt a special tone or deepen the voice to relax the participants. Do not *read* verbatim instructions. Do not *read* instructions out loud at all.

• Giving encouragement by using the phrase "as best you can" rather than the word "try." This phrase emphasizes gentleness rather than striving. For example, " . . . as best you can, bringing your awareness to settle on the breath" rather than "try to bring your awareness to the breath. . . . "

• Doing the practice with the class. When guiding a practice, you are meditating out loud—not "telling people what to do." This means that you are guiding out of your own moment-to-moment experience during the guided meditations. If you usually meditate with eyes closed or gaze lowered, close your eyes or lower your gaze when you guide meditation in the class. It may be helpful to scan the class briefly from time to time, but there is no need to keep your eyes open all the time "to check how people are getting on."

• Allowing for spaces and stretches of silence between your instructions. Give participants the space to "do" the practice for themselves. You do not need to fill the space with speaking. Especially with the shorter practices, you may come to find that speaking consumes time, whereas silence gives time.

Inquiring with Participants

We found that the best timing for reflection on class practice is immediately following it. We adopted the practice of never moving on to the next part of the session without giving people an opportunity to respond to and comment on their experience of the practice that has just ended. We came to see this dialogue within the classes as having two aspects. First, we were interested in people's actual experience during the practice. What sensations, thoughts, impulses, and feelings came up, and what did people notice about them? Second, we wanted to know whether anyone had any *comments* on their experiences (see Chapter 12).

Welcoming and staying attentive to what is offered empowers other group members and contributes to the sense that what they have experienced is legitimate. The instructor's curiosity about participants' experience can invite participants themselves to become curious about their own experience. During the dialogue that took place, therefore, we found it was important to keep close to (and bring the focus back to) participants' actual experience.

The links that class members can see between their own experiences and those of others are very important. We encouraged participants to discuss any difficulties or objections they had. If one person was thinking about them, then somebody else was likely to be thinking about them, too.

Finally, bear in mind that different people may find different aspects of MBCT helpful. The aspect of MBCT that is most helpful for each person cannot be prejudged at the outset. Think of your instructor role as planting seeds. You do not know how long they will take to germinate, and, in a real sense, that is not under your control. As best you can, cultivate instead an openness, a sense of discovery.

THE CORE THEMES
OF MINDFULNESS-BASED COGNITIVE THERAPY

In this section, we sum up, as precisely as we can, what we believe are the central themes of this approach to depression.

Exploring How Best to Prevent the Establishment and Consolidation of Patterns of Negative Thinking

Everything is in the service of preventing the consolidation of self-perpetuating patterns of negative thinking that may escalate negative mood states to depressive relapse. It is not the aim to keep negative mind states out of mind altogether, but rather to prevent their establishment when they occur.

What Drives the Old Habits of Thinking: The Seven Signs of Driven–Doing

The patterns of negative thinking are based on old, well-practiced, automatic cognitive routines (often ruminative). They are motivated (ineffectively) by the goal of escaping/avoiding depression or problematic life situations. These unhelpful routines persist because the person remains in a cognitive mode characterized by a number of features:

1. Living on "automatic pilot" (rather than with awareness and conscious choice).
2. Relating to experience through thought (rather than directly sensing).
3. Dwelling on and in the past and future (rather than being fully in the present moment).
4. Trying to avoid, escape, or get rid of unpleasant experience (rather than approach it with interest).
5. Needing things to be different from how they are (rather than allowing them to be just as they already are).
6. Seeing thoughts as true and real (rather than as mental events that may or may not correspond to reality).
7. Treating oneself harshly and unkindly (rather than taking care of oneself with kindness and compassion).

Each of these are different aspects of the driven–doing mode. Each of them will be foregrounded, session by session, as we move through the program.

What Is the Core Skill?

The *core skill* to be learned is how to exit (step out of) and stay out of these self-perpetuating cognitive routines. The bottom line is *be mindful (aware), let go.* Letting go means relinquishing involvement in these routines, freeing oneself from the need for things to be different that drives the thinking patterns—*it is the continued attempts to escape or avoid unhappiness that keep the negative cycles turning. The aim of the program is freedom*, not happiness, relaxation, and so on, although these may well be welcome by-products.

Kindness Plays an Essential Role

Ensuring that a general attitude of kindness and care pervades all aspects of each class is foundational within MBCT. These qualities of mind help prevent the reinstatement of old habits of thinking, by teaching participants that it is possible to approach unwanted experiences with a gentle curiosity and, in doing so, develop a different relationship to them. They also support the view that mindfulness is not just about paying or shifting attention but more about the *quality* of attention that is being paid. Kindness, initially conveyed by the instructor's personal warmth, attentiveness, and welcoming stance is reinforced throughout the program by the gentle approach taken with participants, especially in the presence of negative affect. This allows participants at first to receive and eventually to practice being kind to their experiences, and gentle with themselves when old habits of mind threaten. A more detailed discussion of this process is provided in Chapter 8.

Experiential Learning

The required *skills/knowledge* can be acquired only through direct experience. Intellectual knowledge may be helpful (it may also get in the way by setting expectations, goals to be attained, etc.) but, by itself, it is wholly inadequate. Acquisition of the skills requires repeated experiences (perhaps many thousands). Getting enough experience can be achieved only if (1) participants accept the responsibility for the 99.9% of learning that will have to occur outside sessions and (2) all experience is grist for the mill—using awareness/letting go of even quite neutral and apparently harmless automatic thoughts–feelings–body sensations to build up skills to deal with depression-related patterns.

Empowerment

Empowerment of participants is absolutely essential if they are to get the required amount of experience in using mindfulness. In the service of empowerment, learning should be based, whenever possible, on participants' own experience rather than lectures from the instructor, and should embody the assumption that participants are the "experts" on themselves, with a fund of relevant experience and skills already.

- Always ask for feedback immediately after any practice or other exercises in session, and from all home practice. This feedback should be the main vehicle for teaching.

- Use open-ended questions and encourage the expression of doubts, difficulties, and reservations.
- Underline the essential learning point that is implicit or explicit in the feedback given by participants. Be concrete and specific in feedback and instructions.
- Keep track, from home practice records, whether home practice is actually occurring and focus in on noncompletion.
- Encourage a clear intentionality (not goal orientation) in participants. Help them relate the practice to a personally valued vision.
- Keep a balance between instructions to "let go" of expectations (which can be demotivating if overemphasized) and the willingness to believe that important changes may occur as a result of doing the mindfulness practice.
- Encourage curiosity as the mode of investigating experience, even when (especially when) such experience appears boring or negative.

What Is to Be Learned?

- *Concentration.* The ability to deploy and maintain attention on a particular focus is central to all other aspects of MBCT. This involves sustained, quality attention that is gathered and focused rather than dispersed and fragmented.

- *Awareness/mindfulness of thoughts, emotions/feelings, impulses to act, body sensations.* This is important because we can't intentionally let go of unhelpful patterns unless we are aware of them; because awareness itself removes processing resources that are required for the self-perpetuation of unhelpful patterns; and because awareness of difficulties (particularly in the body) involves bringing our "best mind" to bear in ways that may allow the process to unfold more creatively.

- *Being in the moment.* Instructors can support a moment-by-moment mode by not "trailering," that is, not giving instructions in advance of the time when participants actually need to act on them.

- *Decentering.* This means to relate to thoughts, feelings, body sensations, and impulses to act as events passing in the mind and body, rather than identifying with them.

• *Acceptance/nonaversion, nonattachment, kindly awareness.* The motivation fueling the automatic cognitive habits is some form of aversion or desire. For this reason, "acceptance of what is" undercuts the power driving these habits. Acceptance and awareness also allow us to see the "bad thing" or "good thing" in a clearer, wider perspective, so we are better able to respond to the totality of a situation rather than to let just one fragment of it instantly "press our buttons." If we can build on this awareness by being kind to ourselves as these reactions unfold, then there is the possibility of learning a new way of relating to aversion when it arises.

• *Letting go.* This is a key skill in both preventing oneself getting into and stepping out of unhelpful cycles. It is a very important part of both the body scan and mindfulness of breath, and one of the key reasons why the very thing people find most difficult (mind wandering) may be one of the most useful; that is, when people are practicing, and their minds repeatedly wander from the breath or the body, then detecting the wandering, and returning, is more important than staying on the breath–body 100% of the time. The outbreath is the natural vehicle used in letting go.

• *"Being" rather than "doing," non-goal attainment, no special state (of relaxation, happiness, peace, etc.) to be achieved.* All the unhelpful patterns are variants of the "driven–doing" mode—concerned with achieving defined endpoints and monitoring current state against expected, desired, or "should" states. Getting the taste for "being" mode, and being able to enter this at will, provides a powerful alternative route when depression-creating "doing" routines are assembling themselves. The practices, and the instructor's own presence and way of being, provide powerful opportunities for direct "tasting" of this mode—hence the importance of the instructor embodying the qualities being developed to whatever degree possible, and, after Session 1, starting each session with a period of practice. Appropriate pacing and punctuation of the session, and having a single focus at any one time, facilitate this mode.

• *Bringing awareness to the manifestation of a problem in the body.* A cornerstone of MBCT practice is to see the body as the key place through which we can learn to relate differently to our experience. As well as providing cues to the presence of aversion, stress, and so on, bringing awareness to the bodily manifestation of a problem provides a way to withdraw processing resources from the automatic, unhelpful (goal-oriented) verbal/analytic routines, while still keeping the problem "in process" (so as not to reinforce aversion). It allows awareness, as a marker of another mode of processing, to get on with the job and let events unfold, undisturbed by the type of thinking that seeks to resolve discrepancies, strive for goals, or solve problems.

CONCLUDING REMARKS

Many psychologists, counselors, and other mental health workers are drawn to their profession by the wish to help people. Such help can take many forms. Most therapies are quite reasonably founded on the principle of getting as clear a view as possible of what has gone wrong in the past and what is going wrong in the present, then helping the person find the resources to cope better. They are based on the idea that assessing and then removing problems is the aim. At best, these attempts empower persons to manage their lives more successfully, and many people have been helped by a number of such treatments.

Our analysis suggests that this will bring temporary relief only, unless people are able to use that respite to find ways to enhance their own well-being, take care of themselves, and relate to their problems in a different way. Both the research data and our clinical experience suggest to us that only when people learn to take a different stance in relation to the "battle-ground" of their thoughts and feelings will they be able in the future to recognize difficult situations early and deal with them skillfully. Taking this different stance involves sampling a different mode of mind from that which we normally inhabit, and which much therapy also inhabits. It involves replacing the old mode of fixing and repairing problems with a new mode of allowing things to be just as they are, in order to see more clearly how best to respond. The aim of the eight sessions described in Chapters 7–17 is to bring about this different way of relating to experience.

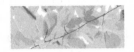

CHAPTER 6

The Preclass Participant Interview

RATIONALE

Because participants' initial encounters with the work in MBCT are experiential in nature, it is important that they arrive at the first session with at least a rough map of what the approach entails. The preclass interview provides the opportunity to develop such an overview. Over the course of a 60-minute, one-on-one meeting or a 90-minute group meeting, participants share what is unique about their experiences with depression and, in return, learn how MBCT can help them. It is also one of the times in the program that participants work individually with the instructor, since once classes begin, less emphasis is placed on the particulars of each participant's story, and more attention is paid to what each has in common (e.g., tendencies to ruminate, or to avoid negative emotion). Participants have Handout 6.1 sent to them beforehand, and Handout 6.2 is provided at the conclusion of the interview.

OVERVIEW OF THE PRECLASS INTERVIEW

As you conduct the interview, make sure to allow enough time for participants to describe what it has been like to live with depression and the extent to which they see themselves as vulnerable to depression returning. It is also important to explore why they feel they are still at risk. You can then outline the cognitive view of vulnerability to recurrent depression,

94

using participants' own examples and experiences, and the role of mindfulness in helping to reduce relapse risk. Toward the end of the interview, make sure to review the expectations placed on those taking the course, address any outstanding questions, and end by making a joint decision about each participant's suitability to start the program at this point in time.

"What Brings You Here?"

One way of opening the interview is to invite participants to say *what has brought them to this point in their lives*. What often comes up is a long history of struggles with depression: a lifetime of episodes, varying in intensity and length, the accumulated effect of which has placed a huge burden on them and their family. In the midst of this description, see if it is possible to *explore a single episode in some detail,* especially one that may have occurred during a sensitive developmental transition point, such as adolescence, midlife, or retirement. In particular, *how has the person reacted to his or her own depression? How does he or she explain the depression?* How do these explanations fit with what others—for example, family members—have said? Have these views changed over time?

Focusing now on the most recent episode, *what triggers did the participants notice* that preceded the onset, and *what was the particular pattern of symptoms* they faced this time? *How did they attempt to deal with it all?* Did they notice a tendency to withdraw, avoid, ruminate, or suppress their feelings? See if it is possible to *explore their habitual ways of coping.*

It is helpful to keep in mind the question "How vulnerable to relapse does this person consider him- or herself to be?" Some participants ascribe depression to entirely external factors, with their risk tied to whether these external factors are still a problem or may return. This might come across in statements such as "I was working far too hard and staying up nights to keep up around the same time that I got depressed. Now that I am no longer in that job, I will be fine." or "My depression occurred when I was in a really bad relationship. My girlfriend was very bossy and was always criticizing me or telling me what to do. We've been broken up for 6 months and so I don't worry much about it." Participants may express other viewpoints that acknowledge personal vulnerability but express passivity when it comes to managing it: "I know my depression is caused by a chemical imbalance so other than taking my medication what more can I do?" or "Depression runs in my family and it seems like it will continue to show up in my life."

What can be helpful in this part of the interview is to discuss how research has shown that even with a predisposition to depression in place, there are things people can do to protect themselves against depression returning. In many ways, this describes the essence of MBCT in a nutshell. You may want to illustrate this by drawing an analogy with Type II diabetes, in which a person has the physiological substrate for the disease, but its expression is effectively managed through diet and exercise.

Last, because studies of motivational interviewing have found that people's sense of urgency about their condition is strongly predictive of commitment to treatment, attendance, and engagement,[77] gathering this information will be helpful in deciding whether now is the right time for enrollment in the program.

How We Understand Recurrent Depression

In discussing participants' own past experiences and explanations, and what they can do to protect themselves against depression's return, it is sometimes worth relating the latest scientific knowledge about the factors that make us vulnerable to depression. In presenting this model, instructors should also ask for participants' ideas, or whether these findings make sense in light of the experiences they have had.

At some point it may be useful to convey some or all of the following:

> "New research shows that during any episode of depression, negative mood occurs alongside negative thinking (e.g., 'I am a failure') and body sensations of sluggishness and fatigue. When the episode has passed, and the mood has returned to normal, the negative thinking and fatigue tend to disappear as well. However, during the episode, a connection has formed between the moods that were present at that time and the negative thinking patterns. This means that when a person feels sad again (for any reason), a relatively small amount of such mood can reactivate the old thinking patterns. Once again, people start to think they have failed, or are inadequate, even if it is not justified by the

current situation. People who believe they have recovered may find themselves feeling 'back to square one,' constantly asking 'What has gone wrong?,' 'Why is this happening to me?,' or 'When will it all end?' They feel that such rumination ought to help them find an answer, but it only succeeds in prolonging and deepening the mood spiral. When this happens, the old habits of negative thinking start up again, getting the person into the same rut, and it can feel a bit like struggling to get out of quicksand. The very struggle to escape from depression makes things worse. As time passes, a full-blown episode of depression may result. One of the main messages of MBCT is that it is possible to learn to step back and find a different way of relating to these thought patterns, and the program is designed to help you find ways to do this."

How Will Mindfulness-Based Cognitive Therapy Be Helpful to You?

Begin by asking whether participants already know something about MBCT or they are coming to it for the first time. They may have read an article about it, found material on the Internet, or even dipped into *The Mindful Way through Depression*.[76] It is also good to ask what are they hoping to get out of the course and whether they have any past experience of cognitive-behavioral therapy (CBT) or meditation. Some participants, while unconcerned about the CBT aspects of the program, may be skeptical when they realize that a core skill in the program is learning how to meditate. As the instructor, there is no need to sell them on the idea at this point; rather, note their reaction and to try and engage their curiosity about doing something that may seem unusual. For example, many participants say that one aspect of their emotional difficulties is that their attention is always being "hijacked" by other concerns: regrets, worries, and preoccupations. This is a great opportunity to say how the first part of the program focuses on training attention (rather in the same way that we go to a gym to train muscles), and that many different practices help to show how we can train our attention, so that we have more choice about our attentional focus.

You might continue like this:

"As for the program itself, MBCT has been shown in a number of clinical studies to reduce significantly the chance of a recurrence of depression. It teaches you to become aware of the workings of your mind and, in so doing, to recognize where there are choice-points to prevent your mind from slipping back into old patterns. One of the main approaches for learning about this is the practice of mindfulness meditation. A number of different practices are covered over the 8 weeks, and you will be helped to discover the ones that are most useful for you. We simply ask that you try all the meditations during the classes and at home. We also emphasize that the classes provide an opportunity to care for yourself during this process by being kind and gentle with any new learning that may occur during this process."

Continuing to Practice at Home

One of the main vehicles for developing mindfulness is doing the practice at home between classes. This, along with other home practice, is assigned at the end of each class and, all added together, may take close to an hour a day to complete. It is important to recognize that while this is a considerable demand on participants' time, it also provides enough exposure to the practice of mindfulness that it can help them decide how best to look after themselves once the course is over. Toward the end of the course, participants are encouraged to identify which, if any, practices they see themselves continuing. Setting the stage for home practice can also make things go more smoothly. For example, participants should consider where to find an hour in the day to practice during the 8-week course, informing family members or others at home what is involved, and getting an audio player for listening to the guided meditations.

Challenges That May Show Up When Taking the Mindfulness-Based Cognitive Therapy Course

Participating in the MBCT course can be challenging for a variety of reasons. It may be helpful even at this early stage to share with each participant the feedback from past participants that it is definitely worth hanging in. The instructor can take a few minutes to review possible challenges and respond to them based on his or her experience with past classes. Challenges may include the following: Not all people feel comfortable with being in a group; some people might feel that they are under pressure to talk; class members may come from very different backgrounds; and it may not always be obvious how the practices will be helpful. As the program continues, people who are used to dealing with their emotions by ruminating extensively or pushing them out of mind may notice that emotional issues are coming up in the class or during their home practice. Although an eventual encounter with this type of material is built into the MBCT program, there may be many times when participants feel like giving up or stop coming to class. Our research has found that *those who are most prone to ruminate and/or to avoid difficult experiences are most likely to drop out early*,[78] and we have found it especially helpful, when we notice these tendencies, to take more time in the preclass interview to *draw out the possible difficulties in staying with and exploring difficult experiences*, the various ways the wish to give up may arise, and the importance of spotting these wishes early and seeing them as an expected part of doing the program.

The Need for Confidentiality

In order for class members to feel safe disclosing personal information, confidentiality is an essential foundation for the class. For some especially vulnerable clients (e.g., those at risk of suicidal behavior), the instructor needs to identify a contact person, such as a primary care doctor or psychiatrist, who can be notified if there is significant concern for the safety/well-being of the participant in cases of immediate risk to themselves or others. Consent to contact needs to be obtained as well.

Practical Arrangements

Instructors should look after the practical details of setting up the group, such as signage, access to parking, start times, and room booking. If participants need to fill out questionnaires, they should arrive a little early to do this. Also, instructors should ask group members to phone when they are not able to attend. They should also ask for permission, if no notification is received, to call the participant to find out how he or she is doing.

Concluding the Interview

By the end of the interview, it is important that the two of you decide whether enrolling in the program is the best course of action. In many cases, this will be self-evident. Some of the time, however, the provision of concrete details about what goes on in the program will lead some participants to express reservations. Participants may be too busy to find the time, or they may not feel sufficiently at risk to warrant the investment of time; they may even want to disengage from, rather than stir up, painful emotions. As the instructor, there also may be times when you have reservations of your own. These can stem from a concern that a participant may be disruptive to group process; has a history of trauma that has not been treated in individual therapy; or is still experiencing acute symptoms of depression, such as difficulties with concentration and decision making. Sometimes a recommendation to explore MBCT as a future option can be a relief to the participant.

Finish the interview with a note of hope, acknowledging the courage that it has taken for the person to get to this point, and the sense of looking forward to the classes.

Preliminary Handout
for Mindfulness-Based Cognitive Therapy

Please read this before we meet.

DEPRESSION

Depression is a very common problem. Twenty percent of adults become severely depressed at some point in their lives. Depression involves both biological changes in the way the brain works and psychological changes—the way we think and feel. Because of this, it is often useful to combine medical treatments for treating depression (which act on the brain) with psychological approaches (which teach new ways to deal with thoughts and feelings).

TREATMENT OF DEPRESSION

When you have been depressed in the past your doctor may have prescribed antidepressants. These work through their effects on the chemical messengers in your brain. In depression, these chemical messengers have often become run down, lowering mood and energy levels, and disturbing sleep and appetite. Correcting these brain chemicals may have taken time, but most people experience improvements in 6 to 8 weeks.

Although antidepressants generally work well in reducing depression, they are not a permanent cure—their effects continue only so long as you keep taking the pills. Your doctor could continue to prescribe antidepressants for months, or even years, since this is now recommended if further depression is to be prevented by this means.

However, many people prefer to use other ways to prevent further depression. This is the purpose of the classes you will be attending.

PREVENTION OF MORE DEPRESSION

Whatever caused your depression in the first place, the experience of depression itself has a number of aftereffects. One of these is a likelihood that you will become

(cont.)

depressed again. The purpose of these classes is to improve your chance of preventing further depression. In the classes, you will learn skills to help you handle your thoughts and feelings differently.

Since many people have had depression and are at risk for further depression, you will learn these skills in a class with up to a dozen other people who have also been depressed and treated with antidepressants. You will meet in eight 2-hour sessions to learn new ways of dealing with what goes on in your mind, and to share and review your experiences with other class members.

After the eight weekly sessions are over, the class will meet again four times over the following few months for reunions, and to see how things are progressing.

HOME PRACTICE:
THE IMPORTANCE OF PRACTICING BETWEEN CLASSES

Together, we will be working to change patterns of mind that often have been around for a long time. These patterns may have become habit. We can expect to succeed in making changes only if we put time and effort into learning skills.

This approach depends entirely on your willingness to do home practice between class meetings. This home practice will take at least an hour a day, 6 days a week, for 8 weeks, and involves tasks such as listening to the recorded meditations and other exercises, performing brief exercises, and so on. We appreciate how it is often very difficult to carve out that amount of time for something new in lives that are already very busy and crowded. However, the commitment to spend time on home practice is an essential part of the class; if you do not feel able to make that commitment, it would be best not to start the classes.

FACING DIFFICULTIES

The classes and the home practice assignments can teach you how to be more fully aware and present in each moment of life. On one hand, this makes life more interesting, vivid, and fulfilling. On the other hand, this means facing what is present, even when it is unpleasant and difficult. In practice, you will find that turning to face and acknowledge difficulties is the most effective way, in the long run, to reduce unhappiness. It is also central to preventing further depression. Seeing unpleasant feelings, thoughts, or experiences clearly, as they arise, means that you will be in much better shape to "nip them in the bud," before they progress to more intense or persistent depressions.

(cont.)

In the classes, you will learn gentle ways to face difficulties, and be supported by the instructor and the other class members.

PATIENCE AND PERSISTENCE

Because we will be working to change well-established habits of mind, you will be putting in a lot of time and effort. The effects of this effort may become apparent only later. In many ways, it is much like gardening—we have to prepare the ground, plant the seeds, ensure that they are adequately watered and nourished, and then wait patiently for results.

You may be familiar with this pattern from your treatment with antidepressants: Often there is little beneficial effect until you have been taking the medication for some time. Yet improvement in your depression depended on your continuing to take the antidepressant even when you felt no immediate benefit.

In the same way, we ask you to approach the classes and home practice with a spirit of patience and persistence, committing yourself to put time and effort into what will be asked of you, while accepting, with patience, that the fruits of your efforts may not show straight away.

THE INITIAL INDIVIDUAL MEETING

Your initial individual meeting provides an opportunity for you to ask questions about the classes or issues related to the points raised in this handout. You may find it useful, before you come for that interview, to make a note of the points you wish to raise.

Good luck!

An Introduction
to Mindfulness-Based Cognitive Therapy

INTRODUCTION

At the introductory interview you had the opportunity to tell us some of your own story, learn about the course, discuss how we understand the problem of recurrent depression, find out about some of the practical arrangements for attending the sessions, and ask any other questions you might have had at that time.

In this brief handout we would like to summarize some of the things we discussed together.

UNDERSTANDING RECURRENT DEPRESSION

You, along with other group members, are here because you have had episodes of recurrent depression and are interested in preventing them from recurring. The work you will be doing in MBCT is based on the latest psychological research on those factors that make people vulnerable to and maintain depression.

First, we would like to share with you our best guess of what these factors are. You have been doing the best you can, and the things you have tried may have worked to a certain extent, but they may not have helped as much as you had hoped. Because you have had no other options, it has felt risky to stop doing what you habitually do. However, some ways of coping are rather like digging to get out of a hole, and just making the hole bigger. We think about this as a vicious circle that works something like this:

- People think more negatively when they are depressed than when they are relatively well.

- During the first episode of depression this negativity takes a while to really build up.

- After repeated episodes of depression, strong associations are formed, meaning that even a small trigger like a dip in mood can be a flash point for depression.

- The spiral of negative thinking that sets in can lead to hopelessness.

- This in turn makes it tempting to withdraw, and to avoid more and more situations.

- It can be difficult to extricate yourself from this, once your old beliefs are activated. It feels a bit like struggling to get out of quicksand.

(cont.)

Instead of another relapse occurring, evidence suggests that it is possible to learn to step back and find somewhere else to go with the problem. We hope to help you find ways to do just this.

HOW WILL THE MINDFULNESS-BASED COGNITIVE THERAPY COURSE BE HELPFUL TO YOU?

Clinical studies of hundreds of patients have shown that MBCT can significantly reduce the risk of your depression returning. Here are some things that participants in past groups have reported:

- I became aware of the workings of my mind.
- I learned to recognize patterns.
- I learned to stay steady, but also to stand back a little.
- I could recognize that I have choices other than slipping back into old patterns.
- I learned to taker a kinder, more gentle attitude toward myself.
- I learned to recognize warning signals and take helpful action.
- I learned how to put less effort into "fixing" things.
- I learned how to focus on the here and now.

During the course, you will find that there are lots of different ways to be mindful. By letting yourself try all the mindfulness practices, you may discover the ones that are most useful for you. The weekly classes also provide the opportunity for you to practice being kinder and gentler to yourself.

HOME PRACTICE

You can expect that there will be home practice every week, often up to 1 hour a day. To help you find the room in your life for this new commitment, it is helpful to consider the following:

- Where in your day will you find the time needed for practice?
- Let others in your family or social circle know what is involved.
- Do you have access to a device on which you can play the guided meditation practices?

(cont.)

- See if you can balance the different motivations that naturally come up, such as being impatient for results versus letting go of your expectations for 8 weeks.
- Treat yourself with kindness throughout this time, especially if you run into some rough spots.

CHALLENGES OF THE COURSE

As we discussed, you might find that taking the MBCT course is challenging for a number of different reasons. We want to assure you that should these challenges arise, your instructor will be able to discuss any potential issues with you. In fact, the feedback that past participants wanted us to convey to those who are just getting started is that it is worth hanging in there, even if it is a struggle. The knowledge and understanding you gain will have an impact on reducing your risk for depression.

CONFIDENTIALITY AND SAFETY

In order to create an atmosphere of trust and sharing within the group, we would like to establish some ground rules in the group.

- Confidentiality will be observed by both participants and instructors.
- If your instructor has a significant concern for your safety or well-being, including immediate risk to yourself or another, he or she will need to contact your general practitioner, or other professional person, but only after consulting you.

PRACTICAL ARRANGEMENTS

- The group starts promptly at _____ and finishes at _____.
- It is a good idea to wear comfortable clothes, and you might like to bring a light blanket.
- We would like to emphasize the importance of attending each session. Please let the instructor know if you can't be there.
- Because the class may be challenging, there may be times when you do not feel like coming. If this happens we would like you to telephone and let us know how you are. We can discuss any problems with you.

It can feel difficult to come back if you miss a session, but it is worth it. You are always welcome to return.

HOW TO READ THE SESSION CHAPTERS

In the chapters that follow, in describing in detail the intentions for each session, we aim to do a number of things: to say what each session includes and describe what may be observed; to let participants themselves speak about their discoveries with the practice; and to speak frankly about where we, as teachers, often find things difficult, and how we may attempt to understand what is going on when such difficulties arise.

The style is somewhat different from that we have used up until now. There are poems, parables, and stories that make the world of the psychology textbook seem even further away. There are many repetitions: The stream of argument sometimes seems to loop back on itself (many times), and it may feel like the stream will never reach the river, nor the river the sea. Our hope is that gradually a more complete picture emerges from the individual parts, just as, for participants in the program, the same message in the context of different sessions makes sense to them the second or third time they hear it, when perhaps they had not even noticed it before.

Although there are a lot of practical details in each chapter, each starts with some general remarks to introduce the theme of the chapter. These are intended to orient the reader, not to be used as introductions to the class sessions themselves (which always start with practice after Session 1), although some of the examples may be useful later in the class as illustrations to help the learning that is taking place. We wish you well as you begin the journey from this reading, through practice, to teaching.

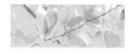 CHAPTER 7

Awareness and Automatic Pilot

Session 1

BACKGROUND

Have you ever opened a packet of sweets, tasted the first, then found yourself with an empty bag? Did someone else eat them, or was it just that you did not notice yourself eating? Or have you driven home along your normal route, only to arrive and realize that you forgot to stop and pick up something at a friend's house as you had intended? In such cases, you may or may not be aware of where your attention has gone—but you end up doing something you had not intended. An older habit has, it seems, taken control.

When asked to describe these kinds of events, many people use the term "automatic pilot" as a way to say that they are just behaving mechanically, without really being aware of what is going on. In automatic pilot mode, it is as if the body is doing one thing, while the mind is doing something else. Most often, we do not *intend* to be preoccupied with this or that—it simply happens. The mind is therefore passive much of the time, allowing itself to be "caught" by thoughts, memories, plans, or feelings. Our attention seems to have been hijacked by something else.

While, many times, we may not be fully aware of what is happening, this state of mind is especially problematic if we have suffered from depression in the past. In automatic pilot, fragments of negative thinking are less likely to be noticed. If unchecked, they may coalesce into patterns

BOX 7.1

Theme and Curriculum for Session 1

THEME

On automatic pilot, it is easy to drift unawares into "doing" mode and the ruminative thought patterns that can tip us back into depression. Habitual doing mode also robs us of our potential for living life more fully. We can transform our experience by *intentionally* paying attention to it in particular ways. We begin to practice stepping out of automatic pilot by paying attention intentionally, mindfully, to eating, to the sensations of the body, and to aspects of everyday experience.

AGENDA

- Establish the orientation of the class.
- Set ground rules regarding confidentiality and privacy.
- Ask participants to pair up and introduce themselves to each other, then to the group as a whole, giving their first names and, if they wish, saying what they hope to get out of the program.
- The raisin exercise.
- Feedback and discussion of the raisin exercise.
- Body scan practice—starting with a short breath focus.
- Feedback and discussion of body scan.
- Home practice assignment:
  o Body scan for 6 out of 7 days.
  o Mindfulness of a routine activity.
- Distribute audio files (via CD, flash drive, or URL) and Session 1 participant handouts (including the Home Practice Record form).
- Discuss in pairs:
  o Timing for home practice.
  o What obstacles may arise.
  o How to deal with them.
- End the class with a short, 2- to 3-minute focus on the breath.

(cont.)

PLANNING AND PREPARATION

In addition to your personal preparation before the class, remember to bring a bowl with raisins and a spoon, as well as copies of body scan audio files.

PARTICIPANT HANDOUTS FOR SESSION 1

Session 1–Handout 1. A Definition of Mindfulness

Session 1–Handout 2. Summary of Session 1: Awareness and Automatic Pilot

Session 1–Handout 3. Home Practice for the Week Following Session 1

Session 1–Handout 4. A Patient's Report

Session 1–Handout 5. Home Practice Record Form—Session 1

that lead to stronger feelings of sadness and more severe depression. By the time the unwanted thoughts or feelings surface, they are often too strong to be dealt with easily. We have more to say about alternative ways of handling such thoughts and feelings later.

First, however, we have to deal with the start of the sequence, the day-to-day "mindlessness" that seems harmless but can be so damaging if a person has a history of emotional problems. In helping recovered depressed patients stay well, an important first step is to find ways to help them recognize, then intentionally step out of, automatic pilot mode. The practice of mindfulness involves becoming more aware of these patterns of the mind, so that we can learn to pay attention intentionally, that is, with awareness.

It is one thing to decide that a fundamental building block of preventing relapse is to teach people to recognize those times when their minds are running on automatic pilot and intentionally to shift their awareness to something else. It is quite another to find a simple way to show this to people early on, in the first session, in a way that does not just add one more "wrong thing" they are doing.

STARTING THE SESSION

When we first visited the Stress Reduction Clinic at UMass Medical Center, we sat in on Session 1 of a new class led by Jon Kabat-Zinn. After a short word of welcome, reminding participants of why they had come, he asked people to introduce themselves, first in pairs and then to the whole class, saying their name, why they had come, and what they hoped to get out of the program. He then introduced a short meditation exercise that went to the heart of the automatic pilot theme. It involved eating a raisin.

Eating is a particularly useful task for this first exercise because it is such an "automatic act," one that is hardly ever done mindfully. It is therefore both a good illustration of the extent to which we are often unaware of what is going on and an example of the changes that can take place when we slow down and focus on such a simple act. This simple eating exercise is a first step in helping participants understand what mindfulness is.

THE RAISIN EXERCISE

How much explanation should be given at the start of this exercise? It is most helpful to keep any explanations very brief: to err on the side of saying too little rather than too much. Our aim from the outset is to teach the course as experientially as possible; as with other practices in this program, participants learn from them by first having the experience and only afterwards trying to make sense of what it means. The transcript illustrates how we guide people through the raisin exercise.

The exercise is an excellent introduction to mindfulness for people who have been depressed. First, it provides an experiential rather than a verbal problem-solving base for learning. It sets a scene in which learning takes place through practice* and feedback from the practice. Practice is central and will become the core of the course. But the raisin exercise is also a very good introduction to the way we, as instructors, can most helpfully respond to what people say following the exercise. We need

---

*We use the word "practice" here to refer to the formal and informal mindfulness exercises that participants will be learning to use in their daily lives. Although it has this meaning, it retains its more usual meaning to convey the idea of a gentle and persistent attempt to learn a skill, or in this case, to become aware of a mode of mind.

BOX 7.2

Transcript: The Raisin Exercise

I'm going to go around the class and give you each a raisin.

Now, what I would like you to do is to see it as an object—just imagining that you have never seen anything like it before, as if you had dropped in from another planet this moment and you had never seen anything like it before in your life.

Note. There is at least a 10-second pause between phrases, and the instructions are delivered in a matter-of-fact way, at a slow but deliberate pace, asking the class to do the following:

Taking the object and holding it in the palm of your hand, or between your finger and thumb. (*Pause*)

Paying attention to seeing it. (*Pause*)

Looking at it carefully, as if you had never seen such a thing before. (*Pause*)

Turning it over between your fingers. (*Pause*)

Exploring its texture between your fingers. (*Pause*)

Examining the highlights where the light shines . . . the darker hollows and folds. (*Pause*)

Letting your eyes explore every part of it, as if you had never seen such a thing before. (*Pause*)

And if, while you are doing this, any thoughts come to mind about "what a strange thing we are doing" or "what is the point of this" or "I don't like this," then just noting them as thoughts and bringing your awareness back to the object. (*Pause*)

And now, taking the object and holding it beneath your nose, and with each in-breath, carefully seeing what you notice—does it have a smell? (*Pause*)

And now looking at it again. (*Pause*)

And now slowly taking the object to your mouth, maybe noticing how your hand and arm know exactly where to put it, perhaps noticing what happens in your mouth as it comes up. (*Pause*)

(cont.)

And then gently placing the object in the mouth, noticing how it is "received," without biting it, just exploring the sensations of having it in your mouth. (*Pause*)

Exploring the object with your tongue, noticing the sensations as you move it around the mouth. (*Pause*)

And when you are ready, very consciously taking a bite into it and noticing what happens—the tastes that it releases. (*Pause*)

Slowly chewing it, . . . noticing what's happening in the mouth, . . . the change in consistency of the object. (*Pause*)

Then, when you feel ready to swallow, seeing if you can first detect the intention to swallow as it comes up, so that even this is experienced consciously, before you actually swallow it. (*Pause*)

Finally, seeing if you can follow the sensations of swallowing it, sensing it moving down to your stomach, any aftertaste, then noticing the absence of the raisin in the mouth—and what the tongue does when it is gone.

Based on Kabat-Zinn.[67]

to embody, in the way we deal with issues raised in the class, the very approach to those issues we hope participants will find helpful. If we do not embody a spirit of genuine curiosity and inquiry about people's experience, or if we tend to rush for a premature explanation of what is going on, how can we expect participants to change the way they approach the tasks they are going to do? The hope is that, in time, a gradual fine-tuning of people's experience might take place, and with it, the realization that one can practice mindfulness by being present in all waking moments, no matter how ordinary or routine.

One way to facilitate this is to ensure that as many questions as possible are open-ended (e.g., "Would anyone like to comment about what we just did?"). This way of using the practice in the class is not easy to learn. Closed-ended questions come all too naturally ("Did anyone feel tired?", "Did your mind wander?"). Such closed-ended questions produce, rather inevitably, a "yes" or "no" response. By contrast, look at the following response to a more open-ended question:

Interviewer: Does anyone want to say anything about their experiences while eating?

Participant: Different thoughts went through my mind, looking at the raisins.

I: Would you be able to say what kind of thoughts went through your mind?

P: I was thinking how strange that something quite so dried up and ordinary looking could taste so good . . . that if we didn't know how it tasted, perhaps we wouldn't bother trying it.

I: So, thoughts associated with the raisin—where did those thoughts take you?

P: Different occasions—dried-up deserts, hot sand . . . holidays with my parents when I was small—different associations.

I: That's interesting; that's really nice. So the task is to actually focus your awareness on the raisin, but the mind isn't having any of that!

P: It goes off in all sorts of directions.

I: It goes from the raisin to reflections on how curious that it should taste nice, and it's sort of dried up, to hot sand, to holidays with your parents. . . . It's a lovely example of the way the mind has its own agenda, if you like. The exercise is one where we're trying to focus our attention in the here and now, in this moment, and there we go—we're traveling back to sandy deserts, to your parents, to other places. The mind's gone off on its own. That's a very important thing to notice. We'll come back to that shortly. Any other comments?

Summary of Intentions for the Raisin Exercise

- Noting the contrast between mindful awareness and automatic pilot.
- Seeing how paying attention in detail can reveal things we had not noticed or had forgotten.
- Paying attention in this way can transform the experience.
- Noticing mind wandering as normal.

Notice that the conversation has already highlighted an important theme: the mind wandering that so easily takes us away from our intended focus. Later, the instructor will be able to relate the participant's experience to the theme of the program: that we are often on "automatic pilot"; that mind wandering during periods of automatic pilot happens all the time; that it is the nature of minds to wander in this way, but that this can be particularly dangerous when mood is sinking, and associations and memories are likely to be depressing. It is therefore good to know what's going on in this stream of associations and to be able to disengage intentionally.

The raisin exercise also offers participants a second opportunity: a direct sampling of *a new way of relating to experience* in contrast to the usual automatic pilot way of doing things. They find that paying attention in this way reveals unexpected little things about a raisin, such as its ridges, the folds in its skin, and the small scar at one end, where it was once connected to something larger than itself, that is, to the vine. Some say they can only think of how they like or dislike raisins. Others say that they are able to see the raisin with greater clarity, or that the raisin has a stronger, more vivid taste. We find that this aspect can be explored further by asking, "Did anyone notice anything different from the way you usually eat? What was the difference?" Participants most commonly point out the difference between the way they ate the raisin during the exercise and their normal way of eating.

P2: You wouldn't even stop to notice it. You'd just throw it in automatically. You wouldn't savor a raisin like that.

I: So you'd be quicker and more automatic? And what do you think would be the key differences between this experience and stuffing it in like that? What would you say you might notice?

P2: The *taste* more . . .

I: You noticed the taste more?

P2: And the texture. They were sort of dry on the outside and then you get into the more juicy bit. . . . I never noticed that before.

Another set of responses clearly shows a growing awareness of the difference between this experience and what normally happens in everyday life.

I: How about the actual experience that you've all had? Any comments on that?

P3: I don't usually eat them; but for some reason, our cat loves raisins, so when I'm cooking, I throw a few down for her. I was thinking, actually, next time I give some to the cat, I think I'll have some. It was really nice doing it really slow. I liked that.

I: How was it different from the normal experience?

P3: Well, because I just normally shovel stuff in my mouth, you know, as quickly as possible, in order to go and do something else, really, like throwing coal onto a fire.

I: OK. So could you say a little bit more about how this was different?

P3: Well I *knew* I was eating it. That probably sounds a bit odd.

I: No, that's interesting. You knew you were . . .

P3: I knew I was eating it.

Note here that it is not clear whether the participant was using the word "know" to mean intellectual, factual knowledge or more direct sensory experience. Given the theme of the program—of moving away from rumination toward direct experience—this was an interesting thing to explore (though not necessarily to develop further at this point).

I: Could you say a little bit more about that?

P3: Well, I just think I was extremely aware of the fact that I was eating something.

I: Right. As a fact or as a sensation?

P3: As a sensation, yeah, definitely.

I: The taste or . . . ?

P3: Yeah, and all that stuff about your arm and everything. I just grab things usually. I don't know what my arms are doing normally; I mean, I know but I don't feel it.

I: That's a really really important distinction. So that, compared to the usual experience, there was much more awareness of direct experience.

P3: Yeah.

I: Direct experience of physical sensations in your arm, direct experience of the taste?

P3: Exactly.

I: OK, that's very helpful. Thank you. Any other comments on the experience?

P4: I guess it was sensual, wasn't it? If I can remember what "sensual" is. (*Laughs.*) Yeah, I think it could be described as being sensual.

I: Can you say a little bit more about what you mean?

P4: Well, I mean, I was thinking: I should do this more often because I'm actually experiencing something far more . . . um . . . in a sort of stronger way than usual awareness. I suppose, yeah, it's sort of a sensual experience.

I: Right, rather than just some automatic experience that passes you by.

P4: Yes.

I: So these are really important points: that intentionally and deliberately bringing awareness to something changes the experience. It actually can enrich the experience, change the nature of the experience, and it makes you aware of things that often you may not have been aware of, like the sensations in your arm. Any other comments before we move on?

Of course, not all participants find the exercise enjoyable. The instructor ensures that these comments are welcome too, emphasizing the importance of noticing these reactions:

P5: I thought it was frustrating. Sitting here thinking . . .

I: That is very interesting. So the sort of thing that was running off in your mind was a sort of "Let's get on with it" kind of thing. "Why are we dragging this all out?" A real sense of frustration?

P5: Because I only eat when I am hungry.

I: OK, so that's interesting. Were you able to notice that and come back to the raisin?

P5: I could just come back and eat the raisin.

I: Good noticing. Anything else?

All these reactions, whether they appear to be positive or negative, are welcome. They can be woven into a more general "pulling together" of all the feedback comments in a way that draws out the relevance of becoming more aware to the aim of relapse prevention:

> "So really, this is a very simple exercise that is just meant to illustrate how, first of all, much of the time we are actually not getting our moment's worth, if you like. You know, all that taste, all that smell, all the visual patterns of the texture, they just disappear in one handful. We are not really there for it. And it also shows what happens when we bring awareness to experiences in a different way. This, for most of us, is slightly different from the way we normally eat raisins. It is interesting that it provides a sort of background against which we can then begin to notice any sense of irritation, urgency, wanting to get on, 'What on earth are we doing this for?' So it's all good noticing.
>
> "This exercise is an example of a lot of what we will be doing. We will practice bringing awareness to our everyday activities, so that we know what is going on and can actually change the nature of the experience. If you are fully aware of thoughts, feelings, sensations in the body, in the sense that you may have glimpsed in this raisin exercise, you can actually change the experience; you have more choices, more freedom. At the moment, this is just theoretical; we need to have more and more experiences of bringing awareness to bear, so that you can see, eventually, in what way it is going to help. And that's why I am asking you, for the moment, to take an interest in what happens when you do something simple like this. At the moment, the connection between slowly eating a raisin and protecting yourself against depression in the future may not be obvious. But the first step, and what we are doing in the first part of the program, is really training awareness.

"So the basic take-home message from that little exercise is that *we're not aware of what's going on a lot of the time.* If we can bring awareness, we become aware of aspects of life that otherwise may just slide by us, both the good and the bad. Missing out on the good means that life isn't as rich as it might be. Not being aware of the bad means that we're not in a position actually to take skillful action ourselves. Depression can creep up on us when our minds are elsewhere.

"*We can't actually control what comes into the mind, but what we can control is what we do next, the next step. And this program is all about being able to move to a place of awareness from which we can choose what the next step is, rather than run off the old habits of mind.*"

In fact, participants in the classes find it relatively easy to use their experiences with the raisin exercise to draw out its relevance to their tendency to fall back into depressive mind states. First, when they start paying attention a little more closely to experience in this way, they discover for themselves quite powerfully how much they normally do automatically; how much of the time the mind is more likely to be in the past or future than in the present; how, in any moment, most of us are only partially aware of what is actually occurring. Whereas many people might sometimes have noticed the effects of being on automatic pilot (e.g., most related easily to the example of driving their car for miles without realizing where their minds had been), it still comes as a discovery for them to see how the same tendency is present for much of everyday life.

Second, the exercise shows how paying attention in a particular way (i.e., intentionally in the present moment and nonjudgmentally to things as they are) can actually change the nature of the experience. By simply paying attention, people find it possible both to wake up from automatic pilot mode and to connect more fully with the present. As participants find when they eat one raisin mindfully, they discover something quite profound: *There is often more that awaits us in the present than we imagine, especially if we have been operating automatically a good deal of the time.* Through exercises such as that with the raisin, participants are able to come to this realization, not because the instructor tells them, but through their own discovery.

TRAINING IN AWARENESS:
USING THE BODY AS A FOCUS

Much emphasis in MBCT is placed on providing participants with opportunities to relate mindfully and directly to their experience. The next stage of Session 1 builds on the raisin exercise, as participants start to explore the awareness of body sensations using a practice called the "body scan." A major aim of the body scan practice is to bring detailed awareness to each part of the body. It is where participants first learn to keep their attention focused over a sustained period of time, and it also serves to help them develop concentration, calmness, flexibility of attention, and mindfulness. It gives an opportunity to practice bringing a particular quality of awareness to things (in this case, the body), an awareness characterized by gentleness and curiosity.

Why use the body as the first object of attention? First, because a greater awareness of the body will be helpful in learning how better to deal with emotion. Powerful feelings such as sadness or hopelessness can be expressed not only as thoughts or mental events but also as effects in the body. Stooped posture, heaviness in the chest, or tightness in the shoulders may at times signal the presence of strong feelings of which we are not fully aware. What happens in the body importantly affects what happens in the mind. Feedback on how the body feels is often an integral part of the loops that sustain old habits of thinking and feeling.

Second, people who have been depressed very often try to *think* their way out of troubling feelings. An alternative is to bring awareness to manifestations of emotion as physical sensations or felt senses *in* the body. In time, this allows a shift of the center of gravity of attention away from "being in the head," toward an awareness of the body. It offers the prospect of coming at emotion from a fresh perspective, tuning in to a new aspect: "How am I feeling this in my body?"

We introduce the body scan as an exercise in awareness, in which we invite people to move their attention intentionally around the body, and to discover what happens when they do so. A helpful way of introducing the body scan is to link it to the raisin exercise that participants have just completed. Just as paying attention has allowed participants to relate directly and in a new way to their experience of eating a raisin, the same can be done with physical sensations. The key issue in doing the body scan is awareness of physical sensations in the body, bringing the same quality of direct awareness as in the raisin exercise.

To prepare for the body scan, we ask participants to lie on their backs, usually on a mat or soft surface (see Box 7.3 for step-by-step instructions). If the room is not large enough, or if some participants prefer, they may do the body scan sitting in a chair. It is usual for the instructor to lie down if most participants are doing so, or to sit on a chair if most are sitting. Next, we spend a few minutes focusing on the movement of the breath into and out of the body. Then, we give the instructions for the body scan: Participants are asked to move their attention through the different regions of the body in turn. The aim is to bring awareness intentionally to each region of the body in turn, exploring the actual physical sensations in that region at that moment. During the body scan, participants have many opportunities to practice its basic instructions—to bring attention to a particular region of the body, to hold that region of the body "center stage" in awareness for a short time, and finally to release and "let go" of that region before shifting their attention to the next region.

Note that in this, as in other practices, rather than "giving instructions" with eyes open, checking how people are doing, the instructor is guiding out of his or her own moment-by-moment practice of the body scan.

CREATING A CONTEXT FOR FORMAL MINDFULNESS PRACTICE: GENERAL COMMENTS

Several general issues arise when starting formal mindfulness practice. Since these begin with the introduction of the body scan, we mention them here. First, there is the issue of success and failure. It is important to mention that there is no success or failure involved. The problem is how to do this in a way that does not put the thought of success into people's heads. An understandable reaction to such practice, particularly for people who have suffered from depression, is to seek social approval and/or "high marks." Many depressive habits of mind revolve around the themes of performance/achievement or social evaluation, so people who have been depressed naturally bring this attitude to bear on any task. The body scan task is not immune to these attitudes, nor is any other practice

BOX 7.3
Body Scan Meditation*

1. Lie down, making yourself comfortable, lying on your back on a mat or rug on the floor or on your bed, in a place where you will be warm and undisturbed. Allow your eyes to close gently.

2. Take a few moments to get in touch with the movement of your breath and the sensations in the body. When you are ready, bring your awareness to the physical sensations in your body, especially to the sensations of touch or pressure, where your body makes contact with the floor or bed. On each outbreath, allow yourself to let go, to sink a little deeper into the mat or bed.

3. Remind yourself of the intention of this practice. Its aim is not to feel any different, relaxed, or calm; this may happen or it may not. Instead, the intention of the practice is, as best you can, to bring awareness to any sensations you detect, as you focus your attention on each part of the body in turn.

4. Now bring your awareness to the physical sensations in the lower abdomen, becoming aware of the changing patterns of sensations in the abdominal wall as you breathe in, and as you breathe out. Take a few minutes to feel the sensations as you breathe in and as you breathe out.

5. Having connected with the sensations in the abdomen, bring the focus or "spotlight" of your awareness down the left leg, into the left foot, and out to the toes of the left foot. Focus on each of the toes of the left foot in turn, bringing a gentle curiosity to investigate the quality of the sensations you find, perhaps noticing the sense of contact between the toes, a sense of tingling, warmth, or no particular sensation.

6. When you are ready, on an inbreath, feel or imagine the breath entering the lungs, and then passing down into the abdomen, into

(cont.)

---

*For ease of reading, we present these written instructions in a "do this, do that" style. However, as stressed on page 86, spoken instructions should avoid such "orders" and instead use present participles, as in the recorded audio tracks.

the left leg, the left foot, and out to the toes of the left foot. Then, on the outbreath, feel or imagine the breath coming all the way back up, out of the foot, into the leg, up through the abdomen, chest, and out through the nose. As best you can, continue this for a few breaths, breathing down into the toes, and back out from the toes. It may be difficult to get the hang of this—just practice this "breathing into" as best you can, approaching it playfully.

7. Now, when you are ready, on an outbreath, let go of awareness of the toes, and bring your awareness to the sensations on the bottom of your left foot—bringing a gentle, investigative awareness to the sole of the foot, the instep, the heel (e.g., noticing the sensations where the heel makes contact with the mat or bed). Experiment with "breathing with" the sensations—being aware of the breath in the background, as, in the foreground, you explore the sensations of the lower foot.

8. Now allow the awareness to expand into the rest of the foot—to the ankle, the top of the foot, and right into the bones and joints. Then, taking a slightly deeper breath, directing it down into the whole of the left foot, and, as the breath lets go on the outbreath, let go of the left foot completely, allowing the focus of awareness to move into the lower left leg—the calf, shin, knee, and so on, in turn.

9. Continue to bring awareness, and a gentle curiosity, to the physical sensations in each part of the rest of the body in turn—to the upper left leg, the right toes, right foot, right leg, pelvic area, back, abdomen, chest, fingers, hands, arms, shoulders, neck, head, and face. In each area, as best you can, bring the same detailed level of awareness and gentle curiosity to the body sensations present. As you leave each major area, "breathe in" to it on the inbreath, and let go of that region on the outbreath.

10. When you become aware of tension, or of other intense sensations in a particular part of the body, you can "breathe in" to them—using the inbreath gently to bring awareness right into the sensations, and, as best you can, have a sense of their letting go, or releasing, on the outbreath.

(cont.)

11. The mind will inevitably wander away from the breath and the body from time to time. That is entirely normal. It is what minds do. When you notice it, gently acknowledge it, noticing where the mind has gone off to, and then gently return your attention to the part of the body you intended to focus on.

12. After you have "scanned" the whole body in this way, spend a few minutes being aware of a sense of the body as a whole, and of the breath flowing freely in and out of the body.

13. If you find yourself falling asleep, you might find it helpful to prop your head up with a pillow, open your eyes, or do the practice sitting up rather than lying down.

From Kabat-Zinn.[67] Copyright 1990 by Jon Kabat-Zinn. Adapted by permission of Dell Publishing, a division of Random House, Inc.

during or after the 8 weeks of classes. Of course, as teachers, we can also recognize this tendency arising in ourselves. Success–failure ("Am I doing this right?") and approval issues ("Will people think this is OK and that I'm all right?") are likely to surface again and again. The task is not to try and stop such thoughts from arising, but to learn to recognize them when they come, so that we might respond to them skillfully.

We therefore find it helpful to mention that "doing it well" is not the issue, through words such as "It is important not to try too hard" and "We are not trying to achieve any special state; we are not even trying to relax." Later in the instructions, the theme is again picked up: "Sometimes the practice may bring up discomfort or boredom. If this happens, it does not mean that you have failed." We offer encouragement by inviting participants to take this chance to discover what such discomfort or boredom feels like in the body, what sensation accompanies each emotion, and their reactions to each emotion.

A second, major general issue is how to respond when difficulties occur. For example, in the body scan, some participants find that they or their neighbor cannot stay awake. Others find that sensations of physical discomfort distract them from the task. Despite this, the spirit embodied by the instructor remains "Whatever happens, whatever comes up, that is OK." Over time, one is able to see such difficulties as opportunities to bring awareness to these feelings and sensations rather than worrying about them, or letting them take control. The essence of the approach is to understand that these reactions are going to come up anyway, since they are part and parcel of life itself. It is how we handle them that makes the difference—whether or not they rule our lives to an inordinate degree.

The instructor has the opportunity to embody this sense of curiosity and adventure in the way he or she handles issues that arise in the class. Right from the start of doing MBCT, we became aware of a wish to make things better for participants, to help them fix their problems, and to reduce the pain of their emotional upset. As instructors from a therapy background, we found it too easy to switch back into therapy mode, with its danger of short-circuiting the cultivation of curiosity. In time, we found that there was no need to rush things, and that allowing pain to be expressed, explored, and held in awareness can itself be transformative. Of course, sometimes it is appropriate to take a very pragmatic approach in dealing with difficulties that arise with the practice; at other times, there is a need to offer (brief) explanations about depression and its nature. But our primary emphasis is on evoking a sense of curiosity in participants, and on developing their intentional awareness of sensations in each moment.

Along with any physical sensations that participants notice in particular body regions, they may also become aware of negative, judgmental thoughts or difficult emotions. Despite our instructions during the practice, some participants found it very difficult to let go of the tendency to check how well they were doing. Thoughts about how they looked, what parts of their bodies they wanted to change, or feelings of embarrassment and awkwardness often came to mind when participants focused on the body in this way. We emphasize that one approach is to acknowledge the feelings and bring to them a sense of curiosity and a willingness to observe. This provides an initial opportunity to relate to thoughts and feelings as mind states rather than to identify with them or take them personally. Such experiences can be used to teach one of the core messages of MBCT, namely, that it is both possible and something of an adventure in self-discovery to learn that through becoming aware, we can relate quite differently to our thoughts, feelings, perceptions, and impulses—in other words, to our experience of being alive.

REACTIONS AND RESPONSES

In the examples that follow, notice how commonly participants inter-preted the instructions as rules to follow (rules that they found themselves or others breaking): rules such as "Don't move or fidget," "Don't go to sleep" (Participant 1); "Don't open your eyes or let your mind wander" (Participant 2); "Relax!" (Participant 3); and "Don't get out of time with the instructions" (Participant 4). Note how each, in his or her own way, moved rapidly from an observation about what was happening to a nega-tive and self-critical judgment.

P: My legs felt really heavy to start with, and then I couldn't keep them still. I wanted to keep moving them all the time. I thought there must be something wrong because I couldn't hear anybody else moving and I was desperate to move my legs. And then I heard somebody beginning to snore gently, and I thought: *Oh, my gosh. This is awful. Somebody has gone to sleep.*

I: Wonderful, wonderful.

P: I was really worried about it because they had gone to sleep. I thought: *Please don't go to sleep.*

I: This is great. I am really glad you are saying all this. This is wonder-ful. Because the whole point of this is that we become aware of what-ever is. So that there isn't a right or a wrong thing to happen. The aim of the exercise is, as best you can (and it is difficult), becoming aware of whatever you are feeling at the time. And for you—your fidgeti-ness and wanting to move—that's great. It's just your experience in that moment. It's not wrong. It's not what shouldn't happen. That is the thing to become aware of. And eventually, you know, with that awareness, you may be able to become aware of the urge to move and make a decision, whether you are going to go with it or not.

P: I tried to suppress it. I wanted to sort of move around.

Note what the instructor has *not* done here. He does not ask why the participant was frustrated, or even try to understand the frustration. Nor does he ask for details of what came with the frustration (e.g., body sensations). Instead, he is interested in drawing out the *reactions* to experi-ence; that is, how the participant is *relating* to her moment-by-moment experience. Another way of saying this is that the instructor is inviting the class to *become aware of the weather patterns of their own minds and the reactions to these weather patterns.* Notice how this is done. First, focusing on the fidgeting, the instructor does exactly the opposite of seeing it as a "problem," saying, "That's great." Why? Because the participant has given a wonderful description of her own reaction to the body scan (heavy legs, wanting to move them, thinking "There must be something wrong"). Then she gives her reaction to hearing someone snoring: *"This is awful."* Here, then, is a series of experiences plus a cascade of reactions following close behind. So giving reassurance about heavy legs could so easily have inadvertently reinforced the message that these things should not really have happened (with the implication that with practice, all will be OK). Instead, the instructor has the opportunity to highlight the central theme of the program: that this is about cultivating awareness of moment-by-moment experience. The words "that is what you really need to know" are centrally important in the passage that follows.

> "OK, well, there is no need to try and fight these things. This is hard, particularly for something as strong as an agitation. But, as best you can, just acknowledge it: 'Right, OK, there you are. I really want to get up and jump around here, and I am fed up with this. It's going too slowly.' Whatever. As best you can, acknowledge all of it. Because that is your experience in that moment, and that is what you really need to know. So you acknowledge it, you don't push it away. Acknowledge it, and then, as best you can, bring your attention back to whatever bit of the body we are working on."

Often, when one participant has raised a point, it encourages others to be bold enough to speak of their own experience. This is indeed what happened next. See how the instructor weaves their experience into the same theme.

P2: My arms felt ever so itchy. I kept getting midges [flies] going round me. There was one on the table and twice it went on my arm, and I opened my eye and had a look. I didn't think I was supposed to do that.

P3: I kept thinking, *I am supposed to be relaxed here.*

I: OK. So this thing that we are going to come across over and over again is this idea of "how things are meant to be" or "how things should be." And it's this tension that causes our distress. It is often something that was put in our minds as children. It may have been useful then, but it may not be useful now. And if we can become aware of this, then we can let go of it and just deal with what is. How do we do this? By becoming aware of the feeling that "I should be doing this right," acknowledging it, and letting go of it. Then we are dealing with reality, with actuality in this moment, rather than all these images about what should be or ought to be, or what we ought to expect.

P4: I find it hard to breathe out when told to. I keep getting it back to front. My breath was not in time with the instructions.

I: Just see if you can be gentle with yourself. See if you can cultivate this attitude, not "It's wrong and naughty; I'm doing it back to front" but "Oh, that's how it is."

In each case, notice how the response of the instructor invites people to acknowledge and become curious about the things that come up for them, to be gentle with themselves rather than blaming themselves for having failed. The task is like that of a cartographer making a map of relatively unexplored land. Whatever the cartographer finds, whether the view is of rolling hills or dangerous-looking precipices, the task is the same: to note as accurately as possible what is there. And "what is there" includes all the self-judgments, impulses to move, restlessness, and boredom. It also includes the persistent running commentaries that tell us we are failing at doing the practice properly.

> "As best you can, acknowledge all of it. Because that is your experience in that moment, and that is what you really need to know."

LEARNING THROUGH HOME-BASED PRACTICE

Home-based practice is a routine aspect of MBCT. The kind of knowledge that we can get from talking about things is of only limited use for our purposes. The real business in MBCT is learning by experiencing for ourselves. This is why the home practice is so central and not an optional extra. We give participants daily, formal meditation practice: recordings of guided meditation instructions, similar to those used in the UMass MBSR program. In our original research, in order to ensure compatibility between sites (Cambridge, Toronto, and Bangor), we used CDs/Tapes Series I and II Meditation instructions recorded by Jon Kabat-Zinn (see Chapter 21). After some years of teaching, we recorded our own guided practice (available for download at *www.guilford.com/MBCT_audio*). The formal home-based practice also includes keeping a written diary of the daily mindfulness practice on the Home Practice Record Form—Session 1 (Session 1–Handout 5; also see other participant handouts for details of the home-based practice for each session).

From the outset, we attempt to convey how serious we are about home practice by making sure that enough time is left toward the end of the session to discuss the assignments for the coming week. We find that allowing sufficient time is important because there are often recordings and handouts to be distributed. All the home-based assignments are listed on handouts, together with a summary of each session. We distribute the relevant handouts during each session rather than giving everything at Session 1. Our reasoning is that "looking ahead" to what is to be done in future classes is not helpful to participants and might undermine the theme of awareness in the present moment.

Recall that all participants have attended individual preclass interviews with the instructor, who has emphasized that because the patterns of mind that we will be working to change have been around a long time, the mindfulness approach depends entirely on willingness to do practice at home between class meetings. Each person has been reminded that the commitment to spend time on home-based practice is an essential part of the class. Participants who were not able to make that commitment were advised not to start the classes at that time. Almost without exception, participants accept the need to do home practice in principle but come up against a range of stumbling blocks once they start actually to do it.

We allow time near the end of Session 1 for participants to *work in pairs to anticipate what difficulties they may discover in doing the home practice, and how they think they will deal with them.* (These points can then be revisited during the home practice review in Session 2—e.g., were the obstacles the predicted ones, or new ones they had not anticipated?)

Some participants have very practical questions, for example, about the best time of day, the best place, and the particular type of equipment to use. Others express a sense that finding time is going to be very difficult, or that the practice will take important time away from their families. We find that a useful general approach is to encourage people to discover what works best for them, without compromising the commitment each has made at the start of the program to do the prescribed practice 6 days a week. We make a point of helping participants create a space for their practice by asking them whether they have a quiet place where they can do the practice. Is there a time when they will not be interrupted? We are very clear about how things might get in the way of doing the home-based practice. For example, how do they intend to continue the home-based practice through weekends, holidays, or when they have visitors?

> "About the home practice, there may be difficulties. Let me say two things. First, you will see in the handouts a report of someone who said, 'I couldn't do this. It went up and down, but eventually something seemed to happen,' so just hang in there. Second, we asked members who had come back for a follow-up meeting, having been through the class themselves for 8 weeks, and with some time to look back on it, what single piece of advice they would offer to this new group starting today. With one voice they said, 'Whatever happens, stick with it.' That may not seem relevant to you now, but it may be at some point. Remember, you do not have to enjoy it, you just have to do it."

MINDFULNESS OF EVERYDAY ACTIVITIES

We give participants daily formal practice to do at home, and we also give some informal assignments. The idea is to enable participants to generalize to everyday life what they learn in the formal practice. For example, we asked people to perform an everyday activity mindfully. This simply involved choosing one routine activity and making a deliberate effort to bring moment-to-moment awareness to the activity, much as was done in the raisin exercise. Any activity—brushing one's teeth, taking a shower, or even taking out the garbage—will do. Participants chose one activity to do—the same one each day until the next class. We stressed the importance of actually bringing oneself back into the moment, of being fully present, feeling the brush on the teeth, or the water as it splashes on the back. The aim of this is not to make these little things pleasant (though they may be), but simply to give participants the opportunity to "wake up" to their actual lives more than they habitually do. (And if it turns out that they forget to do it 1 or more days, then noticing when they realize they have forgotten and any reactions, and using this "waking up" as an opportunity to see what is going on at that moment.)

This type of moment-by-moment awareness helps us to mark the difference between being on automatic pilot and knowing what we are doing while we are actually doing it. Using it with routine activities also illustrates that there is nothing special about mindfulness. We can find it in the middle of whatever we are doing, just by choosing to pay attention.

ENDING THE CLASS

By the end of the first class, participants have been exposed to a lot of new information over a fairly short period of time. In starting work of this kind, they experience many different reactions to the ideas that have been introduced. Some of these reactions have been expressed; many others have not. These and other experiences continue to surface over the coming weeks and, whether judged as "positive" or "negative," become the material around which teaching takes place.

We find that the end of the session is a good time to provide the class with a summary of the session in a way that ties the strands together. We use the Summary of Session 1: Awareness and Automatic Pilot (Session 1–Handout 2) as the structure for this summary, directing participants' attention to the handouts as we summarize.

Finally, we end the class with a short 2- to 3-minute breath focus. Participants are invited to sit with their backs straight (but not stiff), and after a few moments, to focus their attention on their breath as it enters and leaves the body, noticing any sensations associated with it. It is a way to "ground" the class following the discussion, and to provide a foretaste of things to come.

A Definition of Mindfulness

Mindfulness is the awareness that emerges through paying attention

on purpose,

in the present moment,

and

nonjudgmentally,

to things as they are.

—WILLIAMS, TEASDALE, SEGAL, AND KABAT-ZINN (2007)

Summary of Session 1:
Awareness and Automatic Pilot

In a car we can sometimes drive for miles "on automatic pilot," without really being aware of what we are doing. In the same way, we may not be really "present," moment-by-moment, for much of our lives: We can often be "miles away" without knowing it.

On automatic pilot, we are more likely to have our "buttons pressed": Events around us and thoughts, feelings, and sensations in the mind (of which we may be only dimly aware) can trigger old habits of thinking that are often unhelpful, and may lead on to worsening mood.

By becoming more aware of our thoughts, feelings, and body sensations, from moment to moment, we give ourselves the possibility of greater freedom and choice; we do not have to go down the same old "mental ruts" that may have caused problems in the past.

The aim of this program is to increase awareness, so that we can respond to situations with choice rather than react automatically. We do that by practicing to become more aware of where our attention is, and deliberately changing the focus of attention, over and over again.

To begin with, we used attention to eating the raisin to explore how to step out of automatic pilot. We then used attention to different parts of the body as a focus to anchor our awareness in the moment. We will also be training ourselves to put attention and awareness in different places at will. This is the aim of the body scan exercise, which forms the main home practice exercise for next week.

Home Practice
for the Week Following Session 1

1. Do the body scan exercise six times before we meet again. Don't expect to feel any-thing in particular from doing the practice. In fact, give up all expectations about it. Just let your experience be your experience. Don't judge it, just keep doing it, and we'll talk about it next week.

2. Record on the Home Practice Record Form (Session 1–Handout 5) each time you do the practice. Also, make a note of anything that comes up in the home practice so that we can talk about it at the next meeting.

3. Choose one routine activity in your daily life and make a deliberate effort to bring moment-to-moment awareness to that activity each time you do it, just as we did in the raisin exercise. Possibilities include waking up in the morning, brushing your teeth, showering, drying your body, getting dressed, eating, driving, taking out the rubbish (garbage), shopping, and so forth. Simply zero in on *knowing what you are doing as you are actually doing it.*

4. Note any times when you find yourself able to notice what you eat in the same way you noticed the raisin.

5. Eat at least one meal "mindfully" in the way that you ate the raisin.

A Patient's Report

This patient had been hospitalized for depression 4 years before, after which her husband and children left her. There had been no further contact except through lawyers. She had become very depressed and lonely, although she had not been in the hospital again. She was now over the worst of her depression, and started to use the body scan exercise to help prevent her mood from deteriorating. These were her comments looking back after 8 weeks:

"For the first 10 days it was like a burden. I kept 'wandering off' and then I would worry about whether I was doing it right. For example, I kept having flights of fantasy. My mind was all over the place. I tried too hard to stop it, I think.

"Another problem at the start was him saying, 'Just accept things as they are now.' I thought that was totally unreasonable. I thought to myself, 'I can't do that.'

"Eventually, I just put the audio tracks on and expected to go off into a realm of thoughts. I didn't worry if concerns came in. Gradually the 40 minutes passed without me losing him and from then on, the next time was more effective.

"After 10 days I relaxed more, I stopped worrying if I was thinking about anything else. When I stopped worrying about it then I actually stopped the flights of fancy. If I did think of something else, I picked up the audio tracks again when I stopped thinking. Gradually the flights of fantasy reduced. I was happy to listen to him and then I started to get some value from it.

"Soon I had developed it so that I could actually feel the breath going down to the base of my foot. Sometimes I didn't feel anything, but then I thought, 'If there's no feeling then I can be satisfied with the fact there is no feeling.'

"It's not something you can do half a dozen times. It's got to be a daily thing. It becomes more real the more that you try it. I began to look forward to it.

"If people have got to structure the time for the 45 minutes for their recordings, it may be easier to structure other things in their life as well. The recordings would prove an impetus."

Home Practice Record Form—Session 1

Name: _____

Record each time you practice on the Home Practice Record Form. Also, make a note of anything that comes up in the home practice so that we can talk about it at the next meeting.

Day/date	Practice (Yes/No)	Comments
Wednesday Date: _____	Body scan: Everyday mindfulness:	
Thursday Date: _____	Body scan: Everyday mindfulness:	
Friday Date: _____	Body scan: Everyday mindfulness:	
Saturday Date: _____	Body scan: Everyday mindfulness:	
Sunday Date: _____	Body scan: Everyday mindfulness:	
Monday Date: _____	Body scan: Everyday mindfulness:	
Tuesday Date: _____	Body scan: Everyday mindfulness:	
Wednesday Date: _____	Body scan: Everyday mindfulness:	

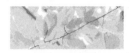

CHAPTER 8

Kindness and Self-Compassion in Mindfulness-Based Cognitive Therapy

In writing the first edition of this book in 2002, we assumed that all of the practices, the inquiry and teaching, both didactic and experiential, should be offered with a spirit of kindness and compassion. The hallmark quality of an MBCT class, in fact, is that participants are treated more as guests than patients, with warm hospitality and respect for the courage that they show, even by turning up. The research evidence that we will return to in Chapter 19 also demonstrates that one of the most important things people learn from an MBCT program is kindness and self-compassion. We regard this as fundamental. *Unless the class takes place within this atmosphere, the MBCT program loses one of its foundational features.*

The truth is that mindfulness cannot be reduced to awareness or attention alone. Whether mindful awareness enables a fundamental shift in how we relate to what is arising in the external or internal world depends on whether friendliness and compassion can be brought to those elements of present-moment experience to which we attend. In fact, attending without kindness can be ineffective or even harmful. Christina Feldman expresses it in this way:

> The quality of mindfulness is not a neutral or blank presence. True mindfulness is imbued with warmth, compassion and interest. In the light of this engaged attention we discover it is impossible to hate or

fear anything . . . that we truly understand. The nature of mindfulness is engagement; where there is interest, a natural, unforced attention follows. (p. 173)[79]

Since we see kindness as foundational to MBCT, the instructor's personal warmth is a necessary condition for implementing any of the more structured elements of the approach. Traditional contemplative approaches for helping people develop these attributes have often used specific meditation practices focused on extending unconditional friendliness to oneself and others.[80] For example, in lovingkindness or *metta* practice, this occurs through the repetition of phrases that help to "incline the mind" toward wishing well to all beings, phrases such as "May I (you, we, they) be safe and protected," "May I (you, we, they) be peaceful and happy," "May I (you, we, they) be healthy and strong," "May I (you, we, they) have ease of being." These phrases, and the underlying intentions they embody, are first directed at oneself then extended to others, moving in succession to a person to whom one feels gratitude and appreciation, a good friend, a neutral person who is neither liked nor disliked, a difficult person who triggers dislike, and finally to all beings everywhere, human and nonhuman. As Sharon Salzberg notes, the connection between this practice and the ability to develop compassion for ourselves in the midst of harsh and critical mind states lies in the recognition that "when we experience lovingkindness, we acknowledge that every one of us shares the same wish to be happy, and often a similar confusion as to how to achieve that happiness. We also recognize that we share the same vulnerability to change and suffering, which elicits a sense of caring" (p. 178).[80] Making this caring available to ourselves can temper the automatic self-blame and rejection that accompany moments of failure or setback.

Some mindfulness programs follow this tradition and also incorporate formal compassion or lovingkindness practices in an 8-week course. We also considered this, but chose not to do so in developing MBCT for those vulnerable to recurrent depression. First, we felt that participants' experiences of kindness should come primarily through the embodiment of these qualities in instructors: in the quality of their welcome, their guidance of meditation practice, and their responses to questions or comments from participants. Second, for someone with a clinical disorder, there is a risk that lovingkindness practices may trigger their vulnerability: For someone who is highly ruminative, the words "happy" or "free from harm" can too easily be understood, narrowly, as a call to *strive to achieve* these qualities, then elicit a cascade of painful emotions based on feelings of failure to do so in the past, or the impossibility of doing so in the future. Third, if the aim of the practice is seen as the development of loving *feelings* (rather than intentions) and one finds oneself unable to do this, it can actually reinforce any preexisting sense of one's inability to love or be loved.

Yet, although there is no explicit practice of lovingkindness or compassion meditation offered in the MBCT for depression program, it is clear that over 8 weeks of cumulative training and a specific orientation to the material, participants nonetheless develop these capacities (see Chapter 20).

INDIRECT ROUTES TO THE PRACTICE OF SELF-COMPASSION

How exactly are kindness and self-compassion expressed in MBCT? Feldman and Kuyken[81] point out that MBCT contains the basic building blocks for cultivating compassion, even though they occur in a different format from that in the traditional approaches. They point to the initial emphasis on developing mindfulness as a vital portal into self-compassion. In their view, the first step in cultivating a mind that is a "friend" rather than an "enemy" is to develop skills of mindfulness that allow one to fearlessly explore the landscape of the mind. To know the mind and its ways is the beginning of befriending the mind. In this process of befriending, qualities of curiosity, kindness, calmness, and steadiness begin to strengthen. They are all part of the fabric of compassion that allows for the beginnings of disidentification with distress. In MBCT programs, clients undertake all these steps.

Jon Kabat-Zinn describes this orientation in writing about the Stress Reduction Clinic: "The entire feeling in the clinic has always attempted to embody lovingkindness. . . . So to my mind, nothing ever needed to be said explicitly about it. Better to be loving and kind, as best we could, in everything that we were and everything that we did, and leave it at that" (p. 285).[82] If the very act of gently turning toward and attending to the present moment is a powerful gesture of kindness and self-care, then all the mindfulness practices in MBSR and MBCT are acts of self-compassion, and there is less need for a single practice exclusively devoted to training this capacity.

THE INSTRUCTOR'S STANCE AND PARTICIPANTS' DEVELOPMENT OF SELF-COMPASSION

If self-compassion in MBCT develops through pervasive indirect, even implicit, instruction, then much of the responsibility for embodying this rests with the instructor. Kindness, initially conveyed by the instructor's personal warmth, attentiveness, and welcoming stance, is reinforced throughout the program by the gentle approach taken with participants, especially in the presence of negative affect such as sadness or anger. In this way, mindfulness and compassion are caught and not taught. This implies that, while the content of each MBCT session is important, the most important "teachings" around kindness are conveyed by the instructor's presence in the classroom. Sometimes, what participants notice may be less *what* is said, than *how* it is said. Seeing kindness in action is the most powerful teaching, whether the instructor is guiding the in-class practices or responding to doubts, anger, or disappointment expressed by participants. Our own personal mindfulness practice as instructors allows us to know this territory through having recognized the times when we have, or have not, responded with kindness and self-compassion to experiences in our own lives.

Self-Compassion during Difficult Teaching Moments

Most instructors have had the experience of leading a practice in which the words said are not what we intended: in the body scan, saying "right knee" when what was intended was "left knee" or in Session 4, going from awareness of the body directly to awareness of thoughts and leaving out mindfulness of sounds altogether. We may become aware of having been less than skillful in dealing with an inquiry, or feel we have been too abrupt in moving on from one part of the curriculum to another. As we sit there, teaching class, we may become aware of our own challenging and self-critical thoughts.

How does the instructor accomplish the dual task of taking care of him- or herself, while continuing to look after the needs of the class? Does one dwell on what felt like a mistake and become critical of oneself, feeling like a fraud? What about the needs of the class? Should one quickly add an extra instruction to correct oneself, or just leave it until the next direction is provided?

In these cases, self-compassion for ourselves as teachers allows space for skillful choices. We do not ignore those places where we feel that other choices would have been more skillful. We can learn from each of them. Neither do we allow self-blame to cloud the clarity of the next moment and the choices that it will provide for us. It may be helpful to realize that even experienced instructors don't have all the answers or may get pulled off their intended focus. Offering this to oneself while the mind is still embroiled in condemning and just watching what happens next may be the kindest thing to do.

Sometimes the difficulties come from what others say to us rather than what we do. How can we embody kindness when responding to a participant who says, "This is a load of rubbish" or "This is not doing me any good at all—if anything, it is making me worse." In fact, these are important teaching moments. Drawing on the fruits of our personal mindfulness practice and knowing well the map of the territory of the suffering of depression, and how hard practice can be at times, the MBCT instructor can feel grounded when moving right into such difficulties expressed in class. Of course, the instructor will probably get an immediate sense of his or her own reaction of "contraction," and it is not unusual for a sense of panic to arise in the back of the mind: "Now what do I say?"

It is not that an experienced instructor does not feel such things, but that such "contraction" is increasingly seen as a sign: It signals the need to take a moment to ground oneself as a preparation for responding skillfully. Can we recall, in that instant (without having to state it explicitly) our own struggles with the practice? Can we remember how judgmental we can often be about our *own* efforts to make space for mindful compassion in our lives? If so, we'll be more likely to feel at one with a participant's expression of frustration. We'll be more willing to see the suffering behind such anger and frustration, and see clearly the courage that it might have taken to express it. Then, out of the compassion and "nonseparation" between instructor and participant can arise an even-handedness in responding, an engaged curiosity that is willing to move "toward the scream" and instead of contraction, aversion, and reactivity comes a greater sense of spaciousness and possibility.

A CAUTION REGARDING UNINTENDED CONSEQUENCES OF SELF-COMPASSION WITH VULNERABLE POPULATIONS

Whether or not explicit lovingkindness practices are used, any kindness—even when embodied implicitly through a compassionate and mindful presence in the classroom—may have an impact on participants that is not uniformly positive. As a phenomenon, this is actually not that unusual when dealing with clinical populations because even the mildest invitation to treat oneself with lovingkindness or self-compassion readily reactivates old and persistent habits of mind in which we view the self as unworthy, unlovable, and imperfect. We know from traditional cognitive therapy that core beliefs have two remarkable qualities: They are resistant to change and very efficient at filtering out disconfirming information. This means that even a kind word or caring remark can lead to a torrent of difficult feelings.

Our research has confirmed that for those who ruminate and brood a great deal, initial attempts to practice lovingkindness may be difficult,[83] and those who habitually ruminate and avoid are more likely to drop out early from MBCT.[78] We therefore allow more time in the preclass interview for participants who recognize these patterns in themselves, or for whom initial assessment has revealed such a pattern. The extra time is given over to talking in more detail about difficulties that might arise with the program and how it can be challenging, and that one of the challenges that may arise is to feel like giving up entirely. We speak of this as a major opportunity for participants to learn something important, so they should look out for it and feel free to talk to the instructor if and when it arises.

Christopher Germer has many valuable things to say about this.[84] He agrees that when any of us start to show ourselves greater kindness we may also notice a rebound back into negative feelings, so that it is useful for an instructor to prepare participants for moments when such bad feelings may arise. The skillful thing for an instructor to do is point this out without inducing undue pessimism; to invite participants to see whether they are able to find a balance point between being kind and the intensity of rebound that is experienced. Sometimes, as we know too well from our own practice, we may strive to increase the internal generation of kindness as a way of battling unpleasant feelings, or we expect kindness to work if we only try hard enough. In this case, it is always possible to move back to the breath as an anchor, or choose to express self-compassion more behaviorally, through enjoying the company of others or doing something special for oneself. This can be more skillful than "battling" with it in formal practice.

At the end of the day, what is important to recognize is that kindness and self-compassion can be held as an intention, even when it is difficult actually to incline the mind in this direction. Having the *intention* to look after oneself, even in the midst of difficult mind states, is itself healing. If we can come to appreciate that kindness is about intention—a practice of *inclining the mind toward* kindness rather *producing feelings of* kindness, then we will likely feel more forgiving toward ourselves at times when we would usually be harsh and condemning.

In summary, what we are saying is this: When we learn or teach mindfulness, we are not learning or teaching a "cold" attentional control that then requires the addition of the further ingredients kindness and compassion. Moments of mindfulness, although we may only be fleetingly aware of them, naturally bring with them kindness, compassion, and a sense of balance and even joy that can surprise us. Kindness and compassion are the ground from which we practice, the ground from which we teach, and the ground that participants may then use in cultivating their own practice.

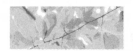

CHAPTER 9

Living in Our Heads

Session 2

The diversity of reactions to the first full week of practice is enormous. For some, the challenge may have seemed too strong. They have had "an awful week," an awfulness compounded by their disappointment that this approach appears not to be helping. They may even think that it is making things worse. For others, it may have "gone very well"; they may have found the body scan very relaxing. How can an instructor remain open and evenhanded in the light of all these different reactions?

When, in 1992, we started wondering whether mindfulness might be combined with cognitive therapy, we were helped to get a flavor of the Stress Reduction Clinic at the UMass Medical Center through a recent Public Broadcasting Service documentary about it. It followed a new class of participants as they attended the eight sessions and learned the mindfulness approach. In Session 1, we saw a sample of the instructor's initial remarks, his introduction of the raisin exercise, and the body scan. The program followed some of the participants home as they did the body scan practice for themselves on a daily basis. For the following week's session, the television program went directly from participants doing their home practice to their arrival for Session 2, and giving their feedback on how the week's practice had gone. We were very interested in seeing how the instructor handled the very different reactions to the first week's practice. Only later, after we had visited and sampled the program for ourselves, did we realize that the inevitable pressure to condense 8 weeks into a 40-minute television program had meant that an important component had been left out of the film—the initial practice at the start of the session.

But not just the constraints of television force the pace in this way. When participants arrive for the second session of any such program, both they and the instructor may feel a strong wish to share their experiences of the week. Before the session starts, the room may be filled with people talking and comparing notes. Participants know a bit more about each other and, of course, they have just spent a week engaged in a new and unfamiliar practice. It is tempting then to follow the television editor and cut directly to discussion of how the week has gone for each of them. Indeed, this would have been an important part of a cognitive therapy approach—set the agenda for the session, then check how the home practice has gone and what has been learned from it. This is a natural way to proceed if the task is to solve problems. Lay out the problems, then work as collaboratively as possible to find solutions.

We discovered that the mindfulness approach is radically different from the approach we might have used before. It does not provide a solution to anyone's problems, including depression. We found from the outset that it is better to start a class not with discussion but with practice. So, first thing, in each session, from Session 2 onward, the instructor leads the class in practice. Formal practice, usually lasting about half an hour, becomes the foundation on which the remainder of the class is built. In the case of Session 2, this is the body scan. Given the importance of allowing participants to become more aware of a different mode, the mode of "being" rather than "doing," the aim of starting with practice is to help participants recognize what mode they are in, and if they find that the more "driven" aspects of the doing mode arise, to see it clearly, disengage from it, and switch to a different mode.

Although the classes explore an alternative to striving for goals, this should not be taken to imply that there is no agenda for each session. There is work to be done, and some effort is required to stay focused enough to use every moment of the 2 hours to give participants opportunities to experience how mindfulness might be relevant to their lives. Box 9.1 shows the agenda for this week's class. First, we do the body scan practice. Second, we review the experience of the practice just completed, then review participants' experience of the formal and informal practice they have done during the week.

BOX 9.1

Theme and Curriculum for Session 2

THEME

In doing mode we "know about" our experience only indirectly, conceptually, through thought. This means we can easily get lost in rumination and worry. Mindfulness of the body provides an opportunity to explore a new way of knowing directly, intuitively—"experientially." Experiential knowing is a way to be aware of unpleasant experiences without getting lost in ruminative thought. Already, most participants will be experiencing some difficulties in their practice. These difficulties offer precious opportunities to practice letting go of thinking and to connect with direct awareness of the body.

AGENDA

- Body scan practice.
- Practice review.
- Home practice review—including difficulty with home practice
- Thoughts and feelings exercise ("walking down the street").
- Pleasant Experiences Calendar.
- Ten-minute sitting meditation.
- Distribute Session 2 participant handouts.
- Home practice assignment:
  o Body scan, 6 out of 7 days.
  o Ten minutes of mindfulness of the breath, 6 out of 7 days.
  o Pleasant Experiences Calendar (one example daily).
  o Mindfulness of a routine activity.

PLANNING AND PREPARATION

In addition to your personal preparation, bring a whiteboard/flipchart and marker pens for the thoughts and feelings exercise.

(cont.)

PARTICIPANT HANDOUTS FOR SESSION 2

Session 2–Handout 1. Summary of Session 2: Living in Our Heads

Session 2–Handout 2. Tips for the Body Scan

Session 2–Handout 3. Mindfulness of the Breath

Session 2–Handout 4. Home Practice for the Week Following Session 2

Session 2–Handout 5. Home Practice Record Form—Session 2

Session 2–Handout 6. Pleasant Experiences Calendar

EXPLORING PRACTICE AS THE FOUNDATION FOR THE CLASS

Responses to the practice are always varied. Some people fold new experiences of the practice just completed into their comments, while others want to discuss their experience of having done the body scan at home over the past week. We find it helpful to start discussion by staying as close as possible to feedback on the practice that has just ended. This involves postponing discussion of the home practice until later.

The themes that commonly emerge from the practice in the session often match very well participants' experience during the week. The most common themes that come out of the practice in the session are "Am I doing it right?", "I got discomfort when I did it," "The conditions aren't right," and "My mind just keeps wandering."

We look out especially for examples—within the practice itself—of how even mildly depressive thoughts and feelings feed off each other to create vicious spirals. The ease with which depressive interpretations can set off such spirals makes them seem hard to deal with if they occur in the practice. Helping participants deal with them involves bringing them to a point where they may see this process occurring more clearly for themselves. We focus on this early in the classes, partly because of its centrality to the prevention of relapse (see Chapter 2), and partly because it might raise participants' level of motivation for persisting with the practice. This is because the old and very familiar mental habits of rumination that commonly arise when doing the practice give us the opportunity to see more clearly the pull they have on our attention.

Let us look at some examples of reviewing practice done in class, before focusing on experiences that link what comes up in class with practice at home.

"The Conditions Weren't Right"

One of the most compelling obstructions to using the approaches we describe in this book is the idea that conditions have to be right: that we may be able to use this approach to deal with things when we are reasonably calm, or have the time, or when there are no distractions, but that otherwise, it just does not work so well.

At one of the first MBCT classes held at Cambridge during the development of MBCT, members of the cleaning staff were working outside the meeting room. The noise of one person calling to another was followed by a vacuum cleaner being switched on, then the drone of the machine as it did its work out in the hallway.

In the review of the practice later on, much of the discussion focused on the noise. Some participants found that they were able to weave the cleaners' noise into the fabric of the awareness of sounds in general. Others, however, experienced the noise as a distraction from the task of sitting quietly. They found it difficult not to get annoyed, thinking that they were being needlessly disturbed.

As the class continued to explore these different perspectives, one thing emerged that seemed important: All who heard the cleaners were also aware of some negative thoughts or reactions. After all, "Didn't they see the sign on the door that indicated a class was in progress?" Some people were able to note these thoughts, let them go, and return to the practice. It was as if they came to see the cleaners' noise as part of it all and were able to let go of the need for conditions to be other than they were. What seemed to fuel other class members' reactions was the expectation that this meditation practice should be a certain way, and that it was turning out to be different than they had hoped. This second, more angry reaction is quite normal; it does not require immediate remedial action, as if these participants are somehow inadequate in their practice. This frustration happens, and it can happen to those who have been practicing for years. The cleaners' noises created a great opportunity to notice what happens when things do not go as planned. We may have no control over either the noise or our initial discomfort or reaction of frustration. The question is: What happens next? Are we able to see our reactivity clearly, acknowledge it without harshness, and return our attention to where we had intended it to be?

No therapy or meditation prevents unpleasant things from happening in our daily lives, and these, together with the mood changes that accompany them, feature as much (perhaps more) when doing the practice as at other times. For people who have been depressed in the past, such occasions are times when the mood could begin to "lock into" the self-perpetuating pattern mentioned earlier. The rumination starts, and the repetitive thoughts may be far more troubling than the vacuum cleaner the participants heard in the class. Distraction caused by external factors and mind wandering are constant themes. Such mind wandering often has a theme of disappointed expectations, including disappointment about the practice itself not proceeding as it should. Many participants believe that it would be easier to deal with any discomfort and other difficulties with the practice if the mind were not so often distracted from the point of focus in the exercise. This raises a more general question that many people bring up again and again: what to do when the mind wanders.

Mind Wandering and Repetitive Habits of Mind

Both in our own experience and in that of others, mind wandering is easily regarded as a "mistake" that needs correction. But "wandering" is what minds do. It is their nature to wander, and we cannot stop them from doing so. The issue is how we relate to their wanderings. When we see our task as trying to empty the mind or to stop our thoughts, or to make the mind blank, and a thought occurs, we tend to see it as something that has gone wrong and needs remedial correction. Here is something that is worth repeating: *Mindfulness meditation is not about clearing the mind.* Even very skilled meditation teachers, who have been practicing for years, find that they have thoughts going through their minds much of the time.

But they describe this as being just like having the radio on in the background. They know it is there, and they know what's on the program if they want to tune in to it, but they can get on with the rest of their lives. So the issue is not learning how to switch thoughts off, but how best we can change the way we relate to them: seeing them as they are, simply, as streams of thinking, events in the mind, rather than getting lost in them. So when the mind wanders, the instruction is to acknowledge that it has wandered, note where it went, then gently return attention to the breath or body. The positive thing about this practice is that wherever your mind may be, you can always start again in the next moment.

> The essence of mindfulness is the willingness to begin over and over and over again.

One of the core skills in mindfulness practice is to disengage from old habits of mind. The body scan provides an opportunity to do this gracefully and gently. It can be seen as a practice of holding momentary experience in awareness, then letting go. This is easy to say. It turns out to be less easy in practice. The practice requires a deliberate decision: to bring the mind intentionally to each region, then either "breathing into and out from it" for a few moments, or focusing on it with the breath in the background, before (again, intentionally) moving the attention on to the next region of the body.

Summary of Intentions for the Body Scan

- Practicing deliberately engaging and disengaging attention.
- Noticing and relating differently to mental states and mind wandering: acknowledging and returning to what you had intended to be focusing on.
- Using breath as a "vehicle" to help direct and sustain attentional focus.
- Allowing things to be as they are.
- Cultivating direct experiential knowing.

HOME PRACTICE:
CULTIVATING MINDFULNESS IN THE REAL WORLD

The first time participants report on their home practice always brings up a variety of responses. These emerge from both the discussion and the review of what participants have written in the diaries they keep on a day-to-day basis. Let us look at some examples of common reactions to doing the body scan practice during the week. We start with the experience of one participant, Louise, giving a little of her background to set the context.

Louise was 38 years old when she was referred to the MBCT program. She had been depressed on and off for many years, with the last episode stretching over 9 months. She came because she feared that her episodes of depression were getting more severe. She was feeling better at the time she was referred to the MBCT trial (recall that MBCT was devised specifically for people who are not depressed at the moment but remain vulnerable to future depression). Louise had a husband and three children, and worked as a school receptionist. When Louise was a child, her parents (who, she said, were very perfectionist) sent her to a convent school (the family was Roman Catholic). Louise often felt she was a poor mother and wife. When she was depressed, her lack of energy confirmed to her how bad she was, and she ruminated endlessly about this.

At her preclass interview, the instructor was able to link some of the core themes of the program to Louise's particular experience. For example, she knew that she judged herself too harshly. She knew this "intellectually" but had not been able to do anything about it. Similarly, she recognized how easily her moods were triggered. Once again, knowledge of this had not altered the pattern. She talked of an "avalanche effect . . . a slippery slope," and the instructor talked about how difficult it can be to see the "warning signs."

At this interview, the instructor had taken time to explain MBCT— the 8-week, 2 hours a week commitment to class meetings. Home-based practice was particularly emphasized. If Louise was not sure she could find the time for this right now, it might be better not to start the classes because the practice between sessions was such an important component. This did not put her off. (It rarely puts anyone off. Most people can see that some work will be necessary, but, once the work starts, they may have very different reactions.)

Attitude toward the Practice: "Am I Doing It Right?"

Louise said that she had been able to concentrate on the body scan in the session much better than she had during the week. As the session progressed, we were able to build up a picture of the nature of this difference. During the week, Louise had done her home practice "religiously." She said she tried to relax, but any distraction made her angry and upset, and this was not the "way it should be." Even worse, Louise found that as she moved attention around her body, she noticed a lot of tension: tightness in the chest, stiffness in the lower back, tension in the shoulders. Her discomfort was compounded by another feeling: If it did not feel pleasant, then she must not be doing it right.

This theme ("Am I doing it right?") connects with what a lot of people in the class feel at some point. For some, it is pain. For others, it is that they fall asleep, lose concentration, keep thinking of other things, or focusing on the wrong part of the body or have no sensations whatsoever. There are a million ways in which people can think they are getting it wrong. The mindfulness approach allows people to experience these feelings in the moment, to acknowledge and register them as events in the mind, and continue with the practice. Recall the instruction given at the end of the first session: "You do not have to enjoy it, just do it!" In Louise's case, there was also a specific problem of pain and discomfort, and it is to this that we now turn.

Painful Sensations

Louise's reaction to her pain is a common one and provides an important opportunity for new learning. The intention in the body scan includes paying attention to physical sensations in the body. When strong sensations are present, the task remains the same, simply, to bring awareness to that region and, as best we can, note carefully the sensations that arise. This involves assuming a different stance from the one we habitually take. A typical reaction is to start thinking *about* the pain. This is what happened to Louise. In answer to a question about what had gone through her mind when she noticed these strong sensations, she said: "It was really uncomfortable. Why am I so tense? Why can't I do anything right?" In the ensuing inner monologue, Louise had, in effect, added concepts to the experience in an understandable attempt to find a way to reduce the discomfort. The problem was that in doing so, she had wandered away from the intended focus and made the experience something other than what it was. What began as an uncomfortable sensation was now an inner monologue about stress at work and tensions with her husband and children, and Louise wondered why she couldn't cope better with it all.

After a number of questions about how long the feelings of discomfort had lasted and whether they had stayed the same or changed over time, the instructor invited Louise, when next she was practicing the body scan and noticed her mind beginning to wander in this way, to bring awareness back as best she could to the part of the body currently under focus in the body scan. In this way, she could use these occasions as opportunities to practice untangling herself from the knots that the monologue was busy creating, not by attempting to undo the knots, but by again and again returning wholeheartedly to the direct awareness of sensations in the body.

"I Couldn't Find Time to Do the Practice"

In each class, some participants report that they have simply not been able to do the home practice, or have only practiced sporadically. Should we let such difficulties pass? Given the central role of home-based practice in the program, it turns out to be more helpful to be explicit when this occurs, to let people know that the lack of home practice will likely affect how much they will get out of the program, but without being critical of them. The task is to use occasions when participants have difficulty doing the home practice as an opportunity to bring curiosity to bear upon what is going on. We refer back to the discussion in Session 1: "Was this one of the difficulties you anticipated, or was it new? What did you discover? How did you handle it?" The participant's task for the next week is to bring an inquiring mind to the very difficulty of finding time for the home practice as it occurs. We find that this approach is more likely to help participants keep the door open to taking a second look at the problem, to bring awareness to the thoughts and feelings that might be blocking home practice activity, and to note what is found.

"I Got Utterly Bored," "I Was So Irritated with the Voice"

These are some of the most compelling types of reactions because they undermine the very motivation to continue with the practice. In class, the instructor, typically, would deal with this feedback matter-of-factly, in an empathetic and accepting way. Such experiences can provide opportunities to work with negative emotions. In this way, the instructor embodies a way of relating to the difficulties that may be novel to participants and quite different from their usual ways of handling these feeling states. Responding to negative thoughts or feelings by being genuinely curious and accepting them as the experience in the moment also provides a compelling first example of a stance toward negative emotions that is a recurring theme in MBCT. Asking questions about the feelings ("At what point did they arise?"; "Were they constant or fluctuating?"; "How long did they last?"; "Did you notice whether other thoughts, feelings, and bodily reactions were drawn in to the picture?"; etc.) assists in getting a better "map of the terrain." These questions are not intended so much to "diagnose a problem" as to invoke a stance of nonjudgmental inquiry.

If participants ask, "What shall I do when I feel this way?", the instructor can maintain the spirit of inquiry by asking what they have already done, and what happened next. Maintaining this curiosity is a more skillful approach than rushing to provide a "solution" based on the instructor's assumptions about a "best method." Often, participants have put tremendous effort into trying to control their bad feelings, and further suggestions (even, apparently, very wise ones) may simply feed their attitude that if only the right technique could be found, all their mood problems would be solved.

Does this mean that all suggestions are banned? No. Rather, the primary stance is to inquire and to question; suggestions, if they come, are borne of such inquiry. For example, one suggestion might be that participants simply choose to note any irritation or boredom as a state of mind. Then, once they register this, participants can bring their awareness back to the part of the body on which they intended to focus. The invitation is that they use the suggestion to notice what happens when they employ this strategy during the body scan. This may provide an example of what happens when they intentionally disengage attention from processing to which the mind has been "automatically" pulled by emotion, and intentionally return it to a chosen object of awareness. Of course, this needs to be implemented over and over again during a period of formal practice. Putting suggestions in the context of inquiry allows participants to see them as part of furthering their discoveries about mind and body rather than as attempts to fix their problems.

"It Was Great, I Fell Asleep," "I Enjoyed It Because I Was Finally Able to Relax," "It Didn't Do Anything for Me, I Just Fell Asleep"

If people find they are less tense or calmer, or if they fall asleep during the practice, they may believe that the body scan "worked" because it helped to induce a pleasant state, or that it "failed to work" because they did not comply with the instruction to be awake and aware. While the negative comments can be handled in the same way as the feelings of boredom we discussed earlier, it is sometimes surprisingly difficult to handle apparently positive comments. Being relaxed and enjoying the practice is often mixed with a feeling that this is the goal of the class. This is understandable from the point of view of participants wanting to get something out of the time and energy they put into this practice. Nevertheless, it will be important at some point to set these feelings in a wider context than mere relaxation:

> "OK, well, that's interesting, isn't it? And obviously we hope that this will eventually become a way of 'falling awake,' of learning how to relax into awareness. But keep in mind that the aim of the body scan is more to aid in the cultivation of awareness than an attempt simply to be relaxed. So we are not fixing any goals at all. It's simply a way of bringing attention to whatever is going on. Our bodies and minds are wonderful things, and if we don't get in the way, then we may sometimes find that they will just settle down into a sort of peaceful, gathered, relaxed state. And it sounds as if that's what has happened here. Just allowing the mind and the body to do those things, we may settle down into a relaxed state, or we may not.
>
> "But the one thing to remember is that it's not a goal or an expectation. We are not sitting down with the intention of being

relaxed by the end and checking to see if we are getting there or not. If you are tense throughout the whole thing and can bring your attention to the physical sensation in the body, then return to the part of the body you intended to focus on, that is it. You've done what you have to do."

The reasons for doing the body scan are more about finding a way to reestablish contact with the body, whether what comes up is pleasant or unpleasant. Looking to the body scan for its positive effects or benefits can get in the way of being with and acknowledging the wider range of reactions that can be revealed through this practice. Moreover, the practice of the body scan is aimed more at waking up than falling asleep. So if someone falls asleep, that is fine. But the instructor might also want to remind the person of the challenge to use it, perhaps, at another time of day, and to wake up to what is happening in his or her body.

At some point, the instructor may give some practical hints about staying awake, such as sitting up, or keeping eyes open, but only after exploring participants' experience and reactions to their sleepiness. Offered too early or as the only response, any "advice" may too easily get into fixing mode and contribute to a feeling in participants that there is a right way to do this and a right way to feel ("and I haven't got it!"). So any practice tips are offered in the spirit of encouraging participants to be curious about their experience and their reactions to their experience.

"I Am Trying My Best and I Still Don't Think I Get It," "I Think I Need to Work Harder at It"

For most people, the experience of depression is aversive enough to motivate them to find ways of preventing its return. We fully expect that participants in MBCT will come to class with specific aims in mind, and many will be willing to work hard to reach these aims. Paradoxically, much of the emphasis in practices such as the body scan is on *not* working or striving for goals. Of that much we can be clear. But putting into words what it is, positively, that we are encouraging is much more difficult. Instead of striving for goals, we might tell people that the emphasis is on "being," "dropping into the experience of the moment," or "allowing things to be held in nonjudgmental awareness, exactly as they are in this moment." Some mindfulness teachers refer to "settling into" each moment. Each of these phrases attempts to capture in words a constellation of meanings and implications. All are trying their best to convey a sense that the practice involves letting go of the impulse to fix or change, to escape or make better, or to be somewhere else in this moment. One way of making sense of this is to recognize that striving and having a goal orientation may work well in certain areas of life. But with emotions, sometimes the best way to change them is not to try to change them, but rather to bring awareness to them in order to see them more clearly. The final wrinkle here is that we must also beware that this is not just another subtle form of fixing.

Participants may be confused by the idea that "you don't need to get anywhere when you practice the body scan." After all, why bother doing this for 45 minutes a day, 6 days a week, if you get nothing out of it? An important point that easily gets lost in striving for outcomes is that, with the body scan, our intention is to be fully present with the physical sensations in each moment. When looked at in this way, there is really nowhere else to go, so efforts to get anywhere else are misplaced and rob us of our power for learning and changing in profound ways.

One way of trying to achieve a balance between these competing demands in the mind (demands that are themselves normal and understandable) is to practice on a regular basis, but to do so without an attachment to specific goals or outcomes. This allows us to recognize that "progress" is possible in one's mindfulness practice and that a "particular" kind of effort is necessary in the practice of the body scan, but it is not a striving to achieve some special state.

"I Just Got Too Upset": Reconnecting with Avoided Emotion

Like many of us, people who have been depressed in the past often live in their heads rather than in their bodies. For one reason or another, they have found that it is "safer" to *think about* emotion (or anything else, for that matter) than to *experience* emotion in the body. In many patients, this strategy may have evolved as a general style for coping with emotion. For others, this retreat from the body to the mind began as a way to avoid intense emotion linked to specific, traumatic bodily experience. Physical or sexual abuse is an obvious example, but medical emergencies can also involve intense affect closely linked to body sensations. Although wholly understandable, habitually withdrawing attention from the body means that "processing" emotional experiences remains uncompleted. Consequently, a continuing effort may be required to avoid having emotion-related body sensations enter awareness.

> Habitually withdrawing attention from the body means that "processing" emotional experiences remains uncompleted.

For such patients, intentionally reconnecting with awareness of body sensations, as the body scan practice requires, may be very difficult, or may even lead to experiences of being quite overwhelmed by previously avoided emotions. It is important in practice of the body scan for the instructor to be vigilant for hints in patients' feedback that they might be experiencing such difficulties. The instructor can then very gently and sensitively guide patients in how to relate skillfully to what might be quite frightening experiences, encouraging patients to walk the often fine line between, on one hand, retreating entirely from bodily awareness and, on the other, being "blown away" by the intensity of their experience. Intentionally returning awareness to the body scan instructions, then following them by focusing on the specified region of the body, as best they can, provides patients with a way to "steady" themselves, while still remaining connected to bodily experience. Putting a "toe in the water" in this way is perfectly OK.

Although difficult, the effects of reconnecting with the body in this way can often be dramatically healing, allowing completion of the unfinished work of emotional processing. Listen to how one patient described this experience, looking backward from the perspective of Session 7:

"I was quite alarmed when I started doing the body scan in the first couple of weeks. It was as if all my past was coming back to haunt me. I got very, very upset.

"Now, I don't feel half as bad. I don't feel so stirred up about it all. I don't know where, but it's all been filed away now, and it's all very much neater and everything. I wish I knew then what I know now, and I might have been a bit more ready for it. It quite worried me that it all happened in the first couple of weeks, and I thought, 'Gosh, you know, it's just going to get worse and worse.' But it actually got better."

"My Mind Wouldn't Stay Still"

Many participants find that when they attempt formal or informal practice, some thought or feeling gets in the way. They may start to experience an inner monologue that runs something like the following:

"What's the point of doing this?"

"It didn't make me feel any better yesterday."

"This is too hard for me."

"I can't see what this has to do with my problems."

"I need more time in my life and this is just wasting time."

One response to this is simply to repeat the message that countless people who have been through this before give to the beginner: "Just do it!" But side by side with that message, important though it is, it is essential to give participants some experience of recognizing the power of thoughts and interpretations in shaping feelings and behavior.

Let us take the example of two participants, Mary and Bob. Mary brought up the unanticipated obstacle of trying to find 45 minutes of free time. This prompted a whole series of thoughts. She wondered what this said about her. Was it simply that she was too busy, or did it mean that she was too concerned with making time for others, leaving little time for herself? We talked in the class about what her original intention had been: What had got in the way of it, and what other options might there be for her? These options could be explored as experiments during the next week.

Bob was able to find the time to practice but was unable to find a place that was quiet or private enough. In discussion in the class, we talked about whether his expectations about needing the "right" type of setting were getting in the way. In cases where it was not possible to have total quiet or privacy, we stressed that whatever space is chosen for practice is designed as much by our intention as by its physical characteristics. Bob decided that he would try an experiment. He would continue to meditate upstairs, despite the fact that the children would be running and playing downstairs, with all the unwanted noise, and rather than see this as a distraction, he would explore how to work with the noise during the practice.

Both of the difficulties brought up by Mary and Bob can also represent an opportunity: They may allow people to observe the thoughts or feelings to which they give rise. This type of observation by participants leads naturally to further exploration of the power that thoughts can have over feelings and behavior. With this in mind, we move to the next exercise, taken from standard cognitive therapy practice.

THOUGHTS AND FEELINGS

Interpretation of events plays a large role in determining moods. Understanding the extent of this can be very helpful for many people in overcoming barriers in practice and in daily life. The link between thoughts and feelings is a basic premise of the cognitive model of emotional disorders, and by making it explicit, we aim to offer participants an additional rationale for the effort being asked of them throughout the program. Of course, one could opt simply to tell people about the connection, but using examples gives people the opportunity for a different sort of learning that connects more strongly to day-to-day experience and therefore has a greater chance of generalizing to everyday life.

Once people have settled into a comfortable position, we ask them to close their eyes and imagine the following scenario:

> "You are walking down the street . . . , and on the other side of the street you see somebody you know. . . . You smile and wave. . . . The person just doesn't seem to notice and walks by. . . . How do you feel? . . . What's going through your mind right now? What do you feel like doing? Any body sensations?"

When participants open their eyes, we invite them to describe any feelings or body sensations they experienced, and any thoughts or images

Situation	Thought	Feeling
Someone you know; passed in the street; did not see you.	He didn't even acknowledge me.	Upset
	What have I done? I must have done something to upset him.	Worried
	Nobody likes me.	I felt isolated, alone.
	You must have seen me. Fine, if that's how you feel. Do what you want.	Angry
	She was probably preoccupied with something. I hope she's OK.	Concern

FIGURE 9.1. Thoughts and feelings scenario: Reactions and responses from a class.

that went through their minds. We list these reactions to the scenario on the whiteboard. Some typical examples of responses are shown in Figure 9.1. For some this scenario really resonates with their experience. "I would be going over this in my head for quite some time. My thinking would be really negative, and every time I went down one branch, there would be three to five negative thoughts coming off that."

Note how the same situation elicits many different thoughts and interpretations, hence many different feelings. This observation can then be used as the basis for discussion of how emotional reactions are often the product of our interpretations of events.

CONNECTING THE COGNITIVE MODEL OF DEPRESSION WITH THE THOUGHTS AND FEELINGS EXERCISE

The main message to draw from this exercise is *that our emotions are consequences of a situation plus an interpretation.* This is the basic ABC model of emotional distress. So often we find ourselves in a situation (A) and end up with a feeling (C). Normally, these are the things of which we are most aware. Often, we are not aware of a thought (B) that links them. It is as if there is this stream of thoughts present all the time, just under the surface, of which we are not aware. These thoughts are often not very obvious, particularly when we are not severely depressed, but they actually determine which emotion we feel, and how strongly we feel it.

In the approach taken in MBCT, dealing with and responding skillfully to this type of inner monologue is easier if it is spotted early enough. Because the inner monologue provides an interpretation of our experiences, it can trigger an entire story about what is going on in our world, without our realizing it.

One minute we are thinking about the friend not noticing us; the next moment, we feel alone. Because of this, it is important to learn to see these automatic thoughts clearly for what they are. By bringing them to awareness, we have greater ability not to be carried away by the cascade of our emotions.

> Spotting the inner monologue early is difficult because it can occur quite automatically and overtake us, without our quite knowing what has happened.

As in the raisin exercise, we may notice new things about our thoughts and feelings that we had not seen before. The teacher needs to be explicit that greater awareness of the (often so rapid) interpretation allows greater freedom and choice, so that we are less likely to become a victim of negative automatic thoughts. Note, again, that our investigations of these processes are borne of curiosity rather than driven by problem solving.

Summary of Intentions
for the Thoughts and Feelings Exercise

- It is not so much what happens, but what we make of it (meanings, interpretations) that determines our reactions.

- This influences other systems (body state, behavior).

- Reactions may reflect old, familiar patterns.

- There is no "right" interpretation—everyone has a different angle. Because of this variability, it is easier to see that thoughts are not facts.

- And the same person may have different reactions at different times (e.g., good day vs. bad day).

- Our interpretations of events, and our reactions in the next moment, are central to what keeps depression in place.

In Session 2, the focus is mainly on the top arrow in Figure 9.2. Later, in Sessions 4 and 6, there will be a chance to be more explicit about the lower (reverse) link between feelings and thoughts, though it is relevant to bring out the influence that mood has on our thoughts and interpretations at this point as well.

At least two other themes emerge from discussion of this exercise. First, by looking at the *variety* of interpretations within the class itself, it is easy to see that our *interpretations of events* (and the feelings they evoke) reflect what we bring to them as much as the "objective" situation does.

> "One thing to notice is that all these different feelings come about because the same event is being given a lot of different interpretations. If you interpret the event as simply the other person not seeing you because of his or her own problems or from being preoccupied, then you feel sorry for the other person. If you interpret the event as being a rejection or a hostile gesture, then you get angry.
>
> "Now ask yourself which of these ways of thinking would be likely to come to mind if this happened when you were depressed: What thoughts would you be most likely to have if you were still depressed?
>
> "As this exercise shows, our thoughts are often powerfully determined by our present mood. The event itself is neutral in

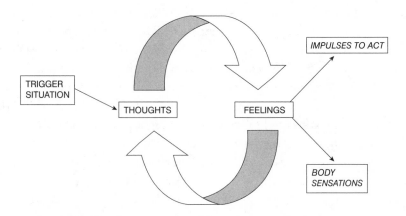

FIGURE 9.2. The ABC model of situation, thoughts, and feelings.

this particular case. All the action is on what you make of it. And what we are trying to do is to become more aware of these intervening thoughts."

The fact that interpretations of the same situation can vary, either over time depending on our mood, or from person to person, begins to show us that *thoughts are not facts.*

Second, *negative thinking is often a warning sign of oncoming depression.* For example, when we look at the list of reactions generated by the class, we can readily identify those statements that might be given by someone who is depressed. Most people agree that there is a strong connection between the types of interpretations listed and how depressed the person is. By comparing depressed and nondepressed thinking we see just how powerfully distorting depression can be. Acknowledging this the next time these reactions pop into the mind enables us to "check in" with ourselves and see to what extent our thoughts and interpretations might have been distorted by depressed mood. This is explored further in Sessions 4 and 6, where there will be an opportunity to explore further why we do not recognize our thoughts as mental events, and why such nonrecognition leads to them being so "adhesive."

AWARENESS OF PLEASANT EXPERIENCES

Becoming more fully aware of the way an experience is sensed as "pleasant" or "unpleasant," and the extent to which our thoughts and moods add an interpretation, may take some practice. Nor is it easy to be aware of all the effects that different situations and events (large and small) have on body sensations, feelings, and thoughts. With this in mind, we use an MBSR exercise for participants to complete as home practice during the week. They are asked to be aware of a different pleasant experience each day (preferably, to become aware of it while it is occurring). The handouts include a calendar (see Session 2–Handout 6) with spaces to write down, as closely as possible in time to any pleasant event, the thoughts, feelings, and body sensations that accompany the event. Participants are encouraged to write down any thoughts as if they were spoken out loud (in the words that actually came), using quotation marks, if that helps. Finally, they are asked to describe feelings and body sensations in as much detail as they can.

Why is it important to incorporate this exercise into an approach for individuals who have been depressed? First, it brings mindful awareness to what may turn out to be a pivotal point in triggering rumination, the early and almost silent sensed reaction—*pleasant* or *unpleasant* or *neutral*. Research on implicit affect cues[85] shows that much of the time we react to incoming stimuli on the basis of whether they feel pleasant, unpleasant, or neutral. These are the trigger points for the mind to begin needing things to be different, or to wander off into thought streams and rumination, and the purpose of this exercise is to make people aware of these pivotal moments. Bringing mindful awareness to bear at these moments may allow people simply to experience and appreciate the moment as it is, without adding further thoughts, such as wishing it would go on forever or wondering why it does not happen more often.

Second, the exercise can help people notice what (even slightly) positive things may be occurring in their daily lives. Although it appears to resemble the pleasant events scheduling that is part of some structured treatments for acute depression, at this point in MBCT, the aim is not to increase the number of pleasant events but simply to become more aware of those that may already be there. For some people, this can be a revelatory experience.

Summary of Intentions
for the Pleasant Experiences Calendar

- Brings mindful awareness to the earliest reaction to moment-by-moment experience as pleasant or unpleasant or neutral—a pivotal point in triggering rumination or avoidance.

- Helps people notice what positive things may be occurring in their daily lives.

- Allows people to become more aware of the thoughts, feelings, and body sensations that accompany pleasant experiences.

- Helps people to tune into the "felt" dimension of experience in a nonthreatening way.

- Helps people to deconstruct fleeting or powerful experiences into constituent elements, such as thoughts, feelings, and body sensations.

Third, the exercise may allow people to become more aware of the thoughts, feelings, and body sensations that accompany such pleasant experiences. Becoming aware of an experience as a constellation of separate elements of thinking, feeling, and sensing rather than as a unitary "thing" can be the beginning of a process of "deconstruction" that can allow us to respond differently, more skillfully, rather than to react automatically with our habitual patterns. The emphasis on awareness of physical sensations is not a prominent feature in cognitive therapy, but it is included in MBCT because body sensations that accompany pleasant and unpleasant experiences can be a sensitive barometer of a person's affective state. In this way, such sensations can provide a signature or readout, in the body, of how a person is feeling from moment to moment.

Fourth, it is a nonthreatening way to begin tuning back into the "felt" dimension of experience. Participants have often developed a protective habit of "experiential avoidance," or tuning out from feelings, as a way to defend themselves from potentially overwhelming feelings. Although it may seem to have been helpful in the short term, the long-term effects of such avoidance are actually to perpetuate, rather than escape, unwanted emotions.[86] The pleasant experiences exercise provides a nonthreatening way to encounter the full range of elements that comprise participants' experience.

Together with the other home practice assignments set for the following week (further formal practice using the body scan, brief mindfulness of breathing, bringing mindful awareness to another routine activity each day; see participant handouts for details), the aim is to link awareness of the body to awareness of the body's reactions and responses to everyday events.

SITTING WITH THE BREATH

At this point, although participants will do a further week's practice with the body scan on a daily basis, we prepare the ground for a transition to a form of meditation in which the attention is kept on a single focus. We therefore finish Session 2 with a brief sitting meditation, lasting 10 minutes, with awareness of breathing as the primary object of attention. Paying attention to a single focus, in this case, the breathing, is the next step in training participants to recognize old mental habits as they arise.

By learning to allow *any* distractions—thoughts, feelings, impulses, and sensations—to come and go in the mind, we cultivate a way of releasing ourselves from the grip of the older, more adhesive mind states that occur from time to time. Distractions are seen most clearly when the mind is given just one thing to do, and placing the attention on the breath is a skillful way to anchor the mind, so the "tug" on the anchor may be felt.

BOX 9.2.
The Breath

Breath is life. You can think of the breath as being like a thread or a chain that links and connects all the events of your life from birth, the beginning, to death, the end. The breath is always there every moment, moving by itself like a river.

Have you ever noticed how the breath changes with our moods—short and shallow when we're tense or angry, faster when we're excited, slow and full when we're happy, and almost disappearing when we're afraid? It's there with us all the time. It can be used as a tool, like an anchor, to bring stability to the body and mind when we deliberately choose to become aware of it. We can tune into it at any moment during everyday life.

Mostly, we're not in touch with our breathing—it's just there, forgotten. So one of the first things we do is to get in touch with it. We notice how the breath changes with our moods, our thoughts, our body movements. We don't have to control the breath. Just notice it and get to know it, like a friend. All that is necessary is to observe, watch, and feel the breath with a sense of interest, in a relaxed manner.

With practice, we become more aware of our breathing. We can use it to direct our awareness to different aspects of our lives, for example, to relax tense muscles, or to focus on a situation that requires attention. Breath can also be used to help deal with pain, anger, relationships, or the stress of daily life. During this program, we will be exploring this in great detail.

Adapted with permission from Karen Ryder, Instructor, Stress Reduction Clinic, University of Massachusetts Medical Center (personal communication).

> Paying attention to a single focus, the breath, is the next step in training participants to recognize old mental habits as they arise.

Since this is the first time that participants practice a sitting meditation, we give instructions on how to sit. We speak of the choices that are available, and the danger of setting goals for the "right" or "proper" way to sit in meditation (often based on images in the media of people meditating). These instructions are also provided in Session 2–Handout 3, including some basic tips on how to check the position of legs, hips, and spine (e.g., whatever one is sitting on, it is helpful for the knees to be below the level of the hips).

Once the sitting posture has been described, we ask participants to choose a comfortable posture that embodies a sense of dignity and alertness, with the back straight but not stiff, the head balanced, and the head, neck, and spine in line, with the shoulders relaxed. After a moment, we ask people to bring their attention to the breathing. The particular focus here involves paying close attention to the physical sensations of breathing: to be fully aware of each inbreath for its full duration, and each outbreath for its full duration. As is bound to happen, the mind will eventually drift to other concerns. Every time people notice that their minds have wandered off the breathing, the instruction is to note what took it away, then gently escort the attention back to the sensation of the breath coming in and out. As often as the mind wanders from the breath, the task remains the same: simply to bring the mind back to the breath each time, no matter what has preoccupied it.

ENDING THE CLASS

As Session 2 draws to a close, note the implicit message that ends it, an idea to which we return again and again: It is just as valuable to become aware that the mind has wandered and to bring it back, as to remain fixed on the chosen object of attention. This is all part of learning how to pay attention in this new way: on purpose, in each moment, and nonjudgmentally.

Summary of Session 2: Living in Our Heads

Our aim in this program is to be more aware, more often. A powerful influence taking us away from being "fully present" in each moment is our automatic tendency to judge our experience as being not quite right in some way—that it is not what should be happening, not good enough, or not what we expected or wanted. These judgments can lead to sequences of thoughts about blame, what needs to be changed, or how things could or should be different. Often these thoughts will take us, quite automatically, down some fairly well-worn paths in our minds. In this way, we may lose awareness of the moment and also the freedom to *choose* what, if any, action needs to be taken.

We can regain our freedom if, as a first step, we simply acknowledge the actuality of our situation, without immediately being hooked into automatic tendencies to judge, fix, or want things to be other than they are. The body scan exercise provides an opportunity to practice simply bringing an interested and friendly awareness to the way things are in each moment, without having to do anything to change things. There is no goal to be achieved other than to bring awareness to bear as the instructions suggest—specifically, achieving some special state of relaxation is *not* a goal of the exercise.

Tips for the Body Scan

1. Regardless of what happens (e.g., if you fall asleep, lose concentration, keep thinking of other things or focusing on the wrong bit of body, or not feeling anything), persist with it! These are your experiences in the moment. See if it is possible to be aware of them all, just as they are.

2. If your mind is wandering a lot, simply note the thoughts (as passing events), then bring the mind gently back to the body scan.

3. Let go of ideas of "success," "failure," "doing it really well," or "trying to purify the body." This is not a competition. It is not a skill for which you need to strive. The only discipline involved is regular and frequent practice. Just do it with an attitude of openness and curiosity, then allow the rest to take care of itself.

4. Let go of any expectations about what the body scan will do for you: Imagine it as a seed you have planted. The more you poke around and interfere, the less it will be able to develop. So with the body scan, just give it the right conditions—peace and quiet, regular and frequent practice. That is all. The more you try to influence what it will do for you, the less it will do.

5. Try approaching your experience in each moment with the attitude: "OK, that's just the way things are right now." If you try to fight off unpleasant thoughts, feelings, or body sensations, the upsetting feelings will only distract you from doing anything else. Be aware, be nonstriving, be in the moment, accept things as they are.

Mindfulness of the Breath

1. Settle into a comfortable sitting position, either on a straight-backed chair or a soft surface on the floor, with your buttocks supported by cushions or a low stool. If you use a chair, it is very helpful to sit away from the back of the chair, so that your spine is self-supporting. If you sit on the floor, it is helpful if your knees actually touch the floor; experiment with the height of the cushions or stool until you feel comfortably and firmly supported. Whatever you sit on, arrange things so that your knees are lower than your hips.

2. Allow your back to adopt an erect, dignified, and comfortable posture. If sitting on a chair, place your feet flat on the floor, with your legs uncrossed. Gently close your eyes.

3. Bring your awareness to the level of physical sensations by focusing your attention on the sensations of touch and pressure in your body where it makes contact with the floor and whatever you are sitting on. Spend a minute or two exploring these sensations, just as in the body scan.

4. Now bring your awareness to the changing patterns of physical sensations in the lower abdomen as the breath moves in and out of your body. (When you first try this practice, it may be helpful to place your hand on your lower abdomen and become aware of the changing pattern of sensations where your hand makes contact with your abdomen. Having "tuned in" to the physical sensations in this area in this way, you can remove your hand and continue to focus on the sensations in the abdominal wall.)

5. Focus your awareness on the sensations of slight stretching as the abdominal wall rises with each inbreath, and of gentle deflation as it falls with each outbreath. As best you can, follow with your awareness the changing physical sensations in the lower abdomen all the way through as the breath enters your body on the inbreath, and all the way through as the breath leaves your body on the outbreath, perhaps noticing the slight pauses between one inbreath and the following outbreath, and between one outbreath and the following inbreath.

6. There is no need to try to control the breathing in any way—simply let the breath breathe itself. As best you can, also bring this attitude of allowing to the rest of your experience. There is nothing to be fixed, no particular state to be achieved. As best you can, simply allow your experience to be your experience, without needing it to be other than it is.

(cont.)

7. Sooner or later (usually sooner), your mind will wander away from the focus on the breath in the lower abdomen to thoughts, planning, daydreams, drifting along—whatever. This is perfectly OK—it's simply what minds do. It is not a mistake or a failure. When you notice that your awareness is no longer on the breath, gently congratulate yourself—you have come back and are once more aware of your experience! You may want to acknowledge briefly where the mind has been ("Ah, there's thinking"). Then, gently escort the awareness back to a focus on the changing pattern of physical sensations in the lower abdomen, renewing the intention to pay attention to the ongoing inbreath or outbreath, whichever you find.

8. However often you notice that the mind has wandered (and this will quite likely happen over and over and over again), as best you can, congratulate yourself each time on reconnecting with your experience in the moment, gently escorting the attention back to the breath, and simply resume following in awareness the changing pattern of physical sensations that come with each inbreath and outbreath.

9. As best you can, bring a quality of kindliness to your awareness, perhaps seeing the repeated wanderings of the mind as opportunities to bring patience and gentle curiosity to your experience.

10. Continue with the practice for 10–15 minutes, or longer if you wish, perhaps reminding yourself from time to time that the intention is simply to be aware of your experience in each moment, as best you can, using the breath as an anchor to gently reconnect with the here and now each time you notice that your mind has wandered and is no longer down in the abdomen, following the breath.

Home Practice
for the Week Following Session 2

1. Do the body scan for 6 days and record your reactions on the Home Practice Record Form (Session 2–Handout 5).

2. At different times, practice 10 minutes of mindfulness of breathing for 6 out of 7 days (*www.guilford.com/MBCT_audio*, track 4). Being with your breath in this way each day provides an opportunity to become aware of what it feels like to be connected and present in the moment without having to *do* anything.

3. Complete Session 2–Handout 6, the Pleasant Experiences Calendar (one entry per day). Use this as an opportunity to become really aware of the thoughts, feelings, and body sensations around one pleasant event each day. Notice and record, as soon as you can, *in detail* (e.g., use the actual words or images in which the thoughts came the precise nature and location of body sensations).

4. Choose a new routine activity to be especially mindful of (e.g., brushing your teeth, washing dishes, taking a shower, taking out garbage, reading to kids, shopping, eating).

Home Practice Record Form—Session 2

Name: _____

Record on the Home Practice Record Form each time you practice. Also, make a note of anything that comes up in the home practice, so that we can talk about it at the next meeting.

Day/date	Practice (Yes/No)	Comments
Wednesday Date: _____	Body scan: Breath: Everyday mindfulness:	
Thursday Date: _____	Body scan: Breath: Everyday mindfulness:	
Friday Date: _____	Body scan: Breath: Everyday mindfulness:	
Saturday Date: _____	Body scan: Breath: Everyday mindfulness:	
Sunday Date: _____	Body scan: Breath: Everyday mindfulness:	
Monday Date: _____	Body scan: Breath: Everyday mindfulness:	
Tuesday Date: _____	Body scan: Breath: Everyday mindfulness:	
Wednesday Date: _____	Body scan: Breath: Everyday mindfulness:	

Pleasant Experiences Calendar

Name: _____

Be aware of a pleasant event *at the time it is happening*. Use the following questions to focus your awareness on the details of the experience as it is happening. Write it down later.

Day	What was the experience?	How did your body feel, in detail, during this experience?	What moods and feelings accompanied this event?	What thoughts went through your mind?	What thoughts are in your mind now as you write this down?
Example: Heading home at the end of my shift—stopping, hearing a bird sing.	Lightness across the face, aware of shoulders dropping, uplift of corners of mouth.	Relief, pleasure.	"That's good," "How lovely [the bird]," "It's so nice to be outside."	"It was such a small thing, but I'm glad I noticed it."	
Monday					

(cont.)

Day	What was the experience?	How did your body feel, in detail, during this experience?	What moods and feelings accompanied this event?	What thoughts went through your mind?	What thoughts are in your mind now as you write this down?
Tuesday					
Wednesday					
Thursday					
Friday					
Saturday					
Sunday					

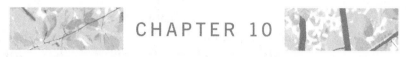

CHAPTER 10

Gathering the Scattered Mind

Session 3

The problem-solving, doing mode of mind is an extraordinary evolutionary achievement. Consider how we perform the simplest of acts, such as taking our favorite coffee cup down from a shelf that is full of cups. How do we not only recognize it as ours but also successfully "navigate" around other cups and pick up our own, without knocking everything over? Research into the cognitive processes that underlie reaching for objects finds that the brain carries out a delicate balancing act between excitation of the object that is to be selected and inhibition (damping down) of the objects that are not to be selected. This balancing act has been finely tuned throughout our evolutionary history. Reaching for desired objects, and avoiding undesired objects, is one of most fundamental building blocks of animal life. Animals whose brains could not carry out the process would soon die: They would fail to pick up food, or they would miss the branch for which they were leaping or the prey on which they were pouncing. Evolution gave the human species these skills long before higher cognitive functions developed, and we see it each time we reach for something.

The computational power needed by the brain to carry out even the simple action of picking up a cup is immense, yet, even for a small child, it soon happens automatically, without awareness. The brain computes the gap between the current position of the hand and the position of the desired object, and the trajectory of the movement needed to close the gap between them. Then it initiates the action of reaching, monitoring the gap as it closes, until the object is grasped successfully, after which the "reaching" can stop; the goal is achieved. Job done.

What happened when humans evolved the ability to solve complex problems "in the head," as well as by trial and error? Evolution did what it usually does: It used the same process that had worked before. So even for complex problem solving, the mind uses the same basic format as the older problem of "reaching for an object." It is called *discrepancy-based processing*. The current situation (A) is compared with the desired state (B), and the various possibilities of getting from A to B are considered.

But what happens when the problem seems to be with our moods? In this case, the "gap" that needs to be closed is not a gap between our hand and an object, but between the *mood in which we find ourselves* and *the mood in which we want to be*. It is natural for us to believe that such discrepancy-based problem solving might also help to solve this emotional problem. It seems plausible enough. The goal is clear: to escape or avoid unhappiness on one hand, and to achieve happiness on the other. In order to see how successful we are at this, we need to monitor how we are getting on.

Such constant monitoring of how we fare against the standards of happiness we have set for ourselves turns out to be very unhelpful. For example, to cope with waking in the morning feeling bad is difficult enough, but if we then match it against some standard, better mood, we worsen the very mood we wanted to get rid of. Soon, we find that the results of this "matching" process create a new train of thought: "I wish I didn't feel this bad in the mornings. Why am I feeling this way? Why do I always feel this way?" We are soon trapped in verbal problem-solving techniques. We imagine that, as in other problem-solving situations, if we could find just the right way to reach for the goal, we would get there in the end.

We can see here how our natural drive for happiness creates brooding and rumination: patterns of thinking, feeling, and behavior that are unhelpful because they simply circle round and round, without producing a resolution, and make us feel worse. Ruminating about a problem feels as if it should bring a solution, but as Nolen-Hoeksema and Morrow found (see Chapter 2), such ruminative brooding most often exacerbates the situation.[57]

> The feeling that our clever problem-solving abilities should be able to sort out all our problems is very compelling and cannot be switched off easily.

We mention this now because we find that, following initial enthusiasm, Session 3 often brings up, with full force, the problems we alluded to in Session 2. In the first two sessions, we have begun to explore how being mindful can help in stepping out of the types of habitual patterns of thinking that can quickly escalate to cause depression. Whether people are able to see the relevance of it for their own lives and their own problems, they are generally prepared to suspend judgment. By Session 3, it becomes clearer that this practice is not going to provide a ready-made set of solutions to their problems, and frustration can set in. There may be many sources for such frustration, but one common source is the feeling that our clever problem-solving abilities should be able to sort out all our problems. This very compelling feeling cannot be switched off easily. In fact, it is unlikely that people would voluntarily give up their old ways of trying to deal with their problems by ruminating about them unless they had sampled an alternative approach.

The mindfulness-based approach does not just involve another, more clever problem-solving technique. Rather, it involves a different mode: a way of "being with" problems that allows people to let go of the need to solve them instantly. In stepping back from the tendency to want instant solutions, we are inviting people to see how much behavior is driven by avoidance of unpleasantness and attachment to pleasantness. Simply being aware of the difficulty, and holding it in awareness, can provide a time-out from getting caught in old mental routines. Mindfulness practice involves sampling the "being" mode, in which we are invited to let go of our usual striving and goal orientation.

In the process of letting go, we may, ironically, become more open to seeing more clearly what is a skillful next step to be taken when a problem arises. All the practices learned during the classes and practiced at home are in the service of sampling and learning to trust this new approach.

> Many problems that arise in practice can be traced to the understandable difficulty in trusting that this new way—letting go of our usual striving and goal orientation—will be sufficient.

The next step in the program therefore involves developing mindfulness of the breath, so that people can deepen their use of breathing as an anchor to gather and steady themselves, while at the same time being open to their experience, whatever it is. Once again, the challenge is to find ways that people in the class can sample this different approach.

Recall that one of the attractions of the mindfulness approach in reducing risk of recurrence in those who are not currently depressed is that it can be applied to any experience, whether positive or negative, important or trivial. That is why we emphasize the combination of formal practice (e.g., the body scan) with informal practice (e.g., bringing awareness to a routine activity such as eating). If our task is to enable people to sample ways of looking at the world that are different from the "analytic" or "intellectual," then it is possible to use even the most basic sensations, such as seeing.

STARTING BY SEEING

Consider the page you are reading right now. In order to read, you must see the marks on the page, analyze them as words and sentences, then fold together the sentences to understand the text as a whole. "Seeing" is most often simply what comes before such analysis in most of our daily lives. The way we "parse" the text happens so automatically that it is difficult to disentangle the processes. It also happens with objects and sounds in the world. Our attention naturally and automatically "parses" the world, categorizing and laying it out, ready to be acted upon. One approach to offering a different way of being is therefore to take this most automatic of situations and renew our acquaintance with the sensations that make up the raw material of experience.

One way to do this is to start Session 3 with a simple 5-minute "seeing" or "hearing" exercise. If there is a window in the room, we ask people to look outside, paying attention to sights as best they can, letting go of the categories they normally use to make sense of what they are looking at; rather than viewing elements of the scene as trees or cars, or whatever, we invite them simply to see them as patterns of color, shapes, and movement. The instruction is that whenever they become aware that they have started to think *about* what is being seen, they gently bring the attention back to simply seeing. If a window is not available, then we substitute a "hearing" meditation, asking people to listen to sounds from inside

BOX 10.1
Theme and Curriculum for Session 3

THEME

The mind is often scattered and lost in thought because it is working away in the background to complete unfinished tasks and strive for future goals. Instead, we need to find a way to intentionally "come back" to the here and now. The breath and body offer an ever-present focus on which we can reconnect with mindful presence, gather and settle the mind, and ease ourselves from doing into being.

AGENDA

- 5-minute "seeing" (or "hearing") exercise.
- 30-minute sitting meditation (awareness of breath and body; how to respond to intense physical sensations—see footnote for alternative).*
- Practice review.
- Home practice review (including body scan, mindfulness of the breath and routine activity, and Pleasant Experiences Calendar).
- 3-minute breathing space and review.
- Mindful stretching and review.
- Setting up Unpleasant Experiences Calendar practice.
- Distribute Session 3 participant handouts.
- Home practice assignment:
  o "Stretch and Breath" meditation (audio track 6) on Days 1, 3, and 5.
  o 40-minute mindful movement (audio track 5) on Days 2, 4, and 6.
  o Unpleasant Experiences Calendar (a different experience each day).
  o 3-minute breathing space, three times daily (audio track 8).

(cont.)

---

*In our MBCT classes in Oxford for those who have experienced recurrent suicidal thoughts when depressed, we teach mindful movement at this point (based on lying down, hatha yoga) and later in the session teach the standing movements, followed at that point by a sitting meditation (focusing on breath and body).

PERSONAL PREPARATION AND PLANNING

In addition to your personal preparation, remember to bring the audio files that (1) combine mindful stretching and the sitting meditation and (2) guide the mindful movement.

PARTICIPANT HANDOUTS FOR SESSION 3

Session 3–Handout 1. Summary of Session 3: Gathering the Scattered Mind

Session 3–Handout 2. The 3-Minute Breathing Space: Basic Instructions

Session 3–Handout 3. Home Practice for the Week Following Session 3

Session 3–Handout 4. Home Practice Record Form—Session 3

Session 3–Handout 5. Unpleasant Experiences Calendar

---

the room and beyond. The class is invited to bring attention to hearing, again, as best they can, letting go of the categories normally used to make sense of what is heard—instead of hearing a chair scraping or a person coughing, to hear the sounds as patterns of pitch, tone, and volume. Every time the mind wanders, the attention is gently brought back just to hearing. In this way, we seek to make a transition from the "doing" mode in which people often arrive at the class, to the being mode, which is further explored in the mindfulness of the breath that immediately follows the focus on seeing or hearing. Once the class has spent 4 or 5 minutes practicing "seeing," we invite participants to move to "sitting."

THE SITTING MEDITATION
AS MINDFULNESS PRACTICE

For centuries, people have used breathing as a vehicle for meditation. Why should it be relevant to people who have been depressed in the past and remain vulnerable to becoming depressed again? Recall that in our analysis, the escalation of negative thoughts in the face of mild states of negative mood was responsible for relapse and recurrence of depression. At times of potential relapse, an evaluation of something as positive or negative, particularly depressed mood itself, can set in motion a rumination ("Why can't I be happier? Why do I always feel like this? What's wrong with me?"). Very soon, the mind is lost in thinking about the past or worrying about the future. Now, think about what the breath is and what it does.

First, it takes place in the present, so that focusing attention on it can help a person to let go of the past and the future, and anchor him- or herself in the present moment. Second, it is always here, and therefore always available for focus as a marker of one's emotional state. Third, the very act of intentionally bringing awareness to the breath involves "taking up space" in the same limited capacity channel that has been filled with ruminative thought. So, although this is not the eventual aim, it can provide a temporary substitute for (or distraction from) the ruminative thinking. As alternative foci of attention go, it is also useful because it is in constant change and flux, ebbing and flowing moment by moment, and requiring some effort to maintain attention. Fourth, attention to the breath involves attending to something that is the opposite of goal orientation. It is not our job to make the breath do its work. It simply does it. This attitude toward the breath embodies a more general attitude toward the self and the world: that in our emotional lives, attention to the simple can be more effective than analysis of the complex. And because each of us has breathed all our lives, it can link with many different situations, thereby giving it the potential to transform many situations.

Finally, the simple act of registering that the mind has wandered, noting where it has gone, and returning to the breath involves just the sort of metacognitive awareness—seeing thoughts as thoughts—that promotes the skills of decentering needed to prevent the escalation of negative thought–affect spirals at times of potential relapse. Most important, such acts also provide repeated practice in intentionally disengaging from one mode of mind and engaging in another—shifting mental gears from a mode that may increase rumination to one that emphasizes direct experience.

We begin by using the instructions for the 10-minute sitting meditation introduced in Session 2. Before they begin the sitting practice, it is important that participants find a sitting posture that embodies a sense of calmness and dignity, combining comfort and stability. If this can be accomplished by sitting or kneeling on the floor, using a cushion or bench for support, or by sitting on a chair, then that is all that is required. So we begin by paying attention to posture, noting how the back is upright but not stiff and aligned with the neck and head, with the shoulders relaxed and the chin tucked in a little. If sitting on a chair, participants may find it useful to use a cushion on the seat of the chair, so that the hips can be slightly higher than the knees.

After a few moments, the instructor brings the focus of attention to the breath. This is going to be the primary focus of awareness for the first half of the practice. The guidance for this practice is clear and simple. *Allow the attention to rest on the breath at the abdomen (or tip of the nose or chest, if the breath is more vivid at these places). Feel the sensations of each breath as it moves in and moves out, without looking for anything to happen. If your mind wanders, briefly notice what it is that took your mind away, then gently bring your attention back to your breathing, without giving yourself a hard time.* The instructions are repeated a number of times throughout the 30-minute sitting meditation, with various reminders to see whether the attention was on the breath at that very moment. About halfway through the practice, participants are instructed to expand the awareness to the whole body (see Box 10.2).

The simplicity of this practice is important. Because it appears, on the face of it, to be so simple, it reveals all the more readily the difficulty that all of us have in putting aside the normal mode in which we operate. For people who have been depressed, the thoughts and feelings that come up may echo themes similar to the ruminations that would normally keep them vulnerable.

PRACTICE REVIEW

As in other sessions, we focus first on the practice just completed in the class, then later explore what came up during the week of home practice. In the discussion of participants' actual experiences with the seeing and sitting meditations, several themes are often raised. We present them here, with an accompanying link back to the themes of the program, but this

BOX 10.2

Sitting Meditation: Mindfulness of the Breath and Body

1. Practice mindfulness of the breath, as described earlier (pp. 171–172), for 10–15 minutes.

2. When you feel reasonably settled on awareness of the breath, intentionally allow the awareness to expand around the breath to include, as well, a sense of physical sensations throughout the whole body. While still aware, in the background, of the movements of the breath in the lower abdomen, change your primary focus, so that you become aware of a sense of the body as a whole and of the changing patterns of sensation throughout the body. You may find that you get a sense of the movements of the breath throughout the body, as if the whole body were breathing.

3. If you choose, together with this wider sense of the body as a whole, and of the breath moving to and from, include awareness of the more local, particular patterns of physical sensations that arise where the body makes contact with the floor, chair, cushion, or stool—the sensations of touch, pressure, or contact of the feet or knees with the floor; the buttocks with whatever supports them; the hands where they rest on the thighs, or on each other. As best you can, hold all these sensations, together with the sense of the breath and of the body as a whole, in a wider space of awareness of physical sensations.

4. The mind will wander repeatedly away from the breath and body sensations—this is natural, to be expected, and in no way a mistake or a failure. Whenever you notice that your awareness has drifted away from sensations in the body, you might want to congratulate yourself; you have "woken up." Gently note where your mind was ("thinking"), and kindly focus your attention back to your breathing and to a sense of your body as a whole.

5. As best you can, keep things simple, gently attending to the actuality of sensations throughout your body from one moment to the next.

6. As you sit, some sensations may be particularly intense, such as pains in the back, knees, or shoulders, and you may find that awareness is

(cont.)

repeatedly drawn to these sensations, and away from your intended focus on the breath or body as a whole. You may want to use these times to experiment with choosing intentionally either to shift posture, or to remain still and bring the focus of awareness into the region of intensity. If you choose to remain still, then, as best you can, explore with gentle and wise attention the detailed pattern of sensations here: What, precisely, do the sensations feel like? Where exactly are they? Do they vary over time or from one part of the region of intensity to another? Not so much thinking about them, as just feeling them. You may want to use the breath as a vehicle to carry awareness into such regions of intensity, "breathing in" to them, just as in the body scan. Breathe out from those sensations, softening and opening with the outbreath.

7. Whenever you find yourself "carried away" from awareness in the moment by the intensity of physical sensations, or in any other way, remind yourself that you can always reconnect with the here and now by refocusing awareness on the movements of the breath or on a sense of the body as a whole. Once you have gathered yourself in this way, allow the awareness to expand once more, so it includes a sense of sensations throughout the body.

8. And now for the last few moments of this sitting, bringing your attention back to focus on your breathing in the abdomen. Tuning in to any and all sensations on this inbreath and this outbreath. And as you sit here and as you breathe, allowing yourself to cultivate this sense of moment-to-moment awareness, and remembering that the breath is available to you at any moment of your day, to allow you to feel grounded, to give a sense of balance and an awareness of accepting yourself just as you are in each moment.

is not intended to imply that an MBCT class becomes a question-and-answer session. Rather, the instructor seeks to explore with participants how each aspect of their experience can teach them something of their "internal geography": how they can learn to "read the map," seeing the connections among their thoughts, feelings, body sensations, and behavior. The difficulties reported in class are welcomed as a possible guide to what normally causes moods to deteriorate or prevents attention from being focused or quiet. By asking questions such as "What are you noticing about the feeling right now?", the discussion is grounded in moment-to-moment experience.

Summary of Intentions for the Breath Meditation

- Brings you back to this very moment—the *here and now*.
- Is always available as an anchor and *haven*, no matter where you are.
- Can actually change your experience by connecting you with a wider space and broader perspective from which to view things.

Mind Wandering

"It's really annoying sometimes. I find that I want my mind to stay in one place, but it just seems to go off and do what it wants to anyway."

To describe the sitting meditation as spending 30–40 minutes with the focus of attention on the breath and body is somewhat misleading. Most people at this stage in the program spend a good deal of time struggling to maintain their attentional focus as it is pulled off the breath by thoughts, feelings, body sensations, or external distractions.

An essential characteristic of this practice is that the aim is not to prevent mind wandering but to become more intimate with its patterns. One important practice in the early stages is systematically and repeatedly to bring the attention back from wherever it may have wandered to the primary object of the meditation. In this way, the practice always gives us the chance to begin again, in this moment, with this breath. A common instruction is "If your mind wanders a hundred times, then simply bring it back a hundred times." This is what the practice is all about. The task is to accept those times when our minds have wandered and *gently* reconnect with our breathing. This allows us to sidestep the judgments and criticisms that may arise from believing that we are failing at it or not doing well enough at keeping our attention locked on the breath. Becoming aware of "struggling to maintain awareness on the breath" is itself helpful. At this stage in the program, such struggling is seen as simply another feeling to become aware of, before gently bringing attention back to the breath. This is a reminder for instructors as well: that one of the central intentions during the first half of the program is to train the skill of deliberate focus of attention. One implication of this is that, whatever comes up, the predominant instruction is to notice and acknowledge what the attention has wandered to (including any *reactions* to this experience), then to bring the mind back to whatever had been its intended focus (sights or sounds, breath or body).

Being Curious* about Where the Mind Wanders to

Note in the earlier quotation the expression of a strong desire for a particular outcome. The person wants the mind to be a certain way, and it doesn't happen. Instead, our thoughts are rather more like monkeys running through trees; they are sort of "all over the place." We become aware of how the mind may have "jumped into some other tree" as soon as we can, then we gently bring our attention back. This is how we come to develop a sense of intimacy with our mind states. It is much more flexible than wanting them to be a certain way. Instead, we just watch the mind as it moves. To bring a spirit of kindly interest or curiosity to what is happening is helpful because it is obviously quite easy for us to get impatient and frustrated with ourselves.

Dealing with Thoughts by Trying to Control Them

"I don't know if anybody else has this problem. When my mind is completely going, I have been thinking of a thousand and one other things. It's very difficult to stop myself going into the future, thinking about things. I try to control it and maybe it works for 2 minutes but then I go off again."

*By the word *curious*, we mean an attitude of alert interest or wise attention. This is, of course, different from the more obsessive "picking over" a problem or intellectually "thinking *about*" a problem. We note that the word *curious* originates in the term "to care for," as in "curator."

Note how easily participants mishear the instructions for the practice. Look again at what has been said. "It's very difficult to *stop* myself. . . . I try to *control* it . . . maybe it *works* for 2 minutes but then. . . . " This approach is not about trying to suppress or control thoughts. If we were to try and push them away or squash them down, then they would be more likely to bounce back even more strongly. The practice involves developing a gentle, skillful way of simply becoming aware, of being able to recognize that "Here is thinking," and as best one can, let go of the thinking and focus back on the breath. It's not so much trying to control our thoughts as actually feeling comfortable with letting things be as they are, then returning to the breath.

Sensations of Physical Discomfort

"I find that if I sit for too long, my legs start to fall asleep and my back aches. I don't really want to move because, I guess, it would disturb my concentration, but it gets too painful not to."

Physical discomfort is actually a good target on which to practice these developing skills because it can be so easily located in the field of awareness and is a strong sensation to bring to awareness. Obviously, the natural reaction to such discomfort is to tense or brace and push it away. Simply becoming aware of the tendency to tense up, and bringing as best we can a friendly interest to it, and exploring it gently, provides a very useful practice. In this case, if the mind is pulled away to intense sensations, this is noted, and attention is returned to the breath, using the breath as an anchor to which to return again and again.

Another possibility is to bring awareness to the sensation of discomfort itself. This requires a level of skill in sustaining nonreactive attention that may not be available to all participants at this stage of the program, and we remind participants that it is always open to them to shift their posture to ease discomfort, noticing the intention to move, the movement itself, and the aftereffects of it. For those who wish to bring awareness to the intensity, the instruction is to focus directly on the discomfort and pain (points 6 and 7 of Box 10.2). Later in the program, participants will have the opportunity to learn further how to focus on the difficult and unwanted.

HOME PRACTICE

After exploring the within-session practice, the instructor asks about the home practice. Many participants for one reason or another feel that they have not done what they intended to do. They may not have practiced for 6 out of 7 days, or, if they have, their experiences were not as they hoped. They hoped that these practices might make them feel better, yet they may feel worse. How on earth could this help if it makes them worse?

The instructor is helped by knowing that these difficulties are just what is expected, indeed may be *needed*, for mindfulness to bring about the reduction of risk in depression. These are the mind states arising within the laboratory of the practice that have unknowingly created and maintained the very vulnerability we are seeking to address. The challenge is to be aware of this, and to meet the mind states with a different stance, so they may be held in a more spacious, compassionate awareness.

"I Haven't Got the Time": Recognizing the Judging Mind

This is one of the most common themes, so it is worth exploring in some detail. Here is one participant's comment:

P1: What's wrong with me? Why can't I find the time to practice the meditation?

We see here the link between the difficulty in finding time to practice and the immediate "judging mind" that pops up: "What's wrong with me?" Our task as instructors is not to try to answer the question "What's wrong?" or to provide reassurance, but rather to explore the participants' experience in a way that helps them to see that this wish to find out "what's wrong?" is the mind doing the best it can, but it is using a problem-solving approach that does not work well in this situation. This is explored further in the next dialogue.

P2: I've got all the time in the world, really, to do it, but I only need one noise, and that takes it away instantly.

Note how this person believes that there is something she "has" that can be "taken away." The instructor asks for more information:

I: What happens when the noise comes?

The open-ended question is important. Notice that the instructor has *not* responded to the initially presented issue of being distracted by noise. It might have been possible—and sometimes this would be appropriate—to give the participant instructions on how to deal with distractions—to note them, then return to mindfulness of hearing. Instead, the open-ended question allows the participant to say a little more. And this reveals that behind the frustration with being distracted by noise is another thought:

P2: I think that I am letting you down, and I know it sounds stupid, but . . . well, I feel that I'm not really contributing like I should.

We can see here the machinery of rumination clanking into action. A noise occurs. It distracts. There is frustration at "losing it," rapidly followed by another thought about letting the instructor down because the participant is not contributing as she should. How does she deal with this negative thought? By telling herself that she sounds stupid! Here is rumination laid bare: a thought–affect spiral with escalating attempts to deal with a negative thought by criticizing the self for having it. The instructor decides to stay with this for a moment:

I: Let's stay on this, if you don't mind, because it's really important: this business about letting me down and not doing it properly, and having a whole set of expectations about what should be going on here. Now this is absolutely the target that we need to look at because our aim here is simply, as best we can, to relate to what is there. The job you have is not to achieve a particular standard, but to be aware, if you like, of the thoughts such as "I have got to do well," " I am letting him down," and so on. As best you can, say "Ah, there go those 'standards' again." As best you can, see them as judgments. It's very easy just to get sucked into those things and not see them for what they are. They are just things in the mind.

P2: I find that I just talk to myself. "Here I go again," you know?

I: So it's ever so easy to get sucked in.

Staying with one person's experience enables other participants to see connections with their own experience. The transcript of the session shows a succession of participants building on the experience of this person:

P3: I'm pleased because it has worried me.

P1: Unless there is absolutely peace and quiet, I can't do it. I've only done the practice once.

Once again, there turn out to be more negative thoughts lurking just in the background. It is not simply the difficulty; it is the self-criticism that comes along with the difficulty that really seems to bring the person's mood down. This highlights an important principle in the work of teaching mindfulness: It is most often the *reaction* to an experience, not the experience itself, that creates extra problems for us.

The participant who spoke first now adds her comments to what's been said.

P1: I am ashamed to have missed it, and I didn't want to come tonight. I failed this week.

We can see clearly here that once rumination starts, it does not stop with mild self-criticism about the practice but escalates rapidly, until it connects with a theme that may have been very familiar to the person for some time:

P1: I think to myself, "I only work. I haven't got a family, I haven't really got a busy life. What's wrong with me? Why can't I fit in?"

At one time, we would have felt drawn into using standard cognitive therapy techniques at this point. This would have involved asking more about the effect of such a thought on mood, and other situations in which the thought occurs. We might then have done some thought answering:

investigating why it might be true that she did not fit in, and why it might be false. We would have worked on some home practice tasks that might have given more evidence for and against the idea that she did not fit in.

But what if, instead, we encouraged people simply to label these thoughts as "judgment" and then, as best they could, return to the focus on the breath? This is what the instructor did in this case:

> "OK. Well, as best you can, just notice this as judgment, and just let it go. It comes from somewhere, and it's no friend of yours, but you know, just treat it as kindly as you can. 'Oh, hello, Mr. Judgment. Here you are again. Have a nice day!' And, as best you can, just bring your mind back to where you intended it to be."

It turns out that using the practice to learn how to relate differently to negative thoughts proves to be one of the most helpful aspects of MBCT.

The challenge in all this work is learning how to observe our experience in a friendly way rather than identifying with it, resisting it, or rejecting it. As we have seen, one way to approach negative automatic thoughts is just to notice them as best we can, label them as "judgment," and simply let them go. The really difficult thing is simply to notice them, without criticizing oneself for having them. The thought, "I wish I did not have these thoughts about so-and-so," too easily turns into "I ought to be over this by now. I must be such a weak and immature person." The aim here is not to try and block them out. Instead, we practice being with them in a different way and letting go of the need to engage with them, answer them back, or reassure ourselves through denying their validity. We can be here, and so can our thoughts, but this does not mean we must be tied up with them in our accustomed ways. Being more aware of how our attention moves around is an important ally in this process.

WHEN STRONG EMOTIONS ARISE

"I often find myself identifying with my emotions, believing that they define my experience. Then I feel trapped and hopeless. How can I work with these feelings?"

How can we hold a strong emotion in awareness without it becoming overwhelming? One way is to acknowledge its presence and its power, to note it by saying to oneself, "Ah, the emotion of anger is here" rather than "I am really fed up with her for talking to me that way," or "Here is the emotion of fear" rather than "I'm terrified of making a mess of this presentation." Notice the language here: noting inwardly "the *emotion* of anger" and "the *emotion* of fear" underlies the disidentification one is seeking and underlines that one is not simply "noticing I am angry."

This allows us to be with the emotion in a way that does not require us to identify with it completely. In time, we also learn that the feeling itself may constantly be changing shape; it can become stronger or lose intensity over short intervals. We might picture the mind as being like a vast, clear sky. All our feelings, thoughts, and sensations are like the weather that passes through, without affecting the nature of the sky itself. The clouds, winds, snow, and rainbows come and go, but the sky is always simply itself, as it were, a "container" for these passing phenomena. We practice to let our minds be that sky, and to let all these mental and physical phenomena arise and vanish like the changing weather. In this way, our minds can remain balanced and centered, without getting swept away in the drama of every passing storm.

FEEDBACK FROM
THE PLEASANT EXPERIENCES CALENDAR

A common theme to emerge from the previous comments is the difficulty in dealing with negative thoughts, feelings, and body sensations. Of course, it is rare that people even make the distinction between these three aspects of mind–body phenomena. In order to make the distinctions, it is helpful to use the feedback on the Pleasant Experiences Calendar, which gives participants the chance to reflect with each other on what happened when they tried to record such moments, and to record exactly the thoughts, feelings, and body sensations that occurred in the moments they describe. We find it is helpful to use a whiteboard to record responses to this exercise, distinguishing between (and listing separately) the different elements that emerge: Was that a thought or a body sensation or a feeling?

What is the intention here? One thing that often emerges first is how apparently trivial moments often contain elements and dimensions of which we are not aware, and that these can be more positive than we might have imagined. Day by day, and moment by moment, we sell ourselves short, taking for granted what we are experiencing. One participant said:

> "Yesterday evening I was with my two young daughters, who were playfully heaping as many sofa cushions on my head as they could while I sat desperately trying to read a paper for work. I managed to muster a smile at their persistence, but in my failure to concentrate on the paper, I found my mind constantly jumping from one thing to the next. This is usually my trigger to have a Mindful moment, so I refocused and gave myself fully to being with my two girls. The next 5 minutes were the most rewarding and most meaningful 5 minutes of being a parent that I can recall for a good several weeks."

The second intention for the pleasant experiences exercise is to experience firsthand the distinctions between thoughts, emotions, and body sensations. This comes as a revelation to many. Such distinctions are so evident to psychologists and other health professionals that it is easy to overlook how they are not readily part of everyday experience. Yet once there is an awareness that experience can be "parsed" into these elements, it is easier to see thoughts *as* thoughts, feelings *as* feelings, and body sensations *as* body sensations. Why is this important? Because it is easier to decenter from mind states when they are seen as *bundles* of separable elements that normally come bound together as an indistinguishable "blob."

Third, the exercise reveals that some people find it particularly difficult to become aware of subtle body sensations. The discovery that the body is sending signals to the brain all the time, signals that are generally ignored most of the time, is hugely important. Why? First, because these body sensations can be used to recognize subtle changes in emotion. Second, because it encourages people to see that there is an alternative to being lost "in the head." Here is a place where we can see things directly rather than through a veil of words. These are some of the reasons why the "body sensations" are recorded in the first column.

GENERALIZING THE PRACTICE:
THE 3-MINUTE BREATHING SPACE

It is not unusual for people who are coping with the demands of developing a formal meditative practice to forget about the need to incorporate
this practice into their daily lives. Some "generalization practice" is important to link what is being learned to a larger range of different situations.
Generalizing what is learned in formal practice is not easy. Of course, we
have already given instructions on how to bring mindfulness to the performance of a routine activity (e.g., brushing teeth, feeding the cat, taking
out the garbage). But we need to go further and bring small parts of the
formal practice into daily life. We have developed a "minimeditation" for
this purpose: the 3-minute breathing space.

The exercise is influenced by cognitive therapy practice, in that it is
very explicit and structured, focusing on how to bring mindfulness into
everyday life. First, we program the breathing space to occur three times
a day at set times. Then we ask people to use it not only at the preprogrammed times but also when they feel they need it; for example, if they
feel stressed (introduced in Session 4). For many participants, the 3-min-
ute breathing space will become an important vehicle for bringing formal
meditation practice into daily life and, by the end of the course, allow
them to deal with problems directly as they are developing (or before they
develop). They also find that it is a way to pause, even in the midst of a
hectic day, and reestablish contact with the present moment. Here in Session 3, we lay the groundwork for this essential "anchor point."

There are three basic steps to the exercise. The first involves stepping
out of automatic pilot to ask, "Where am I? What's going on?" The aim
here is to recognize and acknowledge one's experience at the moment. The
second step involves bringing the attention to the breath, gathering the
scattered mind to focus on this single object—the breath. The third step
is to expand the attention to include a sense of the breath and the body as
a whole (see Box 10.3).

After the practice, participants give feedback. Sometimes such feedback continues themes brought up earlier in the class. Other times, however, new themes come up. The following is an example in which the
theme of length versus brevity came up:

BOX 10.3

Breathing Space: Example of How to Introduce It in Class

"We are going to do a brief meditation now—it is called the 3-minute breathing space. The first thing we do with this practice, because it's brief and we want to come into the moment quickly, is to take a very definite posture . . . relaxed, dignified, back erect but not stiff, letting our bodies express a sense of being present and awake.

"Now, closing your eyes, if that feels comfortable for you, the first step is being aware, really aware, of what is going on with you right now. Becoming aware of what is going through your mind; what thoughts are around? Here, again, as best you can, just noting the thoughts as mental events. . . . So we note them, and then we note the feelings that are around at the moment . . . in particular, turning toward any sense of discomfort or unpleasant feelings. So rather than try to push them away or shut them out, just acknowledge them, perhaps saying, 'Ah, here you are, that's how it is right now.' And similarly with sensations in the body. . . . Are there sensations of tension, of holding, or whatever? And again, awareness of them, simply noting them. OK, that's how it is right now.

"So, we've got a sense of what is going on right now. We've stepped out of automatic pilot. The second step is to collect our awareness by focusing on a single object—the movements of the breath. So now we really gather ourselves, focusing attention in the movements of the abdomen, the rise and fall of the breath . . . spending a minute or so to focus on the movement of the abdominal wall . . . moment by moment, breath by breath, as best we can. So that you know when the breath is moving in, and you know when the breath is moving out. Just binding your awareness to the pattern of movement down there . . . gathering yourself, using the anchor of the breath to really be present.

"And now as a third step, having gathered ourselves to some extent, we allow our awareness to expand. As well as being aware of the breath, we also include a sense of the body as a whole. So that we get this more spacious awareness. . . . A sense of the body as a whole, including any tightness or sensations related to holding in the shoulders, neck, back, or face . . . following the breath as if your whole body is breathing. Holding it all in this slightly softer . . . more spacious awareness.

"And then, when you are ready, just allowing your eyes to open.

"Any questions or comments about that?"

P: My attention wandered, not at the beginning, but about 15 seconds after I was into it. And then I got it together again. Is that because you're aware that it's going to be short?

I: It may be. The idea of being aware for a single breath seems doable; the idea of being aware of your breath for half an hour seems an enormous task. But in reality, you know, you can simply take it breath by breath. It's like having an enormous pile of logs in front of you that you have to move. If you contemplate the whole pile, your heart sinks and your energy fails. But you know if you could just focus on the one you've got to do now, give your full attention to that, then take the next one, then it becomes doable.

Notice how this can link with the sense many of us have that we often exhaust ourselves by anticipating all the things we have got to do, not just for this day, but for the rest of the week and the next month. We carry a burden that doesn't need to be carried. Tuning in just to this moment, and to what is before us right now, allows the energy to come through, to complete just this moment's task.

Scheduling another formal practice in a day, even one as short as 3 minutes, will not happen automatically. The class members are therefore given some time to break up into pairs to discuss how they plan to arrange for three occasions each day to practice the 3-minute breathing space over the coming week.

THE BODY AS A WINDOW ON THE MIND

Many participants report that their practice is sometimes dominated by a struggle to maintain balance in the face of negative ruminations. In time, of course, the aim is to find a way of relating differently to such rumination. Disengaging attention from such habitual patterns of the mind in a way that does not simply suppress or shut them out is subtle and can take a lot of practice. We emphasize that if people find they tend to engage in a battle between one thought ("Why did she say that?") and another ("That's a stupid thought"), then they always have the option of paying attention to how the thoughts and feelings affect their bodies. Bodily awareness helps us sample a different "mode" of being. Bringing awareness to a sensation in the body changes the nature of the emotional experience and gives us more choice about how to respond to what is here now. If we are aware of reacting to something emotionally, then the body may tell us our relationship to these feelings.

Paying attention to the body provides another "place" from which to view things, a different vantage point for relating to thoughts. If we want to get a perspective on our thoughts and feelings, if we can actually "be in" our bodies, then we've got a different place from which to stand and look at the thoughts and feelings, rather than just in our heads. Finally, as we observed in Session 1, the body is often part of the feedback loop that maintains depressed mood (e.g., muscle tension keeps us locked in the loop of anxiety; a wilting posture keeps us in the loop of depression). Intentionally bringing awareness to the body can have two additional effects. First, paying attention to sensations of which we may not have been aware can change the experience of these sensations themselves, just as with the experience of mindfully eating the raisin in Session 1. Second, bringing awareness to the body allows people to choose to alter one of the components of the "mode of mind" that is keeping them locked into an emotional state—by intentionally altering their posture or facial expression.

MINDFUL MOVEMENT

In the first 2 weeks, the body scan has been used to help people become more aware of body sensations. The formal practice of sitting meditation also involves becoming aware of body states. However, many people find it easier to focus on the body if it is doing something: stretching or walking. We therefore assign both breath- and body-based mindfulness practice as home practice following Session 3, varying the day-to-day tasks by combining a short mindful stretching exercise (10 minutes), followed by a formal sitting meditation (for 30 minutes) one day of the week, and, on alternate days, use a longer mindful movement practice based on yoga (for 40 minutes) as the formal meditation practice.

We practice the 10-minute series of stretches in the class.* Even within this short practice, a number of issues arise. First, such practice makes it easy to notice contrasts. For example, the effort required to hold a posture and the release associated with returning to a neutral stance is substantial. Similarly, the tension in the muscles used in raising up the arms and the relaxation that comes from bringing the arms back down to one's sides is significant. The task is simply to pay attention to these contrasts and notice the sensations associated with each phase of the prescribed movements. Practicing this in class also gives us an opportunity to remind people to monitor the attitude with which they do the practices. This itself becomes a discovery for some people:

P: The advice is to focus our attention on the muscles and the feeling as we're doing them, isn't it?

I: Yes, I'm glad you raised that because the point of this is, of course, not physical strengthening. It's just another opportunity to become aware of the body, only it's a bit easier because the body is moving. . . . The spirit in which you do it is important. That's why the guidance will say to do it slowly and attend to the particular sensations that you are focusing on. . . . And with the 45-minute mindful movement, be careful if you have any problems with your back. Be ever so gentle with that. As it says, honor the messages from your body. . . . It's a wonderful opportunity for letting go of standards. It is easy to start imposing standards on yourself and making it torture. Instead, it's that spirit of just doing it lightly rather than making it a performance.

This response illustrates the theme of striking the right balance between just how much effort to put into a stretch, and how much to hold back so as to avoid injuring oneself. We emphasize that the idea is not to hold a posture until it is painful. It is rather to move into and back from the point at which one is aware of these strong sensations, while keeping

---

*For some MBCT programs, such as that developed in Oxford for suicidal patients, 30–40 minutes of the longer mindful movement based on yoga is used as the first formal practice in Session 3, and the shorter standing stretches—followed by a short sitting—is used later in the session. The theme of the session remains that of anchoring the mind in the present moment, using the body and breath as allies.

BOX 10.4

Mindful Stretching

1. First, stand in your bare feet or socks with feet about a hip's width apart, with the knees unlocked so that the legs can bend slightly and with the feet parallel (it's actually unusual to stand with the feet like this, and this, itself, can generate some novel body sensations).

2. Next remind yourself of the intention of this practice: to become aware, as best you can, of physical sensations and feelings throughout the body as you engage in a series of gentle stretches, honoring and investigating the limitations of your body in every moment as best you can, letting go of any tendency to push beyond your limits or to compete with either yourself or others.

3. Then, on an inbreath, slowly and mindfully raise your arms out to the sides, parallel to the floor, and then, after breathing out, continue on the next inbreath raising them, slowly and mindfully until your hands meet above your heads, all the while perhaps feeling the tension in the muscles as they work to lift the arms and then maintain them in the stretch.

4. Then, letting your breath move in and out freely at its own pace, continue to stretch upward, the fingertips gently pushing toward the sky, the feet firmly grounded on the floor, as you feel the stretch in the muscles and joints of the body all the way from the feet and legs up through the back, shoulders, into the arms and hands and fingers.

5. Maintain that stretch for a time, breathing freely in and out, noticing any changes in the sensations and feelings in the body with the breath and as you continue to hold the stretch. Of course, this might include a sense of increasing tension or discomfort, and if so, opening to that as well.

6. At a certain point, when you are ready, slowly, very slowly, on an outbreath, allow the arms to come back down. Lower them slowly, with the wrists bent so that the fingers point upward and the palms are pushing outward (again, an unusual position) until the arms come back to rest along the sides, hanging from the shoulders.

(cont.)

7. Allow the eyes to close gently and focus attention on the movements of the breath and the sensations and feelings throughout the body as you stand here, perhaps noticing the contrast in the physical sense of release (and often relief) associated with returning to a neutral stance.

8. Continue now by mindfully stretching each arm and hand up in turn, as if picking from a tree fruit that is just out of reach, with full awareness of the sensations throughout the body, and of the breath; see what happens to the extension of the hand and to the breath if you lift the opposite heel off the floor while stretching up.

9. After this sequence, slowly and mindfully raise both arms up high, keeping them parallel to each other, then allow the body to bend over as a whole to the left, forming a big curve that extends sideways from the feet right through the torso, the arms, and the hands and fingers. Then come back to standing on an inbreath, and then on an outbreath, slowly bend over, forming a curve in the opposite direction.

10. Once you have returned to standing in a neutral position with the arms alongside the body, you can play with rolling the shoulders while letting the arms dangle passively, first raising the shoulders upward toward the ears as far as they will go, then backward, as if attempting to draw the shoulder blades together, then letting them drop down completely, then squeezing the shoulders together in front of the body as far as they will go, as if trying to touch them together with the arms passive and dangling, Continue "rolling" through these various positions as smoothly and mindfully as you can, with the arms dangling all the while, first in one direction, then in the opposite direction, in a forward and backward "rowing" motion.

11. Then, once you have rested in a neutral standing posture again, play with slowly and mindfully rolling the head around to whatever degree you feel comfortable, and very gently, as if drawing a circle with the nose in midair, allow the circling to move gently in one direction and then the other.

12. And finally, at the end of this sequence of movements, remain still for a while in a standing posture, and tune in to the sensations from the body before moving to a sitting meditation.

attention on the sensations themselves, as best one can. This links back to the main theme of this session of noticing when discrepancy-based processing is arising, those times when we find ourselves striving to achieve some goal and end up desperately trying to create the future we want rather than allow the present we have.

Noticing the sensations themselves, such as burning, trembling, or shaking, the task is to breathe with or into the sensations, letting the thoughts—about what it means to feel these things—just come and go in awareness. It is not unlike the sitting meditation, where we escort our attention back to the breath, but in this case, we focus on sensation and let go of whatever else is there. The skill built by doing this with physical sensations comes into play later in the program, when a similar approach is used for mindfully moving into and out of painful emotions.

Participants discover that they derive a number of benefits from doing this work. First, the physical sensations associated with stretching, pulling, holding, balancing, and other demands enable some people to learn more about their bodies. Second, many participants discover that their bodies become more supple and responsive to day-to-day demands placed upon them, even though they have not set this as a goal. Third, the work allows some to learn to distinguish sensations in one part of the body from those in other parts of the body. The result is that even if they feel tension, such sensations are more likely to be confined to a single area rather than spreading throughout the body.

Finally, through mindful movement, we come to realize the difference between stretching and striving. Respecting the boundaries of what is possible in movement teaches us to do so in everyday life, where there is a similar need to be aware of how we might harm ourselves in the rush to meet deadlines and reach goals. For when we unwittingly strive without awareness, we can overstretch and exceed our limits more than is healthy for us.

Summary of Intentions for Mindful Movement

- Build on the foundation of the body scan in learning how we can bring awareness to and "inhabit" body experience/sensation.
- See old habitual patterns of the mind—especially those that emphasize *striving*.

- Work with physical boundaries and intensity, and learn to accept our limits.
- Learn new ways of taking care of ourselves.

SETTING UP
THE UNPLEASANT EXPERIENCES CALENDAR

The theme of being present in the moment will be picked up again when people complete the Unpleasant Experiences Calendar as home practice during the week following Session 3. The task is similar to last week's task of noticing pleasant events. Here, however, participants notice as clearly as possible the thoughts, feelings, and body sensations associated with *un*pleasantness.

In teaching MBCT classes, we have become increasingly aware of how important this home practice is, for no matter how fleeting or momentary the experience in question, a person's reaction to an unpleasant experience can powerfully determine what happens next: whether the mood deteriorates in a cascade of emotional reactivity or the unpleasant moment is seen more clearly for what it is and held in awareness despite what it is, without the mind adding extra. Of course, some situations may be long-lasting and intense, but the task remains to notice the different aspects of the experience as it is unfolding. This is helped if participants can record such experiences in detail, and as soon as possible, afterward.

When discussing the introduction to the Pleasant Experiences Calendar in Session 2, we saw that focusing on body sensations allows people to identify an important signature of their emotion. In the Unpleasant Experiences Calendar (Session 3–Handout 5), we focus on recognizing two elements: the *unpleasant feelings* themselves and any *reaction* to unpleasantness. This is what is important, for it is here that "aversion" starts to reveal itself. We are exploring the heart of what causes repeated relapses into depression: looking more closely at the very start of the tendency to avoid or push away anything that we do not like. (It is something to which we return in Sessions 4 and 5.) But to see this tendency clearly, we need to identify the conditions out of which such reactions occur—the (sometimes very subtle) sense of "unpleasantness." So the question to focus on with unpleasant events (and this may help to set up the exercise) is: "What is the weather pattern in body and mind when unpleasantness occurs, and what *reactions* to this weather do I notice?"

Gradually, in many various ways, a deeper message is communicated through these practices: that bringing awareness to each situation, especially those in which we label things as good or bad, is the first step in learning to relate differently to them. This takes some courage and much practice. People can become discouraged because nothing seems to be happening. But despite the early skepticism that we ourselves felt when first using this approach, evidence from the classes we have taught has shown us that staying with the practice, rather than rushing for solutions, is justified. The picture that is traditionally used is the bucket put underneath a slowly dripping tap. If you stare at the bucket, it is difficult to see any change at all in how full it is, but it nevertheless fills up. Our experience has been that when people are able to set aside their goals and simply practice day by day, they start to notice unexpected changes. They discover, little by little, that the old way—tackling their moods by ruminating about them—might not be the only way, that the old way—running their lives by shouting at themselves—might be able to give way to a gentler way of living their lives.

Summary of Session 3:
Gathering the Scattered Mind

This week we practiced resting awareness on the breath and the body in movement. The mind is often scattered and lost in thought because it is working away in the background to complete unfinished tasks from the past and strive for goals for the future. We need to find a reliable way intentionally to "come back" to the here and now. The breath and body offer an ever-present focus on which we can reconnect with mindful presence, gather and settle the mind, and ease ourselves from doing into being.

Focusing on the breath:

- Brings you back to this very moment—the *here and now*.

- Is always available as an anchor and *haven*, no matter where you are.

- Can actually change your experience by connecting you with a wider space and broader perspective from which to view things.

SITTING MEDITATION: BASICS

It helps to adopt an erect and dignified posture, with your head, neck, and back aligned vertically—the physical counterpart of the inner attitudes of self-reliance, self-acceptance, patience, and alert attention that we are cultivating.

Practice on a chair or on the floor. If you use a chair, choose one that has a straight back and allows your feet to be flat on the floor. If at all possible, sit away from the back of the chair so that your spine is self-supporting.

If you choose to sit on the floor, do so on a firm, thick cushion (or a pillow folded over once or twice), which raises your buttocks off the floor 3–6 inches. Whatever you are sitting on, see if it possible to sit so that your hips are slightly higher than your knees.

Mindful movement allows us to:

- Build on the foundation of the body scan in learning how we can bring awareness to and "inhabit" body experience/sensation.

- See old habitual patterns of the mind—especially those that emphasize *striving*.

(cont.)

- Work with physical boundaries and intensity and learn acceptance of our limits.
- Learn new ways of taking care of ourselves.

The movements provide a direct way to connect with awareness of the body. The body is a place where emotions are often expressed, under the surface and without our awareness. So becoming more aware of the body gives us an additional place from which to stand and look at our thoughts.

The 3-Minute Breathing Space: Basic Instructions

STEP 1. BECOMING AWARE

Become more aware of how things are in this moment by deliberately adopting an erect and dignified posture, whether sitting or standing. If possible, close your eyes. Then, bringing your awareness to your inner experience and acknowledging it, ask, "What is my experience **right now**?"

- What **THOUGHTS** are going through the mind? As best you can, acknowledge thoughts as mental events, perhaps putting them into words.
- What **FEELINGS** are here? Turn toward any sense of discomfort or unpleasant feelings, acknowledging them.
- What **BODY SENSATIONS** are here right now? Perhaps quickly scan the body to pick up any sensations of tightness or bracing, acknowledging the sensations.

STEP 2. GATHERING

Then redirect your attention to focus on the physical sensations of the breathing itself. Move in close to the sense of the breath in the abdomen . . . feeling the sensations of the abdomen wall expanding as the breath comes in . . . and falling back as the breath goes out. Follow the breath all the way in and all the way out, using the breathing to anchor yourself into the present.

STEP 3. EXPANDING

Now expand the field of your awareness around the breathing so that it includes a sense of the body as a whole, your posture, and facial expression.

If you become aware of any sensations of discomfort, tension, or resistance, take your awareness there by breathing into them on the inbreath. Then breathe out from those sensations, softening and opening with the outbreath.

As best you can, bring this expanded awareness to the next moments of your day.

Home Practice for the Week Following Session 3

This week we are going to use three different formal practices:

1. *On Days 1, 3, and 5*, use the combined Stretch and Breath meditation (audio track 6) and record your reactions on the Home Practice Record Form. This meditation combines a few minutes of gentle stretching exercises and instructions for mindfulness of the breath and body.

2. *On Days 2, 4, and 6*, use the Mindful Movement meditation (audio track 5) and record your reactions on the Home Practice Record Form. **If you have any back or other health difficulties that may cause problems, make your own decision as to which (if any) of these exercises to do, and consult your physician or physical therapist if you are unsure.**

3. *Every day:* Practice using the 3-Minute Breathing Space (using the audio version, track 8, at least once a day) three times a day, at set times that you have decided in advance, and record each time by circling an R on the Home Practice Record Form.

4. *Every day:* Complete the Unpleasant Experiences Calendar (one entry per day). Use this as an opportunity to become really aware of the thoughts, feelings, and body sensations in one unpleasant event each day, *at the time that they are occurring*. Notice and record, as soon as you can, in detail (e.g., put the actual words or images in which thoughts came, and the precise nature and location of body sensations). **What are the unpleasant events that "pull you off center" or "get you down" (no matter how big or small)?**

Home Practice Record Form—Session 3

Name: _____

Record on the Home Practice Record Form each time you practice. Also, make a note of anything that comes up in the home practice, so that we can talk about it at the next meeting.

Day/date	Practice (Yes/No)	Comments
Wednesday Date: _____	Stretch and Breath Mindful Movement R R R	
Thursday Date: _____	Stretch and Breath Mindful Movement R R R	
Friday Date: _____	Stretch and Breath Mindful Movement R R R	
Saturday Date: _____	Stretch and Breath Mindful Movement R R R	
Sunday Date: _____	Stretch and Breath Mindful Movement R R R	
Monday Date: _____	Stretch and Breath Mindful Movement R R R	
Tuesday Date: _____	Stretch and Breath Mindful Movement R R R	
Wednesday Date: _____	Stretch and Breath Mindful Movement R R R	

R, 3-Minute Breathing Space—Regular Version

Unpleasant Experiences Calendar

Name: _____

Be aware of an unpleasant experience *at the time it is happening*. Use these questions to focus your awareness on the details of it as it is happening. Write it down later.

Day	What was the experience?	How did your body feel, in detail, during this experience?	What moods and feelings accompanied this event?	What thoughts accompanied this event?	What thoughts are in your mind now as you write this down?
	Example: Waiting for the cable company to come out and fix our line. Realize that I am missing an important meeting at work.	Temples throbbing, tightness in my neck and shoulders, pacing back and forth.	Angry, helpless.	"Is this what they mean by service?" "They don't have to be responsible, they have a monopoly." "This is one meeting I didn't want to miss."	"I hope I don't have to go through that again soon."

(cont.)

Day	What was the experience?	How did your body feel, in detail, during this experience?	What moods and feelings accompanied this event?	What thoughts accompanied this event?	What thoughts are in your mind now as you write this down?
Monday					
Tuesday					
Wednesday					

(cont.)

Day	What was the experience?	How did your body feel, in detail, during this experience?	What moods and feelings accompanied this event?	What thoughts accompanied this event?	What thoughts are in your mind now as you write this down?
Thursday					
Friday					
Saturday					
Sunday					

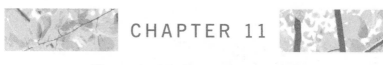

CHAPTER 11

Recognizing Aversion

Session 4

People who have been depressed in the past often spend a great deal of time and energy making comparisons. Perhaps today I feel a little better than yesterday, but am I still feeling worse than last week? Did that person's frown mean he or she feels differently about me? Has he or she lost patience with me? Such people have often suffered many losses and disappointments, together with the sense of rejection and worthlessness that often comes from such events. Long afterwards, mood may remain easily upset by reminders of these bad times. Even when depression is gone, people can feel cheated of the years that the depression has taken out of their lives: "Why didn't my doctor diagnose me earlier?" or "I have lost the best years of my life!" There is a natural tendency to return to the past and sigh, "If only."

Mindfulness approaches are not about thought control or substituting positive for negative images of the past, present, or future. Rather, they offer ways for people to allow these feelings of disappointment and regret to be here. This is very different from how we commonly react to difficult or painful experiences, which is to find a way to get rid of them. We frequently use distraction and denial to shut out painful feelings. On the other hand, when we worry or ruminate about our problems, although we may seem to be addressing the difficulty, such rumination actually takes us further away from a direct sense of what the difficulty is. This happens because rumination involves a judgment about the experience: "I don't want to feel like this." This "not wanting" is like a locknut, holding

BOX 11.1
Theme and Curriculum for Session 4

THEME

The skill of "coming back" needs to be complemented by seeing more clearly what "takes us away" into doing, rumination, mind wandering, and worry. We begin the experiential investigation of "*aversion*," the mind's habitual reaction to unpleasant feelings and sensations, driven by the need not to have these experiences, which is at the root of emotional suffering. Mindfulness offers a way of staying present by giving another way to view things: It helps us take a wider perspective and relate differently to experience.

AGENDA

- 5-minute "seeing" or "hearing" exercise.
- 30- to 40-minute sitting meditation—awareness of breath, body, sounds, then thoughts and choiceless awareness (reading a poem such as "Wild Geese").
- Practice review.
- Home practice review (including sitting meditation/yoga, Unpleasant Experiences Calendar, and 3-minute breathing space).
- Defining the "territory" of depression: Automatic Thoughts Questionnaire and diagnostic criteria for depression.
- 3-minute breathing space + review.
- Mindful walking
- Distribute Session 4 participant handouts.
- Home Practice assignment:
  o Sitting meditation, 6 out of 7 days.
  o 3-Minute Breathing Space—Regular (three times a day).
  o 3-Minute Breathing Space—Responsive (whenever you notice unpleasant feelings).

(cont.)

PERSONAL PREPARATION AND PLANNING

In addition to your personal preparation, remember to read the poem "Wild Geese."

PARTICIPANT HANDOUTS FOR SESSION 4

Session 4–Handout 1. Summary of Session 4: Recognizing Aversion

Session 4–Handout 2. Mindful Walking

Session 4–Handout 3. Home Practice for the Week Following Session 4

Session 4–Handout 4. Home Practice Record Form—Session 4

Session 4–Handout 5. Staying Present

---

in place a mode that is dominated by concept-based thinking—*thinking about* the feelings rather than directly experiencing them. Such ruminative thinking then creates more highly charged feelings, adding further negative thoughts: "My parents never talked about it to me. Nobody ever talked about it to me." These thoughts are, in turn, "not wanted" either. With time, it becomes difficult to separate the raw experience from the judgments about it, and the feeling that the most intimate parts of the self are "rotten to the core."

These reactions, in which avoidance and preoccupation are locked together, arise from a natural desire for things to be different from what they actually are in this moment. We feel compelled to put effort into working out how to change the current state of affairs into "how it should be," in order to avoid having to face the unpleasantness or disappointment of how it actually is. This strategy appears to succeed often enough to reinforce its use. With time, we come to rely on it to take care of things automatically. However, it also locks us into a particular way of coping with unpleasant experiences, leaving little room for change. If unsuccessful, rather than change strategy, we redouble our efforts to use the same sort of avoidance or rumination to deal with the problem.

ATTACHMENT AND AVERSION

Whenever we feel compelled to change the state of affairs in which we find ourselves, that need reflects some very basic habits of mind and heart. Let us look at these habits in more detail. Each experience we have—each sound, sight, smell, taste, body sensation, or thought—automatically evokes a feeling that is pleasant, unpleasant, or neutral. Like a barometer that measures pressure, so the mind–body is constantly registering events—sensations or thoughts—and giving a moment-by-moment automatic "readout" on their pleasantness or unpleasantness, giving a subtle but important "feeling tone" to every event–moment. These feeling tones are usually subtle, and often we are not aware of them; one of the reasons for giving the Pleasant and Unpleasant Experiences Calendars as home practice is to increase awareness of this neglected dimension of our experience and to explore our reactions to it. The feeling tones are an unavoidable dimension of experience; something often happens immediately after registering such a feeling tone. Although they happen quickly and seem to be automatic, these habitual "next-moment" reactions can be dissolved with practice.

Our habitual reaction to pleasant feelings is "attachment"—a need to hang on to the experience that led to them, and to get more and more of such experiences. Our habitual reaction to unpleasant feelings is "aversion"—a need to get rid of the experiences that created the unpleasant feelings, and to do all we can to prevent such experiences happening again in the future. And when the feeling is neither pleasant nor unpleasant (neutral), our habitual reaction is just to lose interest, to tune out and become disconnected from our experience of the moment. We become bored and restless.

In this session, we are particularly interested in the reaction of *aversion*.

> The habitual reaction of aversion is at the root of all the states of mind that underlie relapse in depression. Although aversion has served our species well over the course of evolution, allowing us to escape, avoid, or eliminate *external* threats to our well-being, this deeply rooted habit can backfire disastrously when we look to it to

> save us from unwelcome *internal* experiences. In rumination, the habit of aversion co-opts the mind's capacity to think our way out of problems in an attempt to get rid of feelings of unhappiness. The results are totally counterproductive.

Recognizing aversion and learning to respond more skillfully to it are core aspects of the MBCT program. In this session the focus is mainly on *recognition* of such aversion; in Session 5 we explore in more detail how to *respond skillfully*. Aversion is such a pervasive aspect of all experience that, even if participants do not encounter actual depression over the course of the program, there will be plenty of learning opportunities to see aversive reactions. By recognizing this habit of mind as it is triggered by unpleasant feelings in sessions, in home practice, and in everyday experience, participants will have many opportunities to recognize and then develop skilful ways to relate to it. These skills can then be used with depressed feelings when they arise.

A LIGHTNESS OF TOUCH

A core theme of this program is that the best way to prevent relapse is to stay present with what is unpleasant in our experience. If we can do this mindfully, it allows the process to unfold in ways that let the inherent "wisdom" of the mind deal with the difficulty, and allows more effective solutions to suggest themselves. The idea of "inherent wisdom" can seem strange. By it we mean something analogous to the experience of mathematicians who struggle to find a solution to a puzzle, only to find that the answer comes, as if from nowhere, once they have given up thinking about it. Similarly, people report that when they practice mindfulness, it can feel as if a "process" is unfolding—as if their minds appear to find wiser ways than their thinking to handle difficulties. In particular, the practice of mindfulness allows people to suspend their habitual ways of relating to negative experience, often by seeing more clearly, then decentering from judgments and expectations, so that such reactions lose their usual potency to destroy the quality of the next moment. If the old habits become less powerful, then it gradually becomes easier to take skillful action in response to difficult moods and situations, rather than simply react automatically to them. Having a certain "lightness of touch" in our awareness of thoughts, feelings, body sensations, and behavior evoked by events gives us the possibility of freeing ourselves from habitual, automatic ways of reacting.

But dealing with the negative is not easy. In the sitting meditation participants practice at home during the week, and that is practiced again—and then built on—in Session 4, they may have become aware of negative thoughts and feelings. Simply returning to the breath is often very difficult. Why so difficult? Because we habitually experience *aversion* to such unpleasantness and then feel *the need to do something about it.* At this point in the program, we remain with the simple instruction (but difficult practice!) to become more aware of experience, whatever its quality, to respond mindfully rather than to react automatically, in order to recognize the signatures of aversion.

When we were writing the first edition of this book, the Tate Modern art gallery opened in London. A feature of the gallery on which visitors commented was that it had large spaces, so works of art could be seen from a wide perspective. It was different from the experience people often report after visiting more conventional galleries, where too many people in too small a space means that a picture can be seen only from one angle or too close. By contrast, the new gallery gave viewers a sense of spaciousness.

Becoming more aware of what is occurring in moment-to-moment experience may similarly bring a sense of spaciousness. It involves being flexible in attention, noting when attention is focused on one aspect of experience, while maintaining a sense that this narrow focus can be held within a broader field of view. "Staying present" with awareness of the breath, body, sounds, and thoughts is a way to practice taking this wider perspective in order to see the sequence of reactions in mind and body more clearly.

We see this theme illustrated in different ways as the session progresses: We guide a meditation that starts with seeing or hearing, then moves to focus on breath, body, sounds, thoughts and feelings, and finally, choiceless awareness; we discuss people's experience, particularly any feelings of aversion and attachment in the class and in home practice; we give participants a wider perspective by showing them questionnaires and checklists about the symptoms of depression; and we introduce them to using the breathing space as a way of handling difficult situations.

NARROWING AND WIDENING THE FOCUS OF ATTENTION

The class starts, like Session 3, with a short "seeing" or "hearing" meditation as a way of "arriving/gathering" and coming into the present. Noticing just one feature in the field of sight or sound (e.g., a leaf on a tree or the sound of a car engine) and then expanding awareness out from it can be a powerful way of staying present: changing the mode of mind from "doing" to "being," from "problem solving" to "allowing." The instruction that, if thoughts arise, we just let them go as best as we can and bring our minds back to what we see or hear, reinforces this sense of letting go of any tendency to struggle with such thoughts.

In the same way, the move into the longer sitting meditation (see Box 11.2) provides another opportunity for learning. Once again, awareness of posture is the starting point. The aim is to feel stable and focus attention on being with moment-to-moment experience. The instructions for the sitting meditation begin by focusing attention on the breath. A participant who notices his or her mind wandering simply notes where it went, registers the fact that it has gone, then *gently* brings his or her attention back to the breath.

The longer people sit, the more they find themselves reacting to experience with aversion or attachment. It is helpful, then, to remember that the easiest way to let go is simply to stop trying to make things different. The task remains just to note any thoughts or feelings and return to the breath. Practicing with the breath in this way allows participants to train their attention and observe the movement and patterns of the mind. With time they learn to open awareness to whatever arises in the mind or body, and to use that as a focus.

This is encouraged, at a certain point during the practice, by *expanding* awareness to the *whole body*. If the mind wanders, the task is the same: simply to note where it went and to bring attention back to the current focus—the sense of the body as a whole. We may become aware of sensations throughout the body, particularly noting any regions of intensity or discomfort. We can then intentionally bring awareness to those regions of

BOX 11.2

Sitting Meditation: Mindfulness of Sounds and Thoughts

1. Practice mindfulness of breath and body, as described earlier, until you feel reasonably settled.

2. Allow the focus of your awareness to shift from sensations in the body to hearing. Bring your attention to the ears and then allow the awareness to open and expand, so that there is a receptiveness to sounds as they arise, wherever they arise.

3. There is no need to go searching for sounds or listening for particular sounds. Instead, as best you can, simply open your awareness so that it is receptive to sounds from all directions as they arise—sounds that are close, sounds that are far away, sounds that are in front, behind, to the side, above, or below. Open to a whole space of sound around you. Be aware of obvious sounds and of more subtle sounds, aware of the space between sounds, aware of silence.

4. As best you can, be aware of sounds simply as sensations. When you find that you are thinking *about* the sounds, reconnect, as best you can, with direct awareness of their sensory qualities (patterns of pitch, timbre, loudness, and duration) rather than their meanings or implications.

5. Whenever you notice that your awareness is no longer focused on sounds in the moment, gently acknowledge where the mind had moved to, and then retune the awareness back to sounds as they arise and pass from one moment to the next.

6. Mindfulness of sound can be a very valuable practice on its own, as a way of expanding awareness and giving it a more open, spacious quality, whether or not the practice is preceded by awareness of body sensations or followed, as here, by awareness of thoughts.

7. When you are ready, let go of awareness of sounds and refocus your attention, so that your objects of awareness are now thoughts as events in the mind. Just as, with sounds, you focused awareness on whatever sounds arose, noticing them arise, develop, and pass away, so now, as best you can, bring awareness to thoughts that arise in the mind in just the same way—noticing when thoughts arise, focusing awareness on

(cont.)

them as they pass through the space of the mind and eventually disappear. There is no need to try to make thoughts come or go. Just let them arise naturally, in the same way that you related to sounds arising and passing away.

8. Some people find it helpful to bring awareness to thoughts in the mind in the same way that they might if the thoughts were projected on the screen at the cinema. You sit, watching the screen, waiting for a thought or image to arise. When it does, you pay attention to it so long as it is there "on the screen," and then you let it go as it passes away. Alternatively, you might find it helpful to see thoughts as clouds moving across a vast, spacious sky or as leaves moving on a stream, carried by the current.

9. If any thoughts bring with them intense feelings or emotions, pleasant or unpleasant, as best you can, note their "emotional charge" and intensity, and let them be as they already are.

10. If at any time you feel that your mind has become unfocused and scattered, or if it keeps getting repeatedly drawn into the drama of your thinking and imaginings, you may like to notice where this is affecting your body. Often, when we don't like what is happening, we feel a sense of contraction or tightness in the face, shoulders, or torso, and a sense of wanting to "push away" our thoughts and feelings. See if you notice any of this going on for you when some intense feelings arise. Then, once you have noticed this, see if it is possible to come back to the breath and a sense of the body as a whole, sitting and breathing, and use this focus to anchor and stabilize your awareness.

11. At a certain point, you might like to explore the possibility of letting go of any particular object of attention, like the breath, or class of objects of attention, like sounds or thoughts, and let the field of awareness be open to whatever arises in the landscape of the mind and the body and the world. See if it is possible to simply rest in awareness itself, effortlessly knowing whatever arises from moment to moment. That might include the breath, sensations from the body, sounds, thoughts, or feelings. As best you can, just sit, completely awake, not holding on to anything, not looking for anything, having no agenda whatsoever other than embodied wakefulness.

12. And when you are ready, bring the sitting to a close, perhaps returning for a few minutes to the simple practice of mindful awareness of the breath.

intensity and breathe into them and breathe out from them, as we did in Session 3 (see Chapter 10, Box 10.2).

The awareness is then extended beyond the body to include *sounds*. The instructions invite participants to become aware of sounds from all around, both the obvious and the more subtle sounds, simply as "sensations." This continues the theme explored in the seeing and hearing meditations, a theme introduced as far back as the raisin exercise in Session 1, of direct awareness of the sensory qualities of moment-to-moment experience rather than its meanings or implications.

The next step in the meditation is to let go of awareness of sounds and refocus attention on thoughts—seeing thoughts and images as events in the mind. Just as we invited participants to become aware of sounds as "events" as they arose, stayed around, and ceased, so now the invitation is to bring awareness to thoughts as they arise, stay around in the "space" of the mind, and eventually dissolve.

Some people find it helpful to see thoughts in the mind as if projected on a screen at a movie. You sit, watching the screen, waiting for a thought or image—and any feeling that comes with it—to arise. When it does, the instruction is to pay attention to it so long as it is there "on the screen," then to let it go as it passes away. Alternatively, others find it helpful to see thoughts as clouds moving across the sky. A third metaphor is to observe thoughts as leaves on a stream, being carried past by the current. Any or all of these analogies and metaphors can help.

From time to time, participants may find that their minds get repeatedly drawn into the drama of their thinking and imaginings. This is especially the case when thoughts or images bring with them intense feelings or emotions, pleasant or unpleasant. The instructions invite participants, if this is happening, perhaps also to note what is going on in their bodies at that point, then to come back to the breath and a sense of the body as a whole sitting and breathing, using this focus to anchor and stabilize the awareness before returning, if they choose, to observe the thoughts and feelings as they arise.

Finally, participants may explore what is sometimes called "choiceless awareness": letting go of any particular intentional focus of attention, and instead letting the field of awareness be open to whatever arises in the mind, the body, and the world around them. We then finish the practice by returning for a few minutes to attend to the breath (see Box 11.2).

Notice the change during the practice from *focusing* attention (gathering) in the early stage to *expanding* attention to experience a more *spacious* awareness in the later stage. The intention of the mindfulness approach is ultimately to allow people to become aware that there is a "larger space" in which thoughts, feelings, and sensations may be held in awareness. Being able to hold a larger number of elements in experience at any one time allows us to be sensitive to the wider context, and it contrasts with the narrower focus required at the outset to help "gather" the mind. The instructor may read a poem that explores this sense of spaciousness (e.g., Mary Oliver's poem "Wild Geese"[87]) toward the end of the sitting meditation or later in the session (see Box 11.3).

BOX 11.3

"Wild Geese"

You do not have to be good.
You do not have to walk on your knees
for a hundred miles through the desert, repenting.
    You only have to let the soft animal of your body
        love what it loves.
Tell me about despair, yours, and I will tell you mine.
Meanwhile the world goes on.
Meanwhile the sun and the clear pebbles of the rain
are moving across the landscapes,
over the prairies and the deep trees,
the mountains and the rivers.
Meanwhile the wild geese, high in the clean blue air,
are heading home again.
Whoever you are, no matter how lonely,
the world offers itself to your imagination,
calls to you like the wild geese, harsh and exciting—
over and over announcing your place
in the family of things.

PRACTICE REVIEW

In the inquiry that follows the meditation, attention focuses on not only what happens but also how participants *reacted* to their experience. For example, one participant said:

> "My mind has wandered again. I must be the worst meditator in the world. Why did I ever think this practice would do anything for me?"

We see here that it does not take much for any of us to turn a simple instruction to stay with the breath into a drama of success and failure. It is too easy to believe, deep down, that success is achieved when we are with the breath, and that failure occurs when the mind wanders. The truth is that meditation is the whole process of staying with the breath, moving away, seeing that we are no longer with the breath, then gently returning.

As instructors, time and again we remind ourselves and participants to be gentle when the mind has wandered, and when bringing attention back to the breath. Such gentleness is important because it conveys an attitude of caring both to ourselves and to whatever the experience may be in the moment. The practice is one of noticing, acknowledging, and kindly and gently escorting the mind back to the breath rather than pulling it back abruptly.

What is important is that we come back without blaming, judging ourselves, or feeling that we have failed. And if we find that we have judged ourselves, then the instruction is still the same: simply to note the judgment and bring attention back to the breath or whatever was the focus of attention.

> Meditation is not about clearing the mind. It is the whole process of staying with the breathing, moving away, seeing that we are no longer on the breath, then gently returning.

It is important to remember that we are not trying to teach a method to control the breath. The task is simply to bring full care and attention to the actual physical sensations as the breath moves in and out of the body, allowing the breath to breathe itself. The breath is used as an anchor to reconnect to the present whenever the mind wanders.

REACTIONS TO THE PRACTICE: SEEING AVERSION

"At first when you said to focus on thoughts, nothing came up at all. Then I thought 'I must be doing it wrong,' and I thought of the time when I missed school because I was ill, and all the other kids seemed to know this stuff but I didn't."

This participant reports a very common observation: that when we ask ourselves actually to focus on thinking, no matter how much we have been distracted by our mind wandering up until that point, the mind seems to go blank—just when we wanted to practice observing thoughts. But then something else may happen: We judge our experience against some standard (in this case, "I ought to have some thoughts"), judge ourselves not to be doing very well ("I must be doing it wrong"), and before we know it, we have become enmeshed in memories that echo the sense of failure.

I: So let's see if I have understood; you found your mind blank when you asked yourself to observe your thinking; then came the thought "I must be doing this wrong."

P: Yes . . . and then I felt sort of . . . a bit of a failure—like . . . everyone else seems to be able to do it, but I can't.

I: Then your mind took you down a track of memory?

P: Yeah . . . one time I missed school—I was about 12. I hated missing school because I felt I'd be left behind. It was in Geography. They had all been learning about something called "the Cotswolds," and I hadn't a clue what they were talking about.

I: Your mind was full of this memory. What happened then?

P: I felt sad, I don't know why really.

I: What was happening in your body at this point? Were you aware of anything?

P: (*Pauses.*) . . . a feeling of being "clutched up" about here. (*Indicates center of chest below rib cage.*) (*sigh*) . . . feeling tired.

I: Then what happened?

P: Feeling a bit lost actually . . . just like I did then—out of it; yeah, lost. . . .

Then you said something about going back to the breath if we got lost, and it sort of brought me back. . . .

Notice that this is a wonderful description of how any of us can get caught by something that takes us away—to the distant past, right in the middle of the practice. The instructor focuses on this.

I: Something happened—in this case, the lack of thoughts—then another thought came up about doing it all wrong, then a memory of a time when you felt that others knew something and you did not, and you felt lost. Isn't it amazing how quickly the mind can take us away? And what's really interesting here—did you notice?—was how your body reacted when that unpleasant feeling, then the memory came up? When anything happens that we don't like, the body is a very sensitive indicator, and we see it reacting—like tensing up—ready to fight or run away; or it feels instantly tired and exhausted—a sort of "giving up." It can all happen really quickly.

P: Yeah, it was very powerful.

I: It is great to notice this because these bodily changes are often a sign that the mind–body has seen something it doesn't like, that it wants to be rid of. It is called "aversion," and it can trigger all sorts of other reactions in the very next moment. Often, these reactions prevent us from seeing—and dealing with—the feelings that triggered it in the first place. The body–mind treats our own thoughts and memories as enemies to be eradicated or run away from. But none of us can run fast enough to get away from our own thoughts, so we get stuck—feeling lost, alone, helpless. And this can bring back patterns of mind from way back, as if it was happening all over again, which creates more tension in the body—more "enemies." Did anyone else notice their body reacting in this way?

In this and other ways, participants are encouraged to observe reactions of aversion as they arise in the body (e.g., a sense of contraction or tightness in the face, shoulders, or torso; and a characteristic felt sense of "pushing away" or "not wanting"). They are invited to notice how aversion is a powerful *competitor for attention*, often taking awareness away from whatever had been the intended focus, producing instead a tunnel vision that sees only these seemingly vital thoughts or feelings. The practice of mindfulness can be a powerful ally, allowing us to notice when this has occurred and broadening attention again to regain the ability to choose where we wish to place our attention in this moment. Learning to identify the bodily signatures of aversion gives us a window into the mind's reactivity, and training ourselves to become aware of the very first moment in the sequence brings freedom from the tendency to get drawn into automatic reactions to pleasant and unpleasant thoughts, feelings, and events.

The promise of mindfulness practice is not that reactions of aversion will necessarily be prevented, but that we can learn to extricate ourselves from them in a nonjudgmental way when they do occur. Such freedom is what "staying present" in the face of aversion is all about. People have used many ways to describe this "learning to stay present." Some refer to recovering a sense of balance. Others use the metaphor of a mountain that remains firmly rooted in the earth despite the changing weather conditions around it. It is difficult to find the right words to express such a subtle but deep meaning. But the importance of using the practice itself as a vehicle for this learning cannot be overstated.

PRACTICE REVIEW: HONEYMOONS AND HARD WORK

In reviewing home practice week by week, the instructor gets close to the heart of issues that arise with the practice. Even more important, the home practice review gets close to the heart of the very habits of attachment and aversion that are likely to cause problems. For some people, the "honeymoon" with the program is over and the hard work is beginning.

Here is a participant who was finding it hard work because he had become very *attached* to the practice:

"I find I can really get into the practice now. When I'm sitting, I feel in another world. So much so that if anything interrupts, I get really angry. I feel like a child that has had his ice cream snatched out of his hand."

This person has become strongly attached to the pleasant experiences that can arise as the mind settles. And the attachment is beginning to produce frustration. It may be worth pausing a moment to explore whether the person was focusing on achieving a "special state" and to be very clear about the intention behind the practice. The instructor felt it was important to be as clear as possible about this theme:

"It is really nice to hear that you are getting something out of the practice. When we get such pleasant experiences, it can show us that something is happening. But I'm also going to mention here a word of caution. Pleasant experiences may come and go, and while they last, they are wonderful. But the word of caution is this: Sometimes the pleasant experience will not come. Sometimes you may experience unpleasant feelings when you sit. But this won't mean that you are doing badly. It is still meditation, even when it feels bad or boring or frustrating. The task is the same at these times, too: As best you can, be aware of whatever you are feeling right now, and then return your attention to the breath. So although it's really nice when it seems to be going well, if we get hooked on making it always feel like that, life is going to be a series of ups and downs. We'll have moments of great success, they'll pass, and then what will we do?

"Having this practice gives us a chance to find something that is beyond the ups and downs, beyond the times when things do or don't work out so well for us."

In this case, the instructor invited the participant to look out for similar situations when he felt "attached" to a thought or a feeling, and to note what feelings came up as the situation came and went. Of particular interest is how what is pleasant became a source of frustration (and therefore a negative feeling) the more he tried to cling to what he had judged to be positive.

More often, there is a sense of *aversion* related to the home practice:

P: I have to come clean and be totally honest. I didn't get around to doing any of the home practice. Now I can imagine what R must have felt last week. I felt absolutely terrible myself. You feel as if, you know, you are not even putting the effort in at home, and it's the thin end of the wedge. I feel, you know, I have really let you down.

I: There are two things about that. First is taking responsibility for your own home practice. There is a relationship between how much home practice you do and how you move along—a close relationship. If you don't do it, you reduce the chance of anything happening. This is entirely your responsibility. But second, and the thing I am really interested in, is your feeling of dread and the thoughts about how awful it was going to be coming here. In the course of not doing your home practice, all these thoughts come up: about being no good and letting me down, and not coming up to expectations, and so on. Would you like to say some more about that?

P: Well, sitting here right now, with you talking in your calm voice, it's fine, and I'm really glad I came. But then I get a really funny feeling in my stomach and a tightness in my chest because I think you're thinking I'm a failure.

I: This is really important. It's this contrast between the thoughts that you take to be true, and reality. I can give you the reality: I don't feel let down by you. There are no standards. That is not what it's about. It is actually taking the experience as it is, and letting go of all these comparisons. We are moving to the point where you can begin to recognize these thoughts as mental events. "Here come the self-critical thoughts; here come the guilty thoughts; here is the old tape playing again, creating the same feeling." Clearly, these patterns of thinking come from somewhere. It is possible that at some time, you were severely criticized by somebody for not doing things right. But these are old habits. It doesn't matter where they come from. What we are about is trying as best we can to free ourselves of them. The reason why we use the breath focus, with all the long gaps, is simply to give you lots of chances for these thoughts to come in; to give you a chance to say, "Ah, there you are" and gently go back to the breath.

We should not be surprised that aversion and attachment are such common themes in the practice, as they are our habitual, default reactions to pleasant and unpleasant experiences. Although we all need to keep a wholesome balance of the basic pluses and minuses of our lives, we can find ourselves preoccupied with avoiding harm or achieving reward in unhelpful ways that add to the negativity of the unwanted object or event, or to the frustration of not having the object of our desire.

Many people find the traditional metaphor of the two arrows a helpful way to remind themselves of the way we add negativity to unpleasant experiences: If hit by an arrow we would experience physical pain and discomfort. But, for most of us, it is as if, following this first arrow, we are then hit by a second arrow—the suffering arising from the reactions of anger, fear, grief, or distress that we add to the simple experience of discomfort from the first arrow. And, more often than not, it is this second arrow that causes us the greater unhappiness. The crucial message of this image is that we can learn to free ourselves from the suffering of the second arrow *because we are the very ones who fire it at ourselves!*

REVIEWING
THE UNPLEASANT EXPERIENCES CALENDAR

It is particularly helpful to focus on the theme of recognizing aversion when participants talk about how they got on with the Unpleasant Experiences Calendar (Session 3–Handout 5). Many note that this was easier to complete than the Pleasant Experiences Calendar (Session 2–Handout 6). They noticed many more unpleasant moments each day. Once again, we have a whiteboard available to write down responses, distinguishing thoughts, sensations, and feelings. We highlight any reactions of aversion to each of these aspects of the unpleasant experience. In particular, we see if it is possible to identify patterns of bodily contraction associated with aversion. Participants can then use awareness of these patterns to alert themselves to this habitual reaction arising in the future. We also take this opportunity to explore aversion in the shape of the vicious cycles involved in getting upset about having negative thoughts and feelings (e.g., "I should not be feeling like this. Why am I so stupid and weak?").

The central theme of both attachment and aversion is "needing things to be different from how they are right now." By contrast, the first step in responding skillfully to pleasant and unpleasant experiences, particularly the unpleasant mind states that can trigger rumination, is simply to be present with them. In the fuller space of awareness we may then decide to take further action. And a great ally in "staying present" in this way is to see and to be curious about what is happening in the body. As we cultivate greater curiosity and compassion for how the body is reacting, something settles. We discover that we can actually stop struggling and be present, and this gives us the opportunity to see and relate to our circumstances with greater clarity and directness. It can be enormously empowering to discover that we can simply be with unpleasant experiences without being overwhelmed by them, and that, sooner or later, in their own good time, these feelings will pass. With this insight also comes the possibility of choosing behaviors that are more likely to deal skillfully with the situation before us, rather than having our actions automatically driven by fear or old mental habits.

Reviewing the Unpleasant Experiences Calendar also offers an opportunity to explore the theme that events may not be inherently positive or negative. It is often the mood state that we bring to events that colors them for us, an idea that we pick up further in the next part of the session.

AUTOMATIC NEGATIVE THOUGHTS AND THE SYMPTOMS OF DEPRESSION: GETTING TO KNOW THE TERRITORY OF THE ILLNESS

One of the most valuable aspects of the structured psychotherapies that developed in the 1960s with behavior therapy and continued with cognitive therapy in the 1970s was the therapists' collaborative approach—their willingness to talk openly and in a matter-of-fact way with patients about how mental health problems can arise, and how the aim of therapy is to help them tackle their problems. An important aspect of this was to talk with patients about issues of diagnosis and formulation—about what, in their case, seemed to have caused or maintained the symptoms they were experiencing. Although MBCT does not discuss causes of a particular participant's problems, it retains this important feature: Education about depression is essential if people are going to learn ways to deal with it more skillfully.

At this point, therefore, we move from talking about thinking in general to a more focused discussion of the types of thoughts that are usually reported by people when they are suffering from depression. To help in this work, we hand out copies of the Automatic Thoughts Questionnaire[88] (see Box 11.4). The questionnaire lists a variety of negative statements (e.g., "I can't get things together," "My life is not going the way I want it to," "What's the matter with me?", "I hate myself").

The instructor reads aloud each item, asking participants to reflect on how much they believe the thought, both now and when they were at their most depressed. This provides an opportunity for people in the class to notice whether their degree of belief has changed since the time they were depressed. The instructor also asks if anyone recognizes any of the items on the list. It is common for one person after another to respond along the lines of "Yes, nearly all of them. I used to believe them 100% but now hardly at all." For each participant sitting there, this can provide compelling evidence that these thoughts, which, when depressed, they accepted unquestioningly as personally valid truths about them as individuals, are actually *universal features of the state of clinical depression*—symptoms of an illness, just as much as the more "physical" symptoms of disturbed appetite and sleep.* This alternative way of understanding participants' experience provides another opportunity for the instructor to reinforce a central message of the MBCT program: *Thoughts are not facts*.

> When depressed, we unquestioningly accept negative thoughts as personally valid truths about us as individuals. Yet they are actually *universal features of the state of depression*. They are *symptoms of the illness*, just as much as disturbed appetite and sleep are symptoms of the illness.

---

* Occasionally, describing the symptoms of the "illness" of depression in this way can seem demeaning to people who may have had bad experiences with psychiatric services, some of which may have seemed to use "diagnoses" to explain away a person's experience. The instructor needs to be sensitive to this possibility. The aim here is simply to say that this is what physicians mean when they diagnose major depression. Most participants, however, find that this way of looking at depression demystifies things for them. It also helps them to decenter from negative thoughts, seeing them as universal features of depression, and they are grateful to see that others in the class have experiences similar to theirs.

BOX 11.4

Automatic Thoughts Questionnaire

Listed below are a variety of thoughts that pop into people's heads. Please read the list, and notice what happens as you do so.

Do you recognize any of them? Which thoughts feel most familiar to you?

When you feel very low, how often do thoughts like these occur? And how far do you believe them? How convincing do they seem?

And what about when you are feeling well? How often do the thoughts occur then? And how far do you believe them? How convincing do they feel?

1. I feel like I'm up against the world.
2. I'm no good.
3. Why can't I ever succeed?
4. No one understands me.
5. I've let people down.
6. I don't think I can go on.
7. I wish I were a better person.
8. I'm so weak.
9. My life's not going the way I want it to.
10. I'm so disappointed in myself.
11. Nothing feels good anymore.

(cont.)

12. I can't stand this anymore.

13. I can't get started.

14. What's wrong with me?

15. I wish I were somewhere else.

16. I can't get things together.

17. I hate myself.

18. I'm worthless.

19. I wish I could just disappear.

20. What's the matter with me?

21. I'm a loser.

22. My life is a mess.

23. I'm a failure.

24. I'll never make it.

25. I feel so helpless.

26. Something has to change.

27. There must be something wrong with me.

28. My future is bleak.

29. It's just not worth it.

30. I can't finish anything.

When we feel low, thoughts like these often feel like "the truth" about us. But in fact they are symptoms of depression—just as a high temperature is a symptom of flu. Becoming aware, through mindfulness, that they are just "the voice of depression speaking" allows us to step back from them and begin to choose whether to take them seriously or not. Perhaps, in fact, we can learn simply to notice them, acknowledge their presence, and let them go.

One person's reaction to this exercise was to wonder why her doctor had not recognized her depression earlier. Addressing the instructor, she said: "If you knew that, why don't the general practitioners? Because this has gone on for years." She thought that if such a questionnaire had been used when she was depressed, then at least it would have shown that someone understood: "If it was in this form, it would prove that someone knows what you felt like. . . . It took me a while to realize that it was depression. I just thought I was tired and things were getting me down. . . . You know, that people like me didn't suffer from depression."

The instructor may suggest a number of different ways to see the list of thoughts:

> "Here is one way to look at these negative thoughts. Let's see if you can bring some humor to this exercise by picking out a hit list of your favorites. This can be helpful in reminding yourselves that these are just thoughts, not the truth with a capital T. You might also want to take a minute and compare the extent to which these thoughts seemed to be absolutely true when you were feeling depressed, but, at this point, no longer seem to have the same grip.
>
> "Here is another way to look at it. Let's say a common thought you had when you were depressed was 'I'm never going to get over this depression.' Well, we have got the living proof that you did. So these thoughts are absolutely convincing—they just come into your mind—but they are not true. Those are things that drive your feelings; they drive your actions and they are deadly because, if you think you are not going to get over it, if you think you are useless, if you think there is nothing you can do to make any difference, then you give up.
>
> "So we just need to be able to recognize them over and over again and not get sucked into them. The task now is just to learn to recognize them: 'Here are public enemy numbers 1 to 30.' Then you can just say, 'Ah, there you are. I don't need to get sucked into you right now.'"

The Automatic Thoughts Questionnaire provides a sense of the "territory of depression," a view of the disorder as a whole package. This is then taken further by reviewing the actual symptoms that psychiatrists and psychologists look for when diagnosing major depressive disorder (according to the criteria of the *Diagnostic and Statistical Manual of Mental Disorders* [DSM-IV-TR][28]; see Box 11.5). The reason for going over it is so individuals can recognize that some of the things they may have thought were personal failings are actually well-recognized core features of the syndrome of depression. Once again, the idea is to give participants another perspective on their symptoms. The message is that depression comes as a package of symptoms; the task is to learn how to relate differently to the whole package. Gaining this alternative view of it can go far in preventing people from being trapped in the old, depressive ways of thinking about what it all means.

BOX 11.5

Diagnostic Criteria for Major Depressive Episode

Just as when diagnosing the flu or an ear infection, a psychiatrist or psychologist assessing depression looks for a number of symptoms that occur at roughly the same time and do not resolve on their own. In the case of major depression, the time frame for a diagnosis is a minimum of 2 weeks to a month of a person feeling sad most of the day, or having lost interest in activities they previously enjoyed. It is also important that these changes reduce the person's ability to work or function normally.

If the above are all present, then five of the following symptoms are sufficient to complete the diagnosis: significant weight loss or weight gain, an increase or decrease in appetite, difficulty falling asleep, waking up early or sleeping during the day, feeling slowed down or agitated throughout the day, feeling exhausted, feeling worthless or excessively guilty over past actions, finding it hard to concentrate or being indecisive, and repeatedly thinking about dying or suicide.

Based on DSM-IV-TR.[28]

SOMEWHERE ELSE TO STAND

Note what has happened here. The aim of this fourth session is to explore how to recognize aversion, and to "stay present" in the face of the tendency to chase after the pleasant and avoid the unpleasant. We have seen that staying present involves giving up old habits in order to allow difficult material to come and go in the mind. But we have introduced the Automatic Thoughts Questionnaire and a symptom checklist of depression. What have these got to do with staying present? The answer is that seeing how the signs and symptoms of depression can change when depression changes, seeing how the negative thinking that comes with it (so strongly believed, so overwhelming when in the depressed state) can change gives participants "somewhere else to stand" to see more clearly what their minds can do to them. This links with the practice in which participants have been engaged from the outset of the program: to learn to become more aware of body sensations. Learning to "stay present" in the body also presents people with another place to stand. "Staying present" is rarely easy, but it is easier if a person, when his or her mood starts to shift, has a sense that such moods do not last forever, and that they are part of a recognizable syndrome. The person gains an alternative perspective from which to view his or her experience: Things are not taken so personally.

TAKING A 3-MINUTE BREATHING SPACE DURING CLASS

During the previous session, we introduced the 3-Minute Breathing Space (Session 3–Handout 2) to be used at regular, preset times during the day as a generalization exercise. We now extend this practice by inviting people deliberately to use the breathing space during the week, *whenever they notice unpleasant feelings or a sense of "tightening" or "holding" in the body, or of being overwhelmed*. At such moments, the breathing space might consist of either taking a full 3 minutes of more "formal" practice or momentarily bringing awareness to what is going on in the mind and body, and with the breath, during a period of busyness. In the latter case, it is not always possible for participants to close their eyes and make major adjustments to posture, but the process of intentionally stepping out of automatic pilot remains important. The aim is to use these moments as further opportunities to explore the difference between skillful responding and automatic reacting.

Given this new use of the breathing space, it is helpful to include it during the class at appropriate times, in order to bring to bear another mode or perspective. These might be moments when the class finds itself lost in a lengthy discussion or when strong feelings or reactions surface.

For example, when the class is discussing and analyzing various topics, it is not unusual for everyone's mind (including that of the instructor) to drift away from the present and off into other thoughts, mental routines, and long explanations. For participants, many of these mental routines simply trigger the old habits of depressed thinking. During Session 4 in particular, we find that discussing depressive thoughts and symptoms sometimes produces a sudden sadness in participants. Thinking about depression has the power to activate a lot of negative thinking. At these times, the breathing space can help "shift mental gears" and connect with experience in the present moment.

The following is an example in which someone felt sad after he had read the list of negative thoughts on the Automatic Thoughts Questionnaire:

P: I feel quite sad now, I actually do.

I: About what? Was it reading all this?

P: The thing that got me was . . . because I have spent so much time. My depressions took a lot of years out of my life. That's how I feel. . . . It is easy to get back into it. You could easily get depressed just by looking at this list every day.

I: What we are learning is to how to relate differently to these thoughts and feelings, by practicing over and over again how not to get sucked into them. Why don't we actually do that right now because there is a sadness in this room, with the thoughts about the previous episodes around. So let's do a breathing space because it is one of the ways we have to actually come back into the moment. So to start, we could make a quite definite change in our posture . . . sitting upright. (*The instructor leads a 3-Minute Breathing Space.*)

This is not done in an avoidant way but rather as a means of acknowledging such feelings, creating space for them, and only then moving to focus on the breath and bring awareness to the body as a whole. The task here is a subtle one. We are not using the 3-Minute Breathing Space to achieve a goal, with the idea that doing this will help a person feel better afterward. It is really about (1) acknowledging that there is strong feeling around and (2) seeing what happens if we take a moment to bring awareness to it, simply allowing it to be there without judging it, without trying to chase it away or solve the problem. Using it in this way allows people to "touch base," to return to the anchor of the breath wherever they are, to shift mental gears so that they have a different way of investigating how things are for them right at this moment. As a result it may begin to reveal different possibilities, different ways of responding to the variety of mind states. During the week following this class, participants are encouraged to use the 3-Minute Breathing Space not only at set times during the day but also whenever they feel the need for its help in coping with difficulties—what we call a "responsive breathing space."

MINDFUL WALKING

In Session 3 we introduced formal practices to cultivate greater mindfulness of the body in movement. As with the formal sitting practice, the issue arises as to how this greater awareness of physical sensations in the body can be generalized to daily life. One possibility is to take a physical action that we use every day and slow it down, performing it mindfully, so that the action itself can act as a bridge between practice and daily life. This is what is done in mindful walking.

Mindful walking takes the everyday activity of walking and uses it as a mindfulness practice to become more aware of body sensations (see Session 4–Handout 2). We walk, knowing that we are walking, feeling the walking.

It has been described as "meditation in motion": being with each step, walking for its own sake, without any destination. As with other mindfulness practices in this program, we use the movements and sensations of walking to bring ourselves into the present. The focus is on maintaining moment-to-moment awareness of the sensations accompanying our movements, letting go of any thoughts or feelings about the sensations themselves. This seemingly simple exercise can be a powerful teacher of a core message in MBCT, that our bodies are always available as an anchor to the here and now, at times when our minds ricochet between the past and future. This anchoring allows a greater sense of who we really are in the present moment. Although we don't schedule mindful walking as part of the formal home practice, we encourage any participant who wishes to explore it during the week to do so.

The practice turns out to be especially useful for those who feel agitated and unable to settle. The physical sensation of walking, people comment, tends to enable them to feel more "grounded." To some extent, this can be generalized across all the mindfulness exercises: When the mind is agitated or a person feels pressured, it is easier to be mindful with a practice that involves physical movement than with one that does not.

ENDING THE CLASS

The end of Session 4 represents something of a watershed. Given that we are now coming to the halfway point in the course, it is a good idea to review the whole MBCT model with the class before ending with a brief sitting meditation. Given our theme of "recognizing aversion," this is an opportunity to emphasize the role of breathing in helping us achieve a different stance toward ourselves, our minds, and our bodies.

People who attend the classes are learning a different way of relating to their entire experience. So when, for example, they are ruminating about letting someone down, or feeling angry with someone, they can use that as an opportunity to practice taking a different, more skillful approach. The transcripts of the MBCT sessions show a similar change taking place:

> "For example, I think I started to feel sad because my grandmother is very ill. I kept thinking, 'Oh, I'm getting depressed,' . . . but . . . I was saying this to someone just the other day: 'I am sad, I am tired, but I'm not depressed.' And I don't have to deny the sadness or the tiredness."

"Today, I had a difficult phone call to make and, normally, that would go round and round in my mind. I made the phone call, and I was able to deal with the call, but usually, after a conversation like that, I would be worrying about it for ages. But this time, afterwards, it was great. I stopped thinking about it. It didn't carry on and on. Using the breathing space was amazing to me. It seemed to take the worry right away from me, that would have been churning in my mind all afternoon."

These participants are learning to stop and ask the questions "How are things right now?"; "What is going through my mind here?"; "What is going on in my body?"; and "What is the most skillful response to make right now?" This inquiring stance itself is becoming for them a reminder to step back and observe more carefully what is going on.

This tiny step can make all the difference. As a result of the practice, people are not simply being drawn in to the "bad feeling"; neither do they have to answer back their negative thoughts. Instead, they feel able to see themselves, their thoughts, and feelings within a wider perspective. They are not separating themselves from their thoughts and feelings entirely, but there seems to be more space in which they can work with them. And with a greater sense of space, they are more able to stay present with whatever they find coming into their minds and to be more forgiving with themselves when their best intentions go awry.

Summary of Session 4: Recognizing Aversion

Difficult things are part and parcel of life itself. It is how we handle those things that makes the difference between whether they rule (control) our lives or whether we can relate more lightly to them. Becoming more aware of the thoughts, feelings, and body sensations evoked by events gives us the possibility of freeing ourselves from habitual, automatic ways of reacting, so that we can instead mindfully respond in more skillful ways.

In general, we react to experience in one of three ways:

1. With spacing out, or boredom, so that we switch away from the present moment and go off somewhere else "in our heads."

2. With wanting to hold on to things—not allowing ourselves to let go of experiences we are having right now, or wishing we were having experiences that we are not having right now.

3. With wanting it to go away, being angry with it—wanting to get rid of experiences we are having right now, or avoiding future experiences that we do not want.

As we discuss further in class, each of these ways of reacting can cause problems, particularly the tendency to react to unpleasant feelings with aversion. For now, the main issue is to become more aware of our experience, so that we can respond mindfully rather than react automatically.

Regularly practicing sitting meditation gives us many opportunities to notice when we have drifted away from awareness of the moment, to note with a friendly awareness whatever it was that took our attention away, and to gently and firmly bring our attention back to our focus, reconnecting with moment-by-moment awareness. At other times of the day, deliberately using the breathing space whenever we notice unpleasant feelings, or a sense of "tightening" or "holding" in the body, provides an opportunity to begin to *respond* rather than *react*.

Mindful Walking

1. Find a place where you can walk up and down, without feeling concerned about whether people can see you. It can be inside or outside—and the length of your "walk" may vary perhaps between 7 and 10 paces.

2. Stand at one end of your walk, with your feet parallel to each other, about 4 to 6 inches apart, and your knees "unlocked," so that they can gently flex. Allow your arms to hang loosely by your sides, or hold your hands loosely together in front of your body. Direct your gaze, softly, straight ahead.

3. Bring the focus of your awareness to the bottoms of your feet, getting a direct sense of the physical sensations of the contact of the feet with the ground and the weight of your body transmitted through your legs and feet to the ground. You may find it helpful to flex your knees slightly a few times to get a clearer sense of the sensations in the feet and legs.

4. When you are ready, transfer the weight of the body into the right leg, noticing the changing pattern of physical sensations in the legs and feet as the left leg "empties" and the right leg takes over the support of the rest of the body.

5. With the left leg "empty," allow the left heel to rise slowly from the floor, noticing the sensations in the calf muscles as you do so, and continue, allowing the whole of the left foot to lift gently until only the toes are in contact with the floor. Aware of the physical sensations in the feet and legs, slowly lift the left foot, carefully move it forward, feeling the foot and leg as they move through the air, and place the heel on the floor. Allow the rest of the bottom of the left foot to make contact with the floor as you transfer the weight of the body into the left leg and foot, aware of the increasing physical sensations in the left leg and foot, and of the "emptying" of the right leg and the right heel leaving the floor.

6. With the weight fully transferred to the left leg, allow the rest of the right foot to lift and move it slowly forward, aware of the changing patterns of physical sensations in the foot and leg as you do so. Focusing your attention on the right heel as it makes contact with the ground, transfer the weight of the body into the right foot as it is placed gently on the ground, aware of the shifting pattern of physical sensations in the two legs and feet.

7. In this way, slowly move from one end of your walk to the other, aware particularly of the sensations in the bottoms of the feet and heels as they make contact with the floor, and of the sensations in the muscles of the legs as they swing forward.

(cont.)

---

8. At the end of your walk, stop for a few moments, then turn slowly around, aware of and appreciating the complex pattern of movements through which the body changes direction, and continue walking.

9. Walk up and down in this way, being aware, as best you can, of physical sensations in the feet and legs, and of the contact of the feet with the floor. Keep your gaze directed softly ahead.

10. When you notice that the mind has wandered away from awareness of the sensations of walking, gently escort the focus of attention back to the sensations in the feet and legs, using the sensations as the feet contact the floor, in particular, as an "anchor" to reconnect with the present moment, just as you used the breath in the sitting meditation. If you find your mind has wandered, you might find it helpful to stand still for a few moments, gathering the focus of attention before resuming your walking.

11. Continue to walk for 10 to 15 minutes, or longer, if you wish.

12. To begin with, walk at a pace that is slower than usual, to give yourself a better chance to be fully aware of the sensations of walking. Once you feel comfortable walking slowly with awareness, you can experiment as well with walking at faster speeds, up to and beyond normal walking speed. If you are feeling particularly agitated, it may be helpful to begin walking fast, with awareness, and to slow down naturally as you settle.

13. As often as you can, bring the same kind of awareness that you cultivate in walking meditation to your normal, everyday experiences of walking.

Home Practice for the Week Following Session 4

1. Practice the Guided Sitting meditation (audio track 11) for 6 out of the next 7 days and record your reactions on the Home Practice Record Form. (Alternative option: Alternate Guided Sitting meditation with mindful walking *or* movement. Indicate which on the Home Practice Record Form.

2. 3-Minute Breathing Space—Regular (audio track 8): Practice three times a day, at the times that you have decided in advance. Record each time you do it by circling an R next to the appropriate day on the Home Practice Record Form; note any comments/difficulties.

3. 3-Minute Breathing Space—Responsive (audio track 9): Practice *whenever you notice unpleasant feelings*. Record each time you do it by circling an X for the appropriate day on the Home Practice Record Form; note any comments/difficulties.

Home Practice Record Form—Session 4

Name: _____

Record on the Home Practice Record Form each time you practice. Also, make a note of anything that comes up in the home practice, so that we can talk about it at the next meeting.

Day/date	Practice (Yes/No)	Comments
Wednesday Date: _____	Sitting meditation: R R R X X X X X X X X X X X X	
Thursday Date: _____	Sitting meditation: R R R X X X X X X X X X X X X	
Friday Date: _____	Sitting meditation: R R R X X X X X X X X X X X X	

R, 3-Minute Breathing Space—Regular Version; X, 3-Minute Breathing Space—Responsive Version.

(cont.)

Day/date	Practice (Yes/No)	Comments
Saturday Date: _____	Sitting meditation: R R R X X X X X X X X X X X X	
Sunday Date: _____	Sitting meditation: R R R X X X X X X X X X X X X	
Monday Date: _____	Sitting meditation: R R R X X X X X X X X X X X X	
Tuesday Date: _____	Sitting meditation: R R R X X X X X X X X X X X X	
Wednesday Date: _____	Sitting meditation: R R R X X X X X X X X X X X X	

Staying Present

Remember to use your body as a way to awareness. It can be as simple as staying mindful of your posture. You are probably sitting as you read this. What are the sensations in your body at this moment? When you finish reading and stand, feel the movements of standing, of walking to the next activity, of how you lie down at the end of the day. Be in your body as you move, as you reach for something, as you turn. It is as simple as that.

Just patiently practice feeling what is there—and the body is always there—until it becomes second nature to know even the small movements you make. If you are reaching for something, you are doing it anyway; there is nothing extra you have to do. Simply notice the reaching. You are moving. Can you train yourself to be there, to feel it?

It is very simple. Practice again and again bringing your attention back to your body. This basic effort, which, paradoxically, is a relaxing back into the moment, gives us the key to expanding our awareness from times of formal meditation to living mindfully in the world. Do not underestimate the power that comes to you from feeling the simple movements of your body throughout the day.

CHAPTER 12

Inquiring into Practice
and Practicing Inquiry

In the years since the first edition of this book was published we have been asked many questions about how best to teach MBCT. Some of the most heartfelt and pressing queries focus on "inquiry," the time, either just after a practice or when home practice is reviewed, when the instructor invites participants to describe, comment, or reflect on their experience. It seems that this is the single area of teaching in which both trainees and more experienced instructors are most likely to express concerns about their skills in implementing the program. Yet it is also an area, potentially, in which participants' learning can be enriched enormously. For this reason, this might be a good point to pause and examine this aspect of sessions in some detail.

First, as a way to demystify inquiry a little, it may be helpful to point out that we have looked at many examples of inquiry throughout the book already: Wherever we have quoted, verbatim, the ongoing exchanges between instructor and participants, that is the inquiry process in action. We can think of this dialogue as progressing through three concentric circles and layers of inquiry[90]:

1. In Layer 1, the primary focus is on what participants actually *noticed* in their direct experience of the practice—their description of the thoughts, feelings, and body sensations of which they were aware.
2. In Layer 2, the focus is a continuing *dialogue* about the experiences that were noticed. Through skillful questioning and reflection

those experiences are placed in a personal context of understanding.

3. In Layer 3, the emerging characterization of the experiences is *linked* to the ultimate aims of MBCT (preventing depressive relapse and enhancing well-being) by situating it in a wider context of understanding. This wider context allows the learning to be *generalized*, so that it becomes relevant to all participants in the group, and its implications for further action can be explored.

Kolb's[91] model of adult learning—the "learning circle" (see Figure 12.1)—offers a similar, more dynamic view of the unfolding of experiential learning in the process of inquiry. Inquiry is an ongoing cycle, in which one movement around the circle forms a foundation for the next.

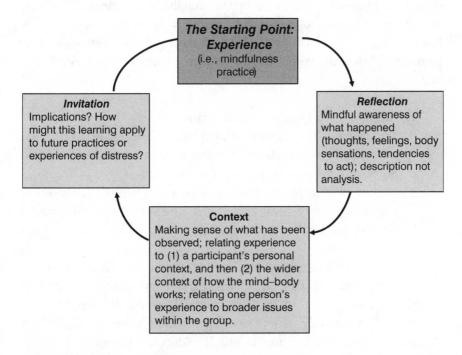

FIGURE 12.1. Kolb's model of adult learning: The learning circle. Kolb, David A., *Experiential Learning: Experience as a Source of Learning and Development*, 1st edition, © 1984. Reprinted by permission of Pearson Education, Inc., Upper Saddle River, NJ.

These general, somewhat abstract descriptions of the inquiry process can be helpful in giving some sense of the overall "shape" of this aspect of the program. However, they do not directly address the question that is the real and pressing concern of most aspiring instructors: "How, actually, do I do inquiry?" We will turn to this vital "How?" question shortly. First, we need to inform that discussion by considering the "Why?" question: What are the aims and intentions of inquiry?

INQUIRY: AIMS AND INTENTIONS

Skillful inquiry serves a surprisingly large range of ends within MBCT.

First, it acts *to tune the way participants bring mindful awareness to their experience.* The simple fact that the instructor, through his or her questioning, shows an interest in the details of experience ("Where, exactly, was the sense of contraction in the body most intense?"; "How did it change, if at all, over time?"; "What thoughts and feelings accompanied it?"; "How did you respond to it?"; etc.) itself conveys a number of key messages:

1. Awareness of experience is important.
2. Mindfulness is about cultivating *a sense of knowing*, in detail, what is happening in experience, moment by moment, rather than simply resting the attention in a particular place.
3. Mindfulness includes knowing what is happening in the mind and body more generally (e.g., how one is reacting emotionally) beyond the specific focus of attention (e.g., the breath).

The way the instructor poses questions and the words he or she uses to respond can also subtly reframe participants' perception of their experience. For example, by focusing separately on the different facets of experience ("What body sensations did you notice? What feelings? What thoughts?") the instructor can reinforce the "deconstruction" or "parsing" of experience into its separate components, which we mentioned in discussing the Pleasant and Unpleasant Experiences Calendars (Session 2–Handout 6 and Session 3–Handout 5, respectively). Equally, by reflecting back participant statements, such as "I was very angry," with the alternative wording, such as "So, there were strong feelings of anger around," the instructor can implicitly support the move to a less personally identified relationship to emotional experience.

Perhaps even more important, the whole stance toward, or relationship with, experience that the instructor embodies in the inquiry dialogue will be a major factor in helping participants themselves embody a new way of relating to experience. This will be particularly important when unpleasant, frightening, difficult, or overwhelming experiences are the focus of inquiry. The instructor who is genuinely curious, open, present, grounded, and unfazed by whatever arises in the course of inquiry is one of the most powerful vehicles for conveying the implicit message: "This too can be experienced fully, held, and worked with; there is no need to escape, withdraw, or numb out." More generally, in the inquiry dialogue the instructor offers the embodiment of the potential for a whole new way of being with experience beyond the program, in all of life.

As well as being a crucial influence on how participants relate to their *experience*, the qualities embodied by the instructor during the inquiry process can also be a significant therapeutic influence in a second area— the way participants relate to *themselves*. As we discussed in Chapter 8, there are good reasons to believe that taking part in the 8-week program increases participants' kindness and compassion toward themselves, and that these changes mediate much of the beneficial effects of MBCT. The fact that these changes can occur in the absence of any specific practices explicitly designed to cultivate kindness suggests that they reflect the implicit, cumulative effects of the program as a whole. Chief among these are the kindness and compassion embodied by the instructor. The inquiry process is probably the main arena in which the instructor has opportunity after opportunity to embody these qualities as participants report experiences they regard as failures, weaknesses, or mistakes, which would ordinarily elicit their harsh self-judgment and self-criticism. For the instructor to embody at such times qualities of respect, warmth, care, and compassion toward participants is a powerful influence in helping them begin to embody these wholesome qualities toward themselves.

WHERE TO BEGIN?

Perhaps the most obvious aim of the inquiry process is to elicit information about participants' experiences with each practice, and in their lives more generally, and to help them understand and see the significance of those experiences in a new light—in ways that will reduce the risk of future depression and increase their capacity to live more fully and freely.

Novice instructors may be helped by knowing that the first part of inquiry, in which participants describe what they noticed during the class or home practice, is itself a critical aspect of the process. Simply to describe their experience out loud can be enormously helpful both to the participant directly involved and to other members of the group, even before the significance of the experience is uncovered more fully in the process of the inquiry dialogue. *For participants it is an invitation and opportunity to "hear" the actualities of their experience, unencumbered by the overfamiliar views, judgments, or habits that too often obscure the points of contact with their direct experience.* For other group members it can be an extraordinary relief to hear another person describe the same difficulties and painful experiences they encountered themselves, assuming "It's just me and my weakness." Seeing the more universal, shared nature of such experiences in this way is an important factor in developing greater compassion for both the self and others. The dialogue within the group helps participants realize that there are common vulnerabilities experienced by all human beings, such as the tendency to add further layers of suffering to unpleasant experiences through our misguided but well-meaning attempts to get rid of them. Equally, hearing others' positive experiences with practice can also reinspire those who may have become disheartened by their own current difficulties. This can be particularly powerful if the persons describing those experiences themselves have previously described going through difficulties in an earlier part of the program.

When a participant has described his or her experience, what then? Recall that *the core aim of the inquiry process lies in the opportunity it provides for the direct experiential learning of new ways of understanding and seeing experience, the ways in which we create suffering, and the ways in which we can free ourselves from that suffering.*

What does this entail for the instructor? It implies that in the course of the inquiry dialogue, he or she gently facilitates a process of discovery and realization through which the participant comes to an experiential appreciation of the core themes and messages of the program, arising directly from his or her own experience. Skillfully conducted, the inquiry can uncover the significance of experiences that might otherwise pass unknown and unacknowledged. For example, at some level, most of us know the obvious "fact" that unpleasant experiences do not last forever, but this does not stop us being convinced, when we are in the grip of a negative mind state, that this particular experience is just going to go on and on for the foreseeable future. On the other hand, sensitively exploring with a participant a difficult experience, which in the moment felt as if it would go on forever but actually passed by the end of the practice period, can offer an opportunity for fresh *experiential* learning. Such experientially based insight and understanding into the transitoriness of experience is likely to have much more liberating potential for the future than the corresponding factual knowledge "all unpleasant experiences pass." Similarly, helping a participant actually to "see" within a specific experience the way that ruminating on unpleasant feelings increased unhappiness, whereas redirecting attention to the breath reduced unhappiness, is more likely to loosen the grip of rumination in the future than the factual, conceptual knowledge that rumination is the cause of persistent depressed mood. Noticing what may be missed by the participant means that the instructor is, in one sense, "listening out for" themes such as tendencies to be judgmental but keeping them very much at the back of the mind, and using them to guide inquiry rather than as "points to be made." For example, look again at the inquiry in Session 2 in which some participants say that they have not done their home practice (see p. 153). It might have been easier to go into the ways we find it difficult to make time in our busy lives for practice, but the teacher instead focuses on the negative patterns of thoughts that the experience of not doing the home practice evokes. Here is not a prescription but an exploration. Exploration comes first, and the instructor then adds some words to contextualize or universalize the experience. But note what is contextualized: not the experience of noncompletion of home practice, but the experience of the way we seem to take every opportunity to blame ourselves for "falling short."

HOW TO LEAD INQUIRY: THE EMBODIED QUALITIES

As we have seen, it is the instructor's embodiment of qualities in relating both to the experiences that participants describe and to the participants themselves that is a powerful influence in engendering those same qualities in group members. More than that, these qualities constitute the essential foundation on which the process of effective inquiry rests. Time and time again, we have noticed that the difference between effective and ineffective inquiry depends not so much on the technical skills with which instructors pose their questions as on the presence of these qualities "in the room." Our impression is that this often is directly related to the depth of personal mindfulness practice of the instructor.

Given the overarching importance of these more general qualities, let us consider them first, before getting down more to the specifics of inquiry.

Genuine, Warm Curiosity and Interest

In the presence of this quality, participants are much more likely to get in touch with and reveal the deeper layers of their experience, and the instructor is much more likely to become aware of, discern, and follow through on the subtler aspects of the experiences being described. It is crucial that the curiosity be both genuine and warm, so in supervision or cosupervision you may want to look out for responses that obscure this genuineness. For example, if we too frequently respond to participants' statements mechanically with the phrase "That's very interesting," then move on to another topic without further comment (inadvertently conveying a *lack* of interest in what has just been described), participants will soon feel unmotivated to share or explore their experience further. Equally, if the interest is genuine but perceived as cool and probing rather than warm and empathic, then participants will be unwilling to risk exposing more sensitive or painful aspects of their experience, and their responses will become diffuse, noncommittal, or evasive.

Not Knowing

Just as in skillful Socratic questioning in cognitive therapy,[92] the inquiry process in MBCT is one of *guiding discovery* rather than *changing minds*; that is, the instructor's questions reflect an openness to discover, in a joint exploration with the participant, the details, significance, and relevance of an experience *without knowing, in advance, what they will be or how the flow of the inquiry process will unfold.* This contrasts with the changing minds approach in which the instructor has a preexisting agenda about the point that he or she wishes to make and uses questioning to "steer" the participant toward that preordained conclusion.

Skillful inquiry therefore involves *letting go of expectations and the sense of a need to guide the inquiry process toward a particular outcome.* The only agenda is that of exploring and understanding the participant's experience in the moment. This necessarily involves a willingness to *surrender* any premature sense of a need for closure, and to *trust the process* and *trust emergence*—that more often than not, if one mindfully and wholeheartedly engages in the inquiry process, something useful, and sometimes surprising, will emerge. As instructors, we do not need to *strive for insights* in or for participants. In this process, we discover again and again that *patience and humility* are key allies. Patience reminds us that we can work with experience only as it is right now, not as we might wish it to be; that things can emerge only in their own time. Humility reminds us that participants themselves are the experts, each on his or her own experience. In this spirit, the instructor will sometimes ask participants' *permission* to continue an inquiry. Even when permission is not explicitly asked, the instructor maintains a keen sense of working with participants on particular topics only as long as they feel OK about investigating—at that moment.

The qualities required of instructors in inquiry are summarized in Box 12.1. Why are these qualities difficult for novice instructors to cultivate in inquiry? Because we know that the overarching aim of the inquiry process is to help participants understand and see the significance of their experience in new ways that will free them from depression and enhance their well-being, we can be impatient to "get the message across." It is wholly understandable, therefore, that we might be tempted to ask questions such as "I wonder whether you can see what this experience has to do with preventing depression coming back?" The problem is that such questions immediately trigger a "shift of mode" from an intuitive connection with direct experience, out of which some felt understanding may naturally emerge, to the conceptual mind "getting on the case" to "find the right answer that the instructor has in mind"—much as one might have done at school. This latter may gain us some intellectual knowledge but has little genuinely transformative power. The subtle but crucial distinction between this approach and asking questions that lead participants

BOX 12.1

Instructor Qualities and Attitudes That Facilitate Inquiry

1. Not knowing—inquiry involves acknowledging to yourself that you don't have all the answers and sometimes even saying this in the group.

2. Curiosity–inquiry involves taking an interest in whatever is being described regardless of valence, and especially the triangle of awareness about thoughts, body sensations, and emotions.

3. Kindness and hospitality—inquiry involves welcoming whatever is present, for example, using attentive and positive nonverbal cues, saying "yes."

4. Embodying the practice—inquiry involves bringing awareness to present-moment experience and not just modeling it.

5. Not fixing—inquiry involves recognizing that solutions are not required when the intention is to foster discovery.

6. Opening the space of dialogue—inquiry involves recognizing possibilities and trusting emergence, for example, "Please say more about that."

7. Asking permission—inquiry involves detecting when a boundary or strong emotion is present and checking in with the participant before proceeding, for example, "May I ask you about that?" or "How is this for you?"

8. Letting go—inquiry involves working with no fixed agenda of where one needs to get to.

9. Asking open-ended questions—inquiry involves maintaining a focus on the participant's experience, for example, "Please say more about that" or "And what happened next?"

10. Humility—inquiry involves recognizing that the other person is the expert on his or her experience, for example, "Did I understand you?" or "I heard you say this—is that correct?"

(cont.)

11. Avoiding attachment to insight—inquiry involves less about "Why do you think this is happening?"—a probe that is more appropriate when providing psychotherapy—and more about "How is this happening?" or "What do you notice about this?"

12. Flexibility and letting go—inquiry involves sometimes choosing to ask follow-up questions and at other times saying "Thank you," then moving on.

quite naturally to a characterization of their experience from which the instructor can, relatively seamlessly, draw out a useful general statement closely linked to direct experience.

HOW TO LEAD INQUIRY: PRACTICAL ISSUES

Let us now look at some very practical issues that might arise in the inquiry.

No Need to Cover Everything

In the context of a 2-hour session of MBCT, the inquiry following a longer, formal practice may take 10–15 minutes, and the inquiry into home practice may be of similar length. If one inquiry takes longer, the other may need to be shorter. This means that many comments made by participants on their experience will not be followed up in any detail by the instructors. Bear in mind that the articulation of what has been experienced is *already* an important process for any individual and a contribution to the class, and that it is perfectly OK for the instructor to thank the participant and let the class fall back into silence to allow someone else to speak. There is no need to expect that all, or even the majority, will speak. This demands a *balancing of individual and group needs*. The instructor balances individual and group processes by drawing out from the particular experiences of an individual the more universal aspects.

Encouraging Expression of Different Experiences

Sometimes it is easy to focus only on difficulties, so that those who have had pleasant experiences find it difficult to speak out. Other times, an inquiry is dominated by pleasant experiences to which others in the class cannot relate. The instructor, alert to this possibility, from time to time asks whether anyone has experienced different reactions and responses to the practice, positive or negative. In this way, the instructor embodies a sense of openhandedness and interest in all experience.

Balancing Delivering the Curriculum and Responding to Whatever Arises in the Group

It is important that as part of their preparation for each session, instructors reacquaint themselves with the aims and intentions for each component of the curriculum. Recall that the MBSR and MBCT programs have deliberately placed particular meditation practices and exercises in particular sessions, so that participants are offered many different possible "gateways" into learning experientially the same fundamental truths: the ways in which we create suffering, and the ways in which we can free ourselves from that suffering. These deliberately unfold in a particular order, session by session. We need to allow the inquiry to reflect and investigate where participants in this class are now—not where the participants in a previous class ended up after 8 weeks. Having prepared well for each session by reminding ourselves of the aims and intentions, it can be helpful to write the session title on the whiteboard as a way to orient the class in a particular way. But then the instructor, with the prepared theme as an "anchor," may also choose to respond appropriately to whatever comes up.

Changing Focus over the Program

Recognizing that the scope of inquiry necessarily changes throughout the program, we see that in the earlier classes, the focus is more on (1) directly observing body sensations, thoughts, impulses (action tendencies), and emotions, and how they are or are not experienced as connected; (2) seeing more clearly the habitual ways we normally relate to these aspects of experience; and (3) recognizing what happens as we bring mindful awareness to our experience. In later classes there is more emphasis on generalizing what is being learned in formal practice to challenges of day-to-day living, using the breathing space to investigate experience and respond wisely to it.

Trusting What Emerges

Because there are multiple gateways into mindful awareness, the instructor can draw out a learning theme from the actual experience of participants only if he or she allows it to emerge, rather than forcing it. There is a real sense that the clearer the plan for a session, the more confidently an instructor is able to let go of the plan, and trust that the learning that needs to happen will happen. As Jon Kabat-Zinn has remarked, "Whatever is going on in mind and body right now *is* the curriculum," and this is true for each of us in meeting the challenges of daily life and as a teacher meeting the challenges and delights of a mindfulness class.

How to Learn

For a new teacher, there is no substitute for sitting in on a class with an experienced MBCT instructor. In sitting in, it is good to pay particular attention to the ways in which the general characteristics we have mentioned are enacted in moment-to-moment teaching in the class.

Types of Questions Asked in Inquiry

An instructor keeps a balance in the types of questions he or she asks. A skilled instructor:

- Uses open questions (e.g., "What did you notice at that point?") rather than closed questions, which require only a "yes" or "no" answer (e.g., "Did you notice any tensing up in your body?").
- Uses questions and statements that open space for discovery (e.g., "Would you be willing to tell me more?"; "Can you say more about that?") rather than questions or statements that close the space, such as "yes" or "no" questions, fixing, or solution-focused statements (e.g., responding to a statement about an experience of

discomfort in a sitting practice by saying, "Many people feel discomfort when they sit," implying that this "goes with the territory" so there is nothing further to be investigated).

- Asks permission to continue where appropriate, so participants feel safe and are in control of when the process ends (e.g., the teacher may say after one or two questions, "Is it OK to ask some more about that?").
- Gives time to each "layer" of the inquiry (each part of the learning circle).

QUESTIONING THAT CAN BE HELPFUL, "LAYER BY LAYER"*

Step 1. Direct Experiencing

Immediately after a formal practice, or when discussing home practice, the first area of inquiry focuses on the *direct experience* of the practice. There is an emphasis on exploration of physical sensations: Thoughts and emotions are explored in connection with how they interconnect and/ or express themselves as sensations. Here are some of the questions often asked at this point (but note that there is no sense of scheduling a particular order of questions or feeling obliged to ask them all).

- "What did you notice?"
  o "Inside your body?"
    ■ "Physical sensations?"
    ■ "Emotions/feelings, and sensations connected to them?"
  o "In your mind?"
    ■ "Thoughts or images?"
    ■ "About now, the past, the future?"
    ■ "Where did these take you?"
    ■ "Outside your body?"
    ■ "Sounds?"

---

*We are grateful for discussions and an unpublished 2007 manuscript (J. Mark G. Williams, Catherine Crane, Judith M. Soulsby, Melissa Blacker, Florence Meleo-Meyer, and Robert Stahl, *The Inquiry Process: Aims, Intentions, and Teaching Considerations*) that informed this section, which also draws from Crane.[90]

- "When your mind wandered, where did it go?"
  - o "Thoughts (memories, worries, planning, time, food)?"
  - o "Body sensations (of restlessness, pain, boredom)?"
  - o "Emotions (sad, angry, fearful, happy, secure, loving)?"
- "What was your reaction, if any, to these experiences? How did you relate to them?"

Step 2a. Exploring the Direct "Noticing" within a Personal Context of Understanding

- "How did you *feel* when your mind wandered?"
- "What did you *do* when your mind wandered (let it wander, get involved in the thoughts, bring it back—did you bring it back with gentleness, firmness, guilt, annoyance, amusement, judgment, etc., and what sensations in the body did you notice came with the gentleness/firmness/guilt/annoyance)?"
- "How did bringing awareness to this experience affect it?"
- "Is this pattern of experience that you describe familiar? If so, in what ways?"

Step 2b. Exploring the Integration of Learning in Layers 1 and 2 into a Wider Context of Understanding

Into this dialogue is woven understanding of the potential relationships between these observations of the individual's experience; the effects of bringing mindful awareness to the processes of the mind; and the understandings about the ways that, for example, "depression mind" is triggered and perpetuates itself. This is sometimes a process of facilitating participants in drawing out these connections and at other times offering teaching which supports this integration. Notice how this is done in the inquiry on pages 264 and 266.

Step 3. Invitation to Investigate Further

An inquiry may end (though not always) with an invitation to explore an experience further in home practice or day-to-day life. This may be relatively formal and offered to the whole class (e.g., the invitation to eat one meal mindfully after the raisin exercise in Session 1, and the invitation to notice moments of autopilot by choosing one routine activity that is usually done on autopilot and see what is noticed when we pay attention to the experience). Or an invitation may be offered to a participant who has commented on particular aspects of mindfulness practice. For example, people who report that when they notice their minds have wandered, always feel that they have failed, may have realized during the inquiry that they do not know what their body feels like at that point. They may be invited to notice, in their home practice, how their bodies react when they discover their minds have wandered and feel they have failed. Notice how the invitation itself can change the spirit of the practice: from that of striving to keep the mind still, to being open to investigate the experience when it is restless. Here a "problem" has been turned into an opportunity. The spirit is one of turning toward any chances to notice that arise— whether mind wandering or anything else—and this "looking out for opportunities" itself conveys a very different attitude to the practice.

Be aware of the edge that is being worked here. The potency of mindfulness-based learning rests on the direct experiential knowing that evolves in participants in its own time. The process of linking this learning with a context of understanding can have the effect of either consolidating and validating this experience or closing things down. It therefore needs to be worked in with skill and sensitivity. As teachers, we remain aware of how much the material for this process is generated by the participants or by the teacher. The experienced teacher allows enough time for the actuality of experience and relationship with experience to be explored before introducing any "learning" elements.

Let us, finally, turn to the inquiries after the raisin practice and body scan as examples to illustrate some of these more general principles.

The instructor poses the first question to the group, asking, "What did you notice about this experience?" or "What did you become aware of during this practice?" and "Would anyone like to comment on their experience?" The intention here is to help participants stay with their direct experience of (in this case) eating the raisin: the reactions in the body, in thoughts and/or feelings. They are helped to see clearly their experience, and perhaps also the sequence of their appearance in the mind–body, then to see what happened in the very next moment—the reactivity that tells us how we are relating to what has come up.

An example might be a participant who reports noticing sensations of sweetness as he or she bit down on a raisin, thinking how lovely this was, then having thoughts about buying raisins as a snack and feeling disappointed that his or her child did not like raisins. The instructor may reflect back what has been said, perhaps asking at what point he or she noticed the mind "going off"—perhaps asking if the mind wandered any further (once it had got into thinking *about* things rather than sensing). At some point, the instructor may gather other similar experiences, then comment, with a lightness of touch, how easily the mind "finds other things to do" when it "thinks it has seen enough" or how easily we get bored, and how the "hurry-up mind" can turn up—how the mind appears to have a mind of its own. Note how the instructor has seamlessly shifted the focus from simple experience to contextualizing or universalizing the experience by reference to *how the mind appears to have a mind of its own.* Here is an implicit invitation for participants to notice this in daily life, and an embodiment of the spirit in which to notice: friendly curiosity rather than harsh judgment.

Similarly, experiences and discoveries about the contrast with the usual way we eat, gathered together, lead naturally to a discussion of the time we spend on autopilot. It is usually not long before someone comments, "This way of eating a raisin is different from how I would ordinarily eat raisins." The question "In what way?" or "Can you say more about that?" may foster reflection on the comparison between doing something mindfully and the more routine or habitual ways we normally engage with the world.

The richness of the scent of the raisin, or its appearance, or its texture, may lead to comments about how slowing things down a little and paying attention can change the nature of our experience in surprising ways—some pleasant and some unpleasant.

Notice what has happened here. The instructor has started with participants' own experiences; invited class members to reflect on it while the experience is still "fresh"; then made full use of the discoveries to contextualize the practice in terms of the themes of Session 1: autopilot; mind wandering as normal, and the way that paying attention—doing one things at a time—can transform the experience in subtle and not-so-subtle ways.

More general learning may be alluded to relatively easily, if briefly: how, if we spend time on autopilot, our moods may escalate without us realizing it is happening; or that when we are brooding about something, life passes us by.

Instructors who are relatively new to MBCT—although they find the inquiry somewhat puzzling or even intimidating—say that they have little problem with the inquiry following the raisin practice. So one way to think of any inquiry is to use the raisin as a prototype: experience–reflection–context–invitation.

Let us take another example. If, in Session 2, participants noticed that their breathing felt shallow, then the instructor might ask when they first noticed that, and whether they noticed any reaction to it. At that point, some participants might report that they simply noticed it, then returned to the focus on sensations. Others at that point might report that they found themselves distracted. In either case, there are choice points here. The instructor may ask how long the distraction lasted, and what happened then (asking for more *reflection* on the experience), commenting that the aim at this stage is to notice the mind "going away" and, wherever it has gone, to bring the attention back to the breath. In these cases, the instructor is choosing to stay with the *learning* that each of us needs to do, again and again, that it is in the nature of the mind to wander; it is not a mistake, and it is possible to wake up to this mind wandering, so that we realize we have many more choices about where the mind is, moment to moment. The *invitation* for the next week's practice—both formal and informal—would then be to see if it is possible to notice how the mind wanders away from where we had intended it to be.

Or, if the instructor chooses and there is sufficient time in the session, he or she may ask participants if they were aware of what had taken them away from the breath—thoughts or feelings (i.e., asking for more *reflection on experience*)? Let us say that the participants comment that they thought that their breath was *too* shallow. The instructor may notice that there is an implicit comparison going on here ("This is not how things should be"). But the instructor noticing this does not mean that anything need be said at this point. It is more helpful to ask: " . . . and then what happened?" Participants may say that they wondered what this might mean: "I thought maybe I was just tense, then I thought it might be the old problem coming back."

Here is another choice point. It can feel tempting to ask about what the "old problem" is. But recall that this might take the class away from the task in hand, to investigate the actual experience of the mind being distracted by thoughts/images about the past, or worries about the future. So *if* the intention of this inquiry is to focus on the patterns of the mind, then the possible *learning* is about the processes of the mind, not its content: how the mind rapidly cascades from (1) sensations to (2) comparisons with how things should be, to (3) asking "Why?" questions, then (4) to past and future thoughts. And all in an instant that can easily be missed. If this is the learning, then this is where the instructor focuses, for the "content" (e.g., "my old problem") will differ from individual to individual. Many different issues take different participants away from their intended focus. But *underneath all these differences in content, there are likely to be common features in process.* One of these is that an implicit comparison ("This is not how things should be") starts a "problem solver" module in the mind that feels very compelling but often takes us down a track that turns out not to be skillful, and may even increase our suffering and distress.

Note that in each case participants may jump to providing a narrative prompted by their experience, and it may be necessary to redirect them gently to stay at the level of process: What sensations, thoughts, and feelings were present? In time, participants learn to see that their reactions and internal experience are actually composed of individual elements of body sensations, thoughts, feelings, and behavioral tendencies. Participants may come to see their automatic tendencies and habits more clearly, and will be helped by hearing from others about common patterns of the doing mode of mind. Class discussion may also reveal the ways in which we all tend to add layers of difficulty to existing problems, anticipate the future, or dwell in the past.

In drawing the discussion together, the instructor may interweave the observations of individual experiences with an understanding of the way that the "ruminative mind" can be triggered and perpetuate itself. Sometimes what is called for is that the instructor facilitate the group itself making these connections, while it might be necessary at other times to offer teaching points that support this integration.

CONCLUDING REMARKS

It is important to acknowledge that in training and in the early days of teaching, most instructors find inquiry challenging. Simply knowing this can be helpful in allowing any sense of difficulty with this aspect of the MBCT program to be seen more as "this is the way it is for everyone" rather than as some reflection of personal deficiency or failure.

On the other hand, it is just as important to stress that it gets easier with practice—by which we do not just mean that inquiry gets more skillful the more often we do it (which, in general, it does). Rather, we also mean that the instructor's continuing and deepening personal practice of mindfulness is a vital support for teaching this aspect of the MBCT program. It is the instructor's practice that enables him or her to embody the qualities of "being"—openness, presence, steadiness, curiosity, patience, kindness, compassion—even in a situation where, quite literally, one may not know what is going to happen from one moment to the next. The situation in the teaching room mimics the situation in our own daily practice, where we also do not know what is going to arise in the next moment. The spirit that the instructor brings to the inquiry is one of *really wanting to know how things unfolded.* This is not a "put-on" or false curiosity, but a genuine exploration of emerging themes that is important for both participants in the dialogue (teacher and participant) because both can learn from it.

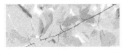 

CHAPTER 13

Allowing/Letting Be

Session 5

There is a story told of a king who had three sons. The first was handsome and very popular. When he was 21, his father built a palace in the city for him. The second son was intelligent and also very popular. When he became 21, his father built a palace in the city for him as well. The third son, neither handsome nor intelligent, was unfriendly and unpopular. When he was 21, the king's counselors said: "There is no further room in the city. Have a palace built outside the city for your son. You can have it built so it will be strong. You can send some of your guards to prevent it being attacked by the ruffians who live outside the city walls." So the king built such a palace and sent some of his soldiers to protect it.

A year later, the son sent a message to his father. "I cannot live here. The ruffians are too strong." So the counselors said, "Build another palace, bigger and stronger, and 20 miles away from the city and the ruffians. With more soldiers, it will easily be able to withstand attacks from the nomadic tribes that pass that way." So the king built such a palace and sent 100 of his soldiers to protect it.

A year later, a message came from the son: "I cannot live here. The tribes are too strong." So the counselors said: "Build a castle, a large castle, 100 miles away. It will be big enough to house 500 soldiers, and strong enough to withstand attacks from the peoples that live over the border." So the king built such a castle, and sent 500 of his soldiers to protect it.

But a year later, the son sent another message to the king. "Father, the attacks of the neighboring peoples are too strong. They have attacked twice, and if they attack a third time, I fear for my life and the lives of your soldiers."

And the king said to his counselors, "Let him come home and he can live in the palace with me. For it is better that I learn to love my son than spend all the energy and resources of my kingdom keeping him at a distance."

People who have been depressed in the past have often spent a great deal of effort trying to avoid or push away negative memories, feelings, and experiences. Avoiding unpleasantness and trying to ensure that we minimize discomfort takes (as the king in the story found out) a great deal of effort. Although it can be exhausting, many people feel that the strategy has worked for them in the past, that the energy is worth the exhaustion. Why, then, should they risk adopting alternative strategies?

The theme of this session is to introduce and cultivate the possibility of a radically different relationship to unwanted experience— that of allowing, and letting be. The work in the first half of the program has enabled participants to become more aware of where their attention wanders, to use this awareness to bring them back to the present, and to rely on the breath as the vehicle for moving attention around in these ways. These efforts have allowed a scaffolding to be put into place that will support the work required in the second half of the program, namely, using these skills in the service of preventing relapse and cultivating a different relationship to life more generally. Central to these attempts is the development of a different relationship to experience.

CULTIVATING A DIFFERENT RELATIONSHIP TO EXPERIENCE

A relationship to experience that is characterized by allowing/letting be is not easy to describe or to cultivate. In preparing ourselves for this task, it is helpful to keep three questions in mind: What is the flavor of allowing/letting be? Why is it important in preventing relapse? How can it best be cultivated or used?

BOX 13.1

Theme and Curriculum for Session 5

THEME

Relating differently to unpleasant feelings and sensations—allowing things to be as they already are. We can disempower aversion by intentionally bringing to all experience a sense of "allowing" it to be, just as it is, without judging it or trying to make it different. Such an attitude of acceptance embodies a basic attitude of kindness to experience. From this clear seeing we can choose what, if anything, needs to change.

AGENDA

- 30- to 40-minute sitting meditation—awareness of breath and body; noticing how we relate to our experiences through the reactions we have to whatever thoughts, feelings, or body sensations arise; introducing a difficulty within the practice and noting its effects on the body and reactions to it.*
- Practice review.
- Home practice review.
- Breathing space (with added instructions) and review.
- Read Rumi's poem "The Guest House."
- Distribute Session 5 participant handouts.
- Home practice assignment:
  - Working with difficulty meditation on Days 1, 3, and 5; use no guided practice on Days 2, 4, and 6 instead, but guide yourself through the same meditation.
  - 3-Minute Breathing Space—Regular (3 times a day).
  - 3-Minute Breathing Space—Added Instructions (whenever you notice unpleasant feelings).

(cont.)

---

*An alternative format is to start with the 30- to 40-minute sitting meditation (as in Session 4), then proceed with the practice and home practice reviews, allowing the discussion of how to relate to the difficult to emerge from these dialogues, then move to a shorter practice to focus on exploring the difficult (see Box 13.3).

PREPARATION AND PLANNING

In addition to your personal preparation, remember to bring the poem "The Guest House" to class.

PARTICIPANT HANDOUTS FOR SESSION 5

Session 5–Handout 1. Summary of Session 5: Allowing/Letting Be

Session 5–Handout 2. Using the Breathing Space: Extra Guidance

Session 5–Handout 3. Home Practice for the Week Following Session 5

Session 5–Handout 4. Home Practice Record Form—Session 5

Session 5–Handout 5. "The Guest House"

What Is the Flavor of Allowing/Letting Be?

Allowing difficult feelings to be in awareness means that we register their presence before making a choice about how to respond to them. This takes a conscious commitment and the deliberate deployment of energy. "Allowing" things is not the same as being resigned to them. Resignation implies passivity and a degree of helplessness. Such difficulty in getting across the flavor of acceptance illustrates the limitations of single words as vehicles to convey the essence of a particular stance or relationship to experience.

Poetry can be used as an alternative vehicle for communicating this different relationship to experience. For example, consider the attitude of active acceptance that is expressed simply and profoundly in the poem "The Guest House" by Rumi, a 13th-century Sufi poet.

We read "The Guest House" in full during Session 5 to illustrate just how radical a shift we seek. Here is someone speaking about assuming a positive relationship to unwanted feelings with phrases and words such as "welcome," "treat each guest honorably," "invite them in," and "be grateful." Is this attitude even possible? Might we actually cultivate a basic friendliness to *all* experiences, including the most difficult and feared?

BOX 13.2

"The Guest House"

This being human is a guest house.
Every morning a new arrival.

A joy, a depression, a meanness,
some momentary awareness comes
as an unexpected visitor.

Welcome and entertain them all!
Even if they're a crowd of sorrows,
who violently sweep your house
empty of its furniture,

still, treat each guest honorably.
He may be clearing you out
for some new delight.

The dark thought, the shame, the malice.
meet them at the door laughing,
and invite them in.

Be grateful for whoever comes,
because each has been sent
as a guide from beyond.

Even if we find such a stance difficult to imagine, making even a tentative first step in this direction can be invaluable and transformative. This involves meeting things, including our strong emotions, as they are, letting go of any attempts to show them the door.

Embarking on the next step, to take a stance of meeting each and every thought, feeling, or body sensation "at the door laughing," is even more radical. It goes against our tendency to distinguish between and react differently to the things we enjoy on one hand, and those we dread on the other. Saki Santorelli echoes this when he writes that "the poem may be suggesting an inner attitude toward whatever we encounter, urging us to consider the possibility of meeting our grief and pain open handedly. This is not our usual way of meeting adversity" (p. 151).[93] Most of the time, the effort we put into our impulse to resist, avoid, or withdraw keeps us from seeing that an alternative approach is possible. This striking presentation of an alternative approach is one of the things that is so valuable about this poem.

Why Is It Important to Cultivate Allowing/Letting Be?

Allowing is so important because, for one thing, its opposite is too risky. An unwillingness to allow negative feelings, physical sensations, or thoughts to be present (due to aversion) is the first link in the mental chain that can rapidly lead to the reinstatement of old, automatic, habitual, relapse-related patterns of mind. We see this every time someone says, "I'm stupid to think like this" or "I should be strong enough to cope with that."

By contrast, to bring *intentionally* an alternative relationship of allowing/letting be to unwanted experiences has effects on a number of fronts. First, by encouraging us to pay attention more intentionally, it serves to offset the tendency for our attention to be automatically "hijacked" by passing thoughts or moods. Second, it shifts the basic stance toward experience. The challenge is to move from a stance of "not wanting" to one of "opening," allowing the chain of automatic reactions to be broken earlier in the process.

> Shifting the basic stance toward experience, from one of "not wanting" to one of "opening," allows the chain of conditioned, habitual responses to be broken at the first link.

Third, it gives us a chance to see that we can be with the feelings and still be OK—that all feelings pass of their own accord if we do not force them. Consider a thought such as "If this goes on any longer, I'm going to scream." Allowing it simply to be there and, as best we can, noticing the effects it has on the body and seeing the moment-by-moment changes in its intensity may offer us the chance to see that the thoughts and feelings may fade. We shall have more to say about how to deal with thoughts in Session 6.

How Can We Cultivate and Use Allowing/Letting Be?

Much of the previous discussion illustrates the difficulty of purely "conceptual" or overeffortful attempts to change our basic stance or relationship to experience. Patients frequently may have been admonished to be more loving, caring, and accepting, but the question remains, how to do it? These qualities are unlikely to be produced merely by an effort of will. In this session, therefore, we examine an alternative route for learning to relate differently: working through the body by bringing our attention/awareness to manifestations of difficult experience.

> Bringing awareness to the body offers us an alternative way for learning to relate differently to difficult experience.

One way to begin "opening to the difficult" is to think of the practice as having two steps. The basic approach remains to become mindfully aware of whatever is most predominant in one's moment-by-moment experience. So, if the mind is repeatedly drawn to a particular place and to particular thoughts, feelings, or body sensations, then the instructions are to bring awareness deliberately and intentionally to whatever is pulling for our attention, noting the sense of being pulled again and again to the same place. That is the first step.

The second step is to bring awareness to how we are relating, *in the body*, to whatever arises in that place. There are different ways we can find ourselves relating to things to which the mind gets repeatedly drawn. We can "be with" an arising thought, feeling, or body sensation, but in a nonaccepting, reactive way. If we like it, we tend to hold on to it, to want it to stay; we become attached to it. If we do not like it because it is painful, unpleasant, or uncomfortable in some way, we tend to contract and to push it away out of fear, irritation, or annoyance; we want it to go. Each of these responses is the opposite of allowing.

Allowing offers a different, more skillful approach: to register that the experiences are here, to let them to be as they are, in this moment, and simply to hold them in awareness. Responding in this way, described as "allowing," "letting be," or "holding in awareness," conveys the core theme of "willingness to experience" difficult feeling states. This is in contrast to automatically reacting to these thoughts or emotions.

DELIBERATELY BRINGING
THE DIFFICULT/PROBLEMATIC TO MIND

At this point, whenever possible, we use problems that arise naturally in the course of the program as opportunities to practice this different way of relating to inner experience. These problems can be excellent "grist for the mill," and this is why we welcome expressions of boredom and irritation from participants earlier in the program. Embodying such a welcoming attitude can itself feed a general shift in one's relationship to the difficult. But if no such experiences arise, then what we ask in this session is that participants intentionally bring a problem to the "workbench of the mind" in order to practice relating differently to it. Again, doing this intentionally creates the implicit message: The purpose is not to get rid of your difficulties.

Accepting experience means simply allowing space for whatever is going on, rather than trying to create some other state. Through acceptance, we settle back into natural awareness of what is present. We let it be—we simply notice and observe whatever is already present. This is a new way to deal with experiences that have a strong pull on our attention.

> Allowing experience means simply allowing space for whatever is going on, rather than trying to create some other state.

The aim of this session is to guide participants, step by step, into this new approach to difficulty, through an "exploring difficulty" meditation (see Box 13.3). The meditation teaches participants how to respond when their awareness repeatedly gets pulled in the same direction, to a particular thought stream, feeling, or set of body sensations. The aim here is to

BOX 13.3

Inviting Difficulty In and Working with It through the Body

Sit for a few minutes, focusing on the sensations of breathing, then widening the awareness to take in the body as a whole (see Box 10.2, Sitting Meditation: Mindfulness of the Breath and Body in Chapter 10).

While you are sitting, if you notice that your attention keeps being pulled away to painful thoughts or emotions, you can explore something different from what we have been practicing up until now.

Until now, when you have been sitting and notice that your mind has wandered, the instruction has been simply to notice where the mind had gone, then gently and firmly escort the attention back to the breath or body, or back to whatever you intended to be focusing on.

Now you can explore a different way to respond. Instead of bringing attention back from a thought or feeling, now allow the thought or feeling to *remain* in the mind. Then, shifting the attention into the body, see if you can become aware of any physical sensations in the body that come along with the thought or emotion.

Then when you have identified such sensations, deliberately move the focus of attention to the part of the body where these sensations are strongest. Perhaps imagine you could "breath into" this region on the inbreath, and "breathe out" from it on the outbreath—just as you practiced in the body scan, not to change the sensations but to explore them, to see them clearly.

If there are no difficulties or concerns coming up for you now and you want to explore this new approach, then, if you choose, you might *deliberately bring to mind a difficulty* that is going on in your life at the moment—something you don't mind staying with for a short while. It does not have to be very important or critical, but something that you are aware of as somewhat unpleasant, something unresolved: perhaps a misunderstanding or an argument; a situation where you feel somewhat angry, regretful, or guilty over something that has happened. If nothing comes to mind, perhaps you might choose something from the past, either recent or distant, that once caused unpleasantness.

Now, once you have focused on some troubling thought or situation—some worry or intense feeling—allow yourself to take some time to tune in to any physical sensations in the body that the difficulty evokes.

(cont.)

See if you are able to note, approach, and investigate inwardly what feelings are arising in your body, becoming mindful of those physical sensations, deliberately directing your focus of attention to the region of the body where the sensations are strongest in a gesture of an embrace, a welcoming.

This gesture might include breathing into that part of the body on the inbreath and breathing out from that region on the outbreath, exploring the sensations, watching their intensity shift up and down from one moment to the next.

Once your attention has settled on the body sensations and they are vividly present in the field of awareness, unpleasant as they may be, you might try deepening the attitude of acceptance and openness to whatever sensations you are experiencing by saying to yourself from time to time: "It is here now. It is OK to be open to it. Whatever it is, it's already here. Let me open to it." Soften and open to the sensations you become aware of, intentionally letting go of tensing and bracing. Say to yourself: "Softening, Opening" on each outbreath.

Then see if is possible to stay with the awareness, exploring these body sensations and your relationship to them, breathing with them, accepting them, letting them be, allowing them to be just as they are.

Remember that, by saying "It's already here" or "It's OK," you are not judging the original situation or saying that everything's fine, but simply helping your awareness, right now, to remain open to the sensations in the body.

You do not have to *like* these feelings—it is natural not to want to have them around. You may find it helpful to say to yourself, inwardly, "It's OK not to want these feelings; they're already here; let me be open to them."

If you choose, you can also experiment with holding in awareness both the sensations in the body and the feeling of the breath moving in and out, as you breathe with the sensations moment by moment.

And when you notice that the body sensations are no longer pulling your attention to the same degree, simply return 100% to sitting with the breath in the body as the primary object of attention.

If, in the next few minutes, no powerful body sensations arise, feel free to try this exercise with any body sensations you notice, even if they have no particular emotional charge.

Adapted with permission from Williams, Teasdale, Segal, and Kabat-Zinn.[76] Copyright 2007 by The Guilford Press.

invite a radically new—and counterintuitive—way of responding when the pull on the attention is strong, and the mind keeps going back to the same place, which happens in ruminative brooding.

We introduce in this session explicit instructions that extend the practice of the previous sessions, inviting participants to explore the possibility of allowing the thought or feeling to remain in the mind as they shift attention to the body to notice where the body is reacting to the difficulty.

What is happening here? When we are able to identify where in the body the physical sensations are the strongest, we are better able to become aware of any aversion present. The physical sensations of contraction or bracing, of ache or tensing, are the signatures of our aversion to distress, the bodily manifestations of such an attitude of aversion. So in this way we are able to see more clearly the physical sense of resisting, holding, pushing away, or tensing and bracing. These body sensations are first brought into awareness, then a sense of "opening" and "softening" on the outbreath is brought to them, in order to work on the second step, *letting go of aversion.*

This is why, once the attention has moved to the body sensations and we have the item in the field of awareness, we invite participants to say to themselves silently, "It's OK. Whatever it is, it's OK. Let me be open to this." The instructions ask people to stay with the awareness of these body sensations and their relationship to them, breathing with them, accepting them, letting them be. We suggest that they experiment with softening and opening to the sensations they become aware of, saying, "Soften, open" on each outbreath. Note that the intention here is not to change the sensations; we are not striving to "soften" the *sensations* themselves, but to soften the way in which they are held in awareness, the way we are relating to them.

In this way, the practice aims to explore the consequences of reversing the habitual tendency of the mind to move *away* from or push away the painful or difficult. This is done through intentionally bringing awareness (a gentle, kindly, friendly awareness) *to* the sense of how the difficult is manifesting *in the body*, including aversion-related physical sensations. Little by little, the practice teaches us how to reverse the habitual rejection of the difficult and the unpleasant, and to cultivate an attitude of acceptance and friendliness. Bringing a gentle curiosity to something is, itself, part of acceptance. Holding something in awareness is an implicit affirmation that we can face it, name it, and work with it. Also, letting go of aversion in the body is particularly relevant to the needs of participants who have been depressed because it provides an alternative to an approach based on thoughts. Focusing on the body may help participants avoid getting caught up in ruminative patterns of thinking.

> Intentionally bringing awareness (a gentle, kindly, friendly awareness) *to* the sense of how the difficult is manifesting *in the body*, including aversion-related physical sensations, we can begin to reverse our habitual rejection of the difficult and the unpleasant, and to cultivate an attitude of acceptance and friendliness.

We find it helpful to support this inner work with detailed suggestions for exploring edges, watching the intensity go up and down, and *breathing into* as ways to carry awareness, supported by words such as "It's OK" and invitations to feel it. These all add up to a package of friendship rather than hostility toward experience. The stance of the instructor is obviously crucial if this is to take place with any authenticity.

BUT IT IS DIFFICULT

Consider the difficulty that one person reported when we practiced this in the class:

P: I find it difficult to say "It's OK" over some things. Because when you say "It's OK," it's not OK. It has to do with noise from the dogs that belong to the people next door. The dogs aren't actually theirs. They belong to their parents-in-law, but they look after them when their in-laws go away. It happened again today. They were barking and barking. They keep them tied up outside when they go out, and even sometimes when they are in, and they bark and howl all day long.

   I tried the breathing and, in the end, I just had to leave the house. It was no use. I kept ringing them up and getting the answering machine. I hammered on the door. Nobody answered. I just had to go out in the end. Now, I find it very difficult with something as invasive as that to say "It's OK." I couldn't deal with it today at all.

I: The words are simply meant to be a way to help you in that particular moment to come to a point of balance. It is not actually the final decision on the state of the world. There's a story in a book written by a famous American teacher of meditation. He was in India, and after a great deal of effort, found himself the ideal little house perched up in the mountains, and he booked it for a few months of absolute peace and stillness for a retreat. The day after he had got himself settled in there, a couple of hundred yards down the hill, a group of Girl Guides arrived and set up loudspeakers on poles all the way around and played pop music full blast from 6:00 A.M. to 10:00 P.M.

P: I bet they had dogs, too!

I: Dogs and pop music; and all through loudspeakers! He suffered the same experience as you. It took days and weeks before he could say, "That's just the way things are just now." Acceptance is not something you can immediately turn on. It's really making some gesture toward not immediately triggering a range of automatic responses.

Clearly, this participant was not only having a difficult time with her neighbors, but also she could not see how coming to the classes was going to help. Note, however, that not only the noise was upsetting but also her own reaction to it. In some ways, the classes were in danger of contributing to the sense that she was not handling it very well.

P: I felt I failed because I hadn't coped with it. I did the breathing, and I did everything else, and then I just had to go out because I couldn't get on with anything. And I thought: "This is a failure, running away from it"; but it was the only thing I could do at that moment.

We can see here that in addition to the problem of the noise, she had noticed her reaction and judged herself harshly for it. She was "failing" by running away from it. The instructor picked up on this point.

I: This is very very important. It may really have been the only thing you could do, but was it a failure? This is the thing to hone in on. The reason for telling you about the man in India was that he couldn't immediately cope with it either. That is just how it is sometimes, so adding "This is a failure" is extra and can create more problems for you.

P: Yes. What was getting to me was that there were several things that I needed to do and to get on with in the house. Every time I called and got the answering machine, a sort of rage came over me.

I: You may not be able to do anything about the noise, I mean, once you have done everything you can, phoned them, knocked on the door, and nothing has happened; but you still have the possibility of doing something about your internal state.

P: I agree. This is why I am still here, to be honest; because I found that doing this breathing exercise meant that the turmoil didn't go on for so long, you know. This is what I found. When I came back, and it was quiet, I wasn't on tenterhooks all the time, thinking, "God, when is it going to start again." That's a good point.

I: You know, acceptance, which is the name of the game we are talking about here, is very difficult to cultivate. But it is something that we may benefit from tremendously if we simply remember to cultivate it as best we can in any moment.

WORKING THROUGH THE BODY

Might the instruction to bring a difficult situation to mind deliberately do more harm than good? Our reasoning for this instruction is that just as yoga practice gives people the opportunity to work with body sensations that have been induced by the stretches, so our participants may need experience at working with negative thoughts and moods (and their consequences in the body) that they have deliberately brought to mind. Feedback from participants suggests that they find this very helpful. Consider how, in a report from a class of our colleague Surbala Morgan, one participant was able (after some struggle) to bring a difficult thing to mind, then to work with it in the body (by bringing awareness to it, breathing into it, and discovering a wider space within which it could exist). We pick up the session where the participant was discussing her reaction to the request to bring to mind a difficult thought.

P: When you said it, I thought, "I'm not sure I'm going to be able to do this. I can't think of anything." And I got worried that I was going to miss out on this exercise. Then, suddenly, something came up into my mind. It was to do with our son, who has been giving us a really hard time recently—staying out all hours, hanging around with people we don't trust. We had a real crisis 2 months ago involving the police. As soon as this came into my mind, I knew it was going to be difficult to get out of my mind again. I try not to think about it at all, but every time I do, I think, "Where have I gone wrong?"

The next instruction, to become aware of what was happening in the body, took her even more deeply into a place she did not want to be.

P: And then, when you said, "How do you feel physically?", that was quite dreadful. And I realized that is exactly how I feel when I think about what's happening in the family. And then you said, "What is your body doing?" At that moment, it was as though my breathing stopped completely. And you were saying, "Recognize what's tense." And I thought, "Yes, it's all tense around here."

Then, a change occurs. The instruction is given to bring awareness to and to breathe into the place in the body that is most tense. This was something of a transformative experience for her.

P: And then when you said to breathe into it, that was really good because it was giving it space. Before, it was like the whole of my body around here was really tight and knotted. And then you said, "Breathe into it," and it suddenly became like a great big empty space . . . with the air coming in and out. You know, sometimes when you come back from holiday, the house is a bit musty, so you open all the doors and windows to let the air blow through. . . . Well, it was like that . . . having doors and windows open, and with curtains blowing and air coming in and out. And it was really amazing. And the tension about my son was still there, you know. I thought, "Oh, you're still there, but never mind, the wind's blowing through and that's all right."

I: So although it was still there, there was more space?

P: Mmm. Yes, and I could sort of look at it. The feeling in my body was still a bit tight, but it was much smaller, and all the air was sort of flowing around it. At the beginning, it was the whole thing. Because I was so tight, you know, there was nothing else there.

The instructor was then able to use this participant's experience to illustrate one of the central themes of the mindfulness approach, and the participant responded by giving a graphic description of the reduced size of the problem, and indicated an increased willingness in the future to explore an alternative to pushing difficult things away.

I: This is exactly what we're about here. This is a really good example. Because it's not about trying to get rid of these states. There's always going to be something going on. There's always going to be something distressing or difficult. And it's not about not having the feelings that go along with those difficult states, but it's exactly as you described—having more space around the feelings, so that there's the discomfort, the distress, and there's more of you, and there's breathing there as well.

P: To begin with, it was like a solid mass of rock. It was huge. It was so solid that you couldn't get around it, but then it shrank to a small stone. It was still stone . . . but it was small. It's really good. Because I think, probably I have been pushing the issue away and sort of sitting on it, and not letting it come up fully to the surface. I haven't allowed it before to simply be there. I thought it would just overwhelm me.

I: It felt as if it would take you over or . . . ?

P: Yes, I think so. Yes, it probably would take me over. It was too much to let in and so my natural reaction, well, before this course, would have been just to tense and push it away, and not even to face it.

I: And now . . .

P: And now—now I've got all this air under there.

I: This is lovely, isn't it? So in a sense, it's less scary that these things are there. It's still not pleasant, you know. It would be nice if you could get rid of all the negatives. But it's not possible. But you're now more able to allow them to be here and not feel crushed by them.

P: Yes, and I started thinking, "Oh, I might like to do that again, just to try it again," which is quite amazing because in the past I would never think, "Ah, I'll have that feeling again."

I: Mmmm. It's very different then. Remember the poem about welcoming each guest across the threshold? It's like you're becoming more welcoming to all different sorts of states.

P: Yes.

IS THIS "ALLOWING"
OR A CLEVER WAY TO FIX THINGS?

One of the most subtle and difficult issues is how to bring an allowing attitude to something without having the hidden agenda of "fixing" it. The distinction between fixing and allowing is a difficult one to grasp, perhaps because when people talk about allowing something, often they go on to describe positive and deep changes that they have noticed as a result. Allowing is then linked to positive outcomes, so it is natural then to try to reproduce such a positive outcome and use "allowing" as part of "doing" mode, as a means of achieving the goal of relaxation or happiness. In the following transcript, we read that Katie, a professional fund-raiser, sees herself as making progress in dealing with some work-related stress. At first it seems that an old style of coping, by distraction and pushing away, seems to have made things easier for her. Rereading the transcript with the theme of this session in mind, however, it is clear that, at some level, she used the focus on the breath to fix a difficult situation, without any real shift toward a relationship of acceptance.

> "There was this person at work doing some rather silly things. I work for a fund-raising business. He was drafting a job description for a new post, but he hadn't given it to the personnel

department to look at. I was trying to explain the procedure he must go through; otherwise, we don't have the authority to advertise the post. He could not see this. I was getting more and more worked up, and I thought to myself, 'No, I've got to try and just concentrate, and get my mind off it and concentrate on my breath.' And I did that, and my mind went back on it again, and I said, 'No, come on back,' and it went back. And it was like a shuttle service! But I did notice this, which rather pleased me. Instead of it going on for an hour winding up, it didn't. This is what I was quite pleased with. It took a while (don't get me wrong), but then I thought to myself, 'No, I'm not thinking about that anymore. It's not continually going on.'"

The danger is that using the breath to escape, fix, or avoid things tends not to make for a lasting change. Consider the following comment:

"Concentrating on the breath again, it took me away from the bad feelings, and then I started thinking, 'Oh, I've got a lot of things that really cause my depression,' and I moved to all of them very quickly and I started feeling a bit 'ugh.'"

At other times, however, it is clear that the practice can change some more fundamental aspect of how a person relates to difficult experiences. In going to visit his father following a routine surgical procedure, Michael reported:

"I was going to visit my father in the hospital last Monday. You never know what you are going to find when you get there . . . you get so many mixed messages. So early Sunday morning, I woke up feeling really apprehensive and panicky. So I thought, 'Unpleasant event, unpleasant event, unpleasant event,' right, which I haven't actually done before. I thought, 'Breathe in to relax.'"

Note that, up to this point, Michael appears to be using the breath to relax, to fix his stress. Then a change occurs:

" . . . but in fact, I thought, 'Now, what are you really feeling?" I was really pleased because I was thinking, 'My tummy's churning, my hands are clenched. I'm having difficulty with breathing.' "

By making use of the "acknowledging" step of the breathing space, bringing awareness intentionally to body sensations, Michael was able to bring a more gentle, friendly attitude to what was going on.

" . . . and then I started breathing . . . and it didn't progress on . . . it didn't progress on. I was really pleased because what it does is make you feel that everything isn't out of control. After all, it doesn't solve everything straightaway—those things were still there—but it did help. It did help."

BREATHING SPACES

We can see by these comments that some people begin to explore the 3-minute breathing space as a way to pause and gather themselves in the midst of troubling situations. It begins to allow some people the chance of seeing a problem (and what might best be done about it) more clearly, rather than getting caught up in older, more depressive ways of viewing things. Our intention for the breathing space is that, if possible, it should always be more than taking a time-out. By encouraging people to step out of automatic pilot, to become aware of the "here and now" of their breath and body sensations, there can be a change in the quality of the awareness of feelings or thoughts: a freshness of perspective that allows people to take a wider view of their experience rather than getting caught up in it.

Once again, the idea is to focus on awareness of body sensations that accompany any intense thought or emotion. This makes it more likely that, should a thought or feeling seem overwhelming, the person would be able to bring awareness to what is most difficult *as it is felt in the body*. From now on, therefore, participants are encouraged to add a sense of "opening to the difficult" after the usual three steps of the breathing space. In addition to the basic instructions for Step 3, the following, further instructions might now be added:

> "Allow your attention to expand to the whole body—especially to any sense of discomfort, tension, or resistance. If these sensations are there, then, bring your awareness there by 'breathing in to them' on the inbreath. Then, breathe out from those sensations, softening and opening with the outbreath. Say to yourself on the outbreath, 'It's OK to feel this. It's OK, whatever it is, it's OK to be open to it.'"

Session 5–Handout 2 offers a breathing space with these added instructions that participants can use following Session 5. Notice that it also offers additional instructions in Steps 1 and 2. These may also help when participants are feeling overwhelmed by things that are happening to them, and they wish to ground themselves using a breathing space.

A NOTE OF CAUTION

Participants vary in the ways in which they use the coping breathing space. Some people see it as an "escape hatch," a brief moment when they can retreat and relax before advancing again into the busyness of their lives. Others see it as an opportunity to bring awareness to what is going on at that moment, to notice and step out of the routine they have become caught up in, so that they might relate differently to the difficulty awaiting them. There is some evidence that the first strategy, though it gives short-term benefits, is not helpful in the long run, perhaps because it does not alter the person's perspective on what gives rise to the feeling of stress and pressure. The second strategy proves to be a more skillful approach to using the breathing space. What is going on here?

An example might help. Most of us have at some time been caught in a severe downpour of rain and have run for shelter, perhaps in a telephone booth or shop doorway. Sometimes we have simply been glad to be out of the rain. We stand for a while, hoping it will stop. We are dry at the moment, but as the rain continues, we know that sooner or later we are going to have to face it; the thing we tried to escape is still there. We may go back out into the rain, cursing it gently as it drenches us. At other times, we may take shelter in a different way. We stand for a while, aware of being wet and not liking it much. We notice that we are hoping it will stop but see that it shows no sign of stopping, and realize that we are going to get wet. We note that being upset about it only adds to our discomfort. We stop clinging to the hope that it will stop raining. Doing this allows us to look more closely at the rain itself. There is something rather compelling about the way it is splashing off everything it hits. We go back out into the rain. It has not stopped, but our relationship to it has changed the whole experience.

Does this mean that if we take the first approach, and find ourselves cursing the rain, we have "failed the test"? Not at all, because nobody is immune to such feelings. They are just the next opportunity to see how best to relate to experience. Just as we can welcome difficult things at the door of the guest house, we can also put out the red carpet for feelings of failure—even failure to welcome the last guest! This is a shameless red carpet! Learning to relate differently in this way takes a great deal of practice, however.

The idea that a practice such as the breathing space is simply a more subtle way of fixing things is very persistent. One participant describes her experience:

P: Last week, when we were talking about breathing into the difficult, I was trying to fix it. That's what I was trying to do. In one way, it's physical, but the mental part, if you like, is "OK, it's a pain; OK, that's what's going on." If you extend that into things like depression and anxiety, and take a kindly interest, then it's a fine line between acknowledging that's what it is and not making it worse by fighting it, and finding a way of breathing into it, but without the intention of getting rid of it.

In reading this transcript, it is clear that here is someone who is getting right to the heart of one of the most radical challenges that MBCT presents.

I: You've put your finger on it. I mean, that is absolutely what it's about, and it's difficult. The most natural tendency in the world is to pretend: "I won't tell that I'm doing this; I'll just take a kindly interest in it; I'm not really going to fix it." But . . . we end up trying to fix it anyway.

She had hit on one of the main themes underpinning the entire program: that inasmuch as we tend to try to fix our problems (however subtly), we run the risk of getting caught in the loop in which we match ourselves against some ideal standard, then find ourselves (and our attempts to fix things) falling short. If this occurs, it puts us back in the "doing" mode and we are likely simply to end up ruminating about how, if meditation doesn't "work," perhaps we have reached the end of the road and had better give up everything. MBCT is based on the radical (in the sense of going to the root) notion that the best way "to get somewhere" is not to try and get anywhere at all, but to open to the way things actually are in this moment; that direct perception and observation will show us new ways of navigating outside the "box" of our habitual patterns of reacting, seeing, and thinking about things.

MINDFULNESS AND CHRONIC PAIN

When MBSR was developed at UMass, much of the program was designed to meet the needs of those referred to the clinic with chronic and unremitting pain. Perhaps this explains why the program was so readily adapted for recurrent depression. When mindfulness is used for physical pain, the main change for patients is not that pain is actually eliminated, but that the *distress* from the pain is reduced. Similarly, for those suffering from recurrent depression, the themes of "allowing" and "letting be" are critical. The key phrase in all this is "relating differently" to what's arising, moment by moment. It's saying, "OK, you're here. Let me turn toward you, even though it scares me." So we move in close. We open the guest house to what we fear; we roll out the red carpet.

How can we do this? The first step is always seeing the mental pain clearly, and also seeing our *reaction* to the experience of it. We notice that, as well as the pain itself, there is in the background a (very natural) wish that it weren't here—we don't want it around. In the "not wanting" and "not liking" the pain gets worse.

So instead we are invited to see clearly what is happening, then to remind ourselves that we do not have to *like* or *want* these feelings. In fact, we might say to ourselves, "It's OK not to like them—it's OK not to want them around." As we explore what happens when we step outside the struggle that arises out of "not wanting," little by little we are learning acceptance, how to relate differently to mental pain and anguish. And we may also discover something profoundly important: that this first step—to let go of trying to force ourselves to like or want things that are inherently unpleasant—is often enough to see the physical sensations more clearly *as* physical sensations; to see our rumination *as* rumination. Out of this new perspective we may see the mental pain change or dissolve by itself, revealing more clearly what action will be most helpful to take as a next step in dealing skillfully with our distress.

ENDNOTE

The story of the king and his three sons, with which we began this chapter, did not say how things ended. The king had realized that keeping his son at a distance used up too many of his resources. That was the first step. But we are left wondering whether he was simply resigned to having to tolerate his son, or whether he had made a fundamental shift toward "welcoming" the difficult, altering radically his relationship with those things in his life that caused him pain and hardship. The ambiguous ending invites the question: Which of these possible attitudes was more likely to bring the king lasting peace?

Summary of Session 5: Allowing/Letting Be

TURNING TOWARD THE DIFFICULT

In Session 5 we extended our formal practice to begin deliberately to turn toward and approach painful experiences with kindness. The basic guideline in this practice is to become mindfully aware of whatever is most predominant in our moment-by-moment experience.

So, the *first step*, if the mind is repeatedly drawn to a particular place, to particular thoughts, feelings, or body sensations, is deliberately to take a gentle and friendly awareness to whatever is pulling for our attention, noting the sense of being pulled again and again to the same place.

The *second step* is to notice, as best we can, how we are relating to whatever is arising in the body or mind. Our reactions to our own thoughts and feelings may determine whether they are passing events or persist. Often we can be with an arising thought, feeling, or body sensation but in a nonallowing, reactive way. If we like it, we may become attached to it, and try to hold on to it. If, on the other hand, we dislike it because it is painful, unpleasant, or uncomfortable in some way, then we may experience fear or irritation, tense up and contract, or try to push it away. Each of these responses is the opposite of allowing.

LETTING GO AND LETTING BE

The easiest way to relax is, first, to let go of trying to make things different. *Allowing experience means simply allowing space for whatever is going on, rather than trying to create some other state.* Through cultivating a "willingness to experience," we settle back into awareness of what is already present. We let it be—we simply notice and observe whatever is already here. This is the way to relate to experiences that have a strong pull on our attention, however powerful they seem. When we see them clearly, it helps prevent us from getting pulled into brooding and ruminating about them, or trying to suppress or avoid them. We begin the process of freeing ourselves from them. We open up the possibility of responding skillfully and with compassion rather than reacting, in knee jerk fashion, by automatically running off old (often unhelpful) strategies.

(cont.)

A NEW PRACTICE

In the class, we explored together this new way of approaching the difficult. If we noticed that our attention kept being pulled away from the breath (or another focus) to painful thoughts, emotions, or feelings, the first step was to become mindfully aware of any physical sensations in the body that were occurring alongside the thought or emotion; we then deliberately moved the focus of awareness to the part of the body where those sensations were strongest. We explored how the breath could provide a useful vehicle to do this—just as we practiced in the body scan, we can take a gentle and friendly awareness to that part of the body by "breathing into" it on the inbreath, and "breathing out" from it on the outbreath.

Once our attention had moved to the body sensations, and they were in the field of awareness, the guidance was to say to ourselves, "It's OK. Whatever it is, it's OK to allow myself to be open to it." Then we just stayed with the awareness of these body sensations and our relationship to them, breathing with them, accepting them, letting them be. It may be helpful to repeat "It's OK. Whatever it is, it's OK. Let me be open to it," using each outbreath to soften and open to the sensations. "Allowing" is *not* resignation—it allows us, as a vital first step, to become fully aware of difficulties and to respond to them skillfully.

Using the Breathing Space: Extra Guidance

You have been practicing the breathing space regularly, three times a day, and whenever you need it. Now we suggest that whenever you feel troubled in body or mind, the first step is always to take a breathing space. Here is some extra guidance that may help at these times.

1. AWARENESS

We have already practiced bringing the focus of awareness to your inner experience and noticing what is happening in your thoughts, feelings, and body sensations. Now, you may find it helpful to describe and identify what is arising—to put experiences into words (e.g., say in your mind, "A feeling of anger is arising" or "Self-critical thoughts are here").

2. REDIRECTING ATTENTION

We have already practiced gently redirecting your full attention to the breath; following the breath all the way in and all the way out. In addition, try noting "at the back of your mind": "Breathing in . . . breathing out" or counting breaths from 1 to 5, then starting over again: "Inhaling, 1 . . . exhaling, 1; inhaling, 2" . . . and so forth.

3. EXPANDING ATTENTION

We have already practiced allowing the attention to expand to the whole body. So now we become aware of our posture and facial expression. We hold in awareness all the sensations in our bodies right now, just as they are . . .

Now extend this step, if you choose, especially if there is any sense of discomfort, tension, or resistance. If these sensations are present, bring your awareness to them by "breathing into them" on the inbreath. Then, breathe out from the sensations, softening and opening with the outbreath. Say to yourself on the outbreath, "It's OK. . . whatever it is, it's already here. Let me feel it."

As best you can, bring this expanded awareness to the next moments of your day.

Home Practice for the Week Following Session 5

1. Practice Working with Difficulty meditation on Days 1, 3, 5 (guided practice audio track 12) and Sitting with Silence (unguided practice) for 30–40 minutes on Days 2, 4, 6 and record your reactions on the Home Practice Record Form.

2. 3-Minute Breathing Space—Regular (audio track 8): Practice three times a day at times that you have decided in advance. Record each time by circling an R next to the appropriate day on the Home Practice Record Form; note any comments/difficulties.

3. 3-Minute Breathing Space—Responsive (audio track 9), if you choose (see Session 5—Handout 2): Practice *whenever you notice unpleasant feelings*. Record each time by circling an X for the appropriate day on the Home Practice Record Form; note any comments/difficulties.

Home Practice Record Form—Session 5

Name: _____

Record on the Home Practice Record Form each time you practice. Also, make a note of anything that comes up in the home practice, so that we can talk about it at the next meeting.

Day/date	Practice (Yes/No)	Comments
Wednesday Date: _____	Working with Difficulty meditation—guided: R R R X X X X X X X X X X	
Thursday Date: _____	Working with Difficulty meditation—self-guided: R R R X X X X X X X X X X	
Friday Date: _____	Working with Difficulty meditation—guided: R R R X X X X X X X X X X	
Saturday Date: _____	Working with Difficulty meditation—self-guided: R R R X X X X X X X X X X	

R, 3-Minute Breathing Space—Regular; X, 3-Minute Breathing Space—Responsive.

(cont.)

Day/date	Practice (Yes/No)	Comments
Sunday Date: _____	Working with Difficulty meditation— guided: R R R X X X X X X X X X X	
Monday Date: _____	Working with Difficulty meditation— self-guided: R R R X X X X X X X X X X	
Tuesday Date: _____	Working with Difficulty meditation— guided: R R R X X X X X X X X X X	
Wednesday Date: _____	Working with Difficulty meditation— self-guided: R R R X X X X X X X X X X	

"The Guest House"

This being human is a guest house.
Every morning a new arrival.

A joy, a depression, a meanness,
some momentary awareness comes
as an unexpected visitor.

Welcome and entertain them all!
Even if they're a crowd of sorrows,
who violently sweep your house
empty of its furniture,

still, treat each guest honorably.
He may be clearing you out
for some new delight.

The dark thought, the shame, the malice.
meet them at the door laughing,
and invite them in.

Be grateful for whoever comes,
because each has been sent
as a guide from beyond.

From Barks and Moyne.[94] Copyright 1995 by Coleman Barks. Reprinted by permission.

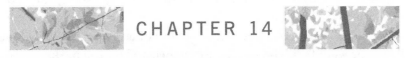

CHAPTER 14

Thoughts Are Not Facts

Session 6

John was on his way to school.

He was worried about the math lesson.

He was not sure he could control the class again today.

It was not part of a janitor's duty.

What do you notice as you read these sentences? Most people find that as they move from one to the next, they have to "update" the scene in the mind's eye. First of all, it is a little boy going to school, worried about the math lesson. Suddenly, the scene changes. For most people, the "mental model" changes to a teacher, before it finally changes into the janitor. It illustrates clearly the fact that we make an implicit inference around the bare facts we are reading. We are actively "making meaning" out of the sensory input all the time, and we are barely conscious that we are doing so, until someone comes along and plays a trick on us, as in this series of sentences. It is almost as if the mind creates a running commentary on all the events that take place in our awareness.

It is easy to see how these inferences, these "commentaries" that occur in our minds, may create or maintain emotional reactions. Once we have made the inference, the emotion follows close behind it. A phone call from a friend might be interpreted as "She needs me" or "She's using me," and our reaction will be completely different depending on which it is. Or imagine the following domestic scene: A husband and wife are in the kitchen. "Would you like fish or soup for supper?", says one. "I

299

don't mind," says the other. Now we shall leave to one side the inference we have all already made about who is asking the question and who is giving the answer! But imagine that they go for counseling because they have some marital difficulties. She remembers that event as "I asked him whether he would like fish or soup for supper, and he said he didn't care." He remembers that event as "She asked me what I wanted, and I said that I would like anything that she cooked for me; I was trying to be helpful." Note again how easily the same event can have different interpretations.

This problem in separating events from interpretation of events can cause a big problem for many people. People who are vulnerable to depression often interpret events in ways that are self-denigrating. Their thoughts become like propaganda directed against themselves. Facts are mixed with self-deprecating thoughts in a very destructive way, resulting in conclusions such as "I am worthless" or "I am a failure" or "If people knew what I was really like, no one would want to know me." And once such an internal propaganda stream has started, it is very difficult to undermine it, for all future events tend to reinforce it: Contrary information is ignored; consistent information is noticed.

DEALING WITH THOUGHTS IN COGNITIVE THERAPY AND MINDFULNESS-BASED COGNITIVE THERAPY

Until the advent of cognitive therapy for depression in the 1970s, the role of such self-directed, negative propaganda in causing and maintaining depression had been ignored by many therapists. The fact that depressed people had such negative thoughts was obvious, but clinicians assumed that they were caused *by* the depression—the result of underlying biological, psychodynamic, or behavioral processes. Cognitive therapists thought differently: Unremitting negative thoughts could cause depression. Interpreting events in the most pessimistic and hopeless way had a number of psychological consequences: It reduced self-esteem, increased guilt, interrupted concentration, and undermined social interaction. In addition, such thinking could have biological consequences (poor appetite, disrupted sleep patterns, agitation, or retardation). Once in place, these symptoms themselves would provide even more evidence for the negative self-propaganda, more evidence of the person's stupidity, weakness, or worthlessness.

Cognitive therapy revolutionized the treatment of depression. Its core feature was to help patients take their thoughts and interpretations seriously, to "catch" their thoughts and write them down, then gather evidence for and against them with an open mind. These procedures, applied systematically with home practice exercises to give extended practice at the skills, were found to reduce depression in ways that would have been astounding to clinicians in the 1950s and 1960s.

In both its rationale and its practice, cognitive therapy puts an explicit emphasis on the content of thoughts. For example, a depressed woman who believes 100% that "my friends are sick of me" will be encouraged by the therapist to think of this as an idea (a hypothesis) that may be true or false but needs to be tested against the evidence of recent events and future home practice experiments. Eventually, she may be able to "answer back" the negative thought. In this case, she may be able to say, "I haven't seen my friends because both I and they have been really busy, not because they are sick of me" or "I had meant to see Nicky last weekend, but I was out of town."

A critical test of whether the reality testing has worked is the degree of belief in the thought before and after the evidence has been examined. But our analysis of how cognitive therapy has its lasting effects (see earlier chapters) suggests that this patient would be less likely to relapse if, during the course of her therapy, she changed the *relationship* to her thoughts; that is, although the *explicit* emphasis of cognitive therapy would be on changing the content of her thoughts through challenging them, answering them back, seeking evidence for and against their truth value, we suggest that changes needed to take place at another level. This level had always been present in cognitive therapy but left *implicit*. Our analysis suggests that unless, through the cognitive and behavioral techniques within cognitive therapy, the patient had begun to shift her *relationship* to thoughts, to recognize her thoughts *as* thoughts, she would remain vulnerable to relapse and recurrence.

SITTING WITH THOUGHTS AS THOUGHTS

What is implicit in cognitive therapy is made explicit in MBCT: this need for a change in relationship to one's thoughts and the entire process of thinking. A key objective of Session 6 is to help participants find ways of reducing their degree of identification with what they are thinking, to encourage them to see thoughts as thoughts (even the ones that say they are not). Our aim is to enable participants to shift their relationship, so that they no longer relate *from* their thoughts but *to* their thoughts, as objects of awareness. The intention is that participants come to see their thoughts as "mental events" that arise with, and are fueled by, depressed mood, but do not have to be taken personally. In preventing future depression, this shift is critical, yet it is very hard to make because the thoughts are so demanding, so adhesive—and seem to tell the truth about oneself.

By this point in the MBCT program, the message of "thoughts as mental events" has been conveyed implicitly hundreds of times. Participants have had a lot of practice noticing their minds wandering, labeling what is going on in their minds as "thinking." They have, many times, gently brought the focus of attention back to the breath, or body, or whatever the intended focus. Sometimes the thoughts were trivial, other times not so trivial. It is now time to address the relationship with thoughts more explicitly. In particular, we need to consider why the message of "thoughts as mental events" is so difficult to take in: Why do we get so enmeshed in thoughts that we do not see them taking control of our lives? Why *are* our thoughts so adhesive? This is a central aim of Session 6.

Many thoughts, noticed during practice in the class or at home, are compelling simply because they seem to demand immediate action: "I ought to phone Mary before I forget," "Was that someone at the door?", "Will I remember to give Bob that report tomorrow?"

The more "adhesive" thoughts seem compelling because they "mesh" with a prevailing negative mood and as a result seem to be absolutely true: "I can't do this. I may as well give up," "When he said that, I know he meant something more by it," "There's so much to do at work, I'll never get it all done." Throughout the first four sessions of the program, the instruction was the same: to note where the mind had gone and gently bring it back to the breath. The message was implicit: This is just a thought. In this way, participants have learned to step back, to decenter from the content and just notice the thoughts. Thoughts themselves have been discussed not only in class dialogues about mind wandering, but also more explicitly in Session 2 in the Thoughts and Feelings Exercise (Figure 9.2), and again in Session 4 in the Automatic Thoughts Questionnaire (Box 11.4) as part of the "territory of depression." In Session 5, another dimension has been added: dealing with compelling and ruminative thoughts by deliberately

BOX 14.1
Theme and Curriculum for Session 6

THEME

Relating differently to thoughts. We free ourselves from the ruminative doing mode when we clearly see negative moods as passing states of mind, and negative thinking as the distorted products of those mind states. It is enormously liberating to realize that our thoughts are merely thoughts, even the ones that say they are not, and to recognize the contexts out of which they are born.

AGENDA

- 30- to 40-minute sitting meditation—awareness of breath, body, sounds, and thoughts/feelings, particularly noticing how we relate to thoughts that arise.
- Practice review.
- Home practice review (includes sitting meditation without recorded guidance and breathing spaces).
- Mention preparation for end of course.
- Moods, thoughts, and alternative viewpoints exercise.
- Breathing space and review.
- Discuss breathing space as the "first step" before taking a wider view of thoughts.
- Discuss relapse signature.
- Distribute Session 6 participant handouts and audio meditations of 10 minutes, 20 minutes, and bells with silence.
- Home practice assignments:
  o Practice with a selection of guided meditations for a minimum of 40 minutes a day.
  o 3-minute breathing space–regular (three times a day).
  o 3-minute breathing space–responsive (whenever you notice unpleasant feelings).

(cont.)

PREPARATION AND PLANNING

In addition to your personal preparation, remember to bring materials for the alternative viewpoints exercise and audio, including 10- and 20-minute meditations and bells plus silence to class.

PARTICIPANT HANDOUTS FOR SESSION 6

Session 6–Handout 1. Summary of Session 6: Thoughts Are Not Facts

Session 6–Handout 2. Ways You Can See Your Thoughts Differently

Session 6–Handout 3. Relapse Prevention

Session 6–Handout 4. Working Wisely with Unhappiness and Depression–I

Session 6–Handout 5. Homework Practice for the Week Following Session 6

Session 6–Handout 6. Home Practice Record Form—Session 6

Session 6–Handout 7. Stepping Back from Thought

Session 6–Handout 8. The Train of Associations

shifting attention to the body to see how the thought (and any reaction to it) is manifest in physical sensations.

Now in Session 6, we return to an explicit focus on thoughts themselves and our relationship to them: We put thoughts in the foreground of our practice. In the sitting meditation that starts the session, we take the opportunity to pay particular attention to observing and recognizing thoughts as thoughts, to bring awareness to them as discrete mental events, and to see each thought as simply a thought, an idea in the mind. We use the phrase "thoughts are not facts" to suggest that we don't have to believe everything we think or take it as absolute truth. This phrase does not imply that thoughts are inherently untruthful or unreliable. The whole reason why we depend on our thinking so much is that it is most often a reliable guide to how things are—so we do not question its validity. But it remains true that every thought is a mental event that contains a seed of reality surrounded by a shell of inference.

There are many images that convey this idea and can help the practice of seeing thoughts as thoughts. For example, we might become aware of the thoughts that are arising in our mind, imagining ourselves sitting in a cinema. We are watching an empty screen, just waiting for thoughts to come. When they come, can we see what exactly they are and what happens to them? Some of them will vanish as we become aware of them.

Joseph Goldstein offers another helpful analogy:

> When we lose ourselves in thought, thought sweeps up our mind and carries it away, and in a very short time we can be carried far indeed. We hop a train of association not knowing that we have hopped on, and certainly not knowing the destination. Somewhere down the line we may wake up and realize that we have been thinking, that we have been taken for a ride. And when we step down from the train, it may be in a very different state of mind from where we jumped aboard. (pp. 59–60)[89]

As in Session 5, toward the end of the meditation practice in this session, we encourage participants deliberately to bring to mind some concern, difficulty, or unpleasant memory—to become aware of and briefly bring to mind any *thoughts* that go along with it. Some participants find the metaphor of the cinema screen very helpful, but others find different metaphors and analogies useful. Some see "thoughts" come onto an empty stage and exit through the opposite wing. Others find it helpful to think of their minds as the sky, with clouds moving across it at varying speeds. Sometimes the clouds might be small; other times, they are dark and looming, covering the entire sky. But the sky remains. Once a difficult situation has come to mind and any thoughts that go with it have been observed, then participants are invited to shift attention to the body to see where the thoughts are affecting the body (as in Session 5).

STANDING BEHIND THE WATERFALL

So far, the emphasis has been on seeing thoughts as mental events. This can be challenging enough for any of us. But sometimes participants may find that thoughts come with such an emotional charge that it is very difficult not to get pulled into the vortex of the story created by the strong feelings. If this happens repeatedly, then the instructions are to shift attention into the body, as practiced in Session 5: to stay with the difficulty (known both by its intensity and its adhesive, "undismissable" quality) by exploring it through the physical sensations in the body. Indeed, it would not be too much of an exaggeration to say that MBCT uses the shift into the body as the predominant strategy—from now on always the first step—in learning to decenter from ruminative thinking and the feelings that create and sustain them.

> "If there is a place in the body that is experiencing intense sensation, then bringing your awareness to that region. Surrounding the physical sensations with a sense of friendly interest.
>
> "Perhaps, on each outbreath, saying, 'It's OK. Whatever it is, it's OK.' Soften and open to the sensations you are experiencing. Particularly if there's any sense of resistance, bringing gentle awareness to it, on each outbreath, opening and softening as best you can, rather than tensing or bracing.
>
> "When it feels comfortable, returning the focus to the breath or to the body as a whole."

These instructions, offered as part of the in-session guided meditation, remind participants that they can learn to distinguish between two ways of relating to thoughts and feelings: relating to thoughts and feelings from "inside the mind state," so to speak, with little sense of perspective; or relating to them so that they are held in a more spacious awareness, seeing them, as it were, from "behind the waterfall."

How can this new perspective be taught within the session itself, for example, in the dialogue that comes after a practice, or in the discussion about home practice? In the inquiry, there will be many reports of times when things get bad; when thoughts, closely tied to particular feelings, come in a rush, with great intensity. Recall that in Session 2 the focus was on the way in which thoughts and interpretations have a direct effect on the feelings about an event (e.g., being ignored by someone we know in the street). The main purpose of that session was to focus on the top arrow in Figure 14.1. Now it is helpful to spend some time focusing on the lower (reverse) link: between feelings and thoughts.

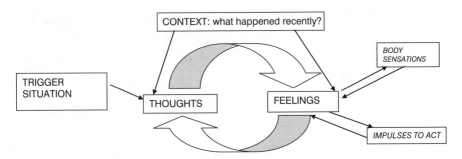

FIGURE 14.1. Thoughts and feelings. In Session 6 we focus especially on the bottom arrow, how feelings can give birth to thoughts.

> We invite ourselves to focus directly on the *feeling* that gives birth to the thought: Instead of getting tangled in thoughts, we explore the option of asking, "What is this I am feeling now, specifically, in this moment?" When we do this, we may discover more feelings than were apparent earlier.

For example, if the thought is "I'm so useless at everything; I never finish anything," we risk being dragged down by a powerful waterfall of ruminations about what such failure says about us as people. Focusing on the feelings that partly drive the vicious cycle of thoughts may give us another place to stand. We may find ourselves standing behind the cascading waterfall of negative thoughts and feelings, and able to see their force more clearly without being dragged down by them.

An example of the way this might sometimes help came in the experience of Louise, the participant we mentioned in Session 2 (Chapter 9). She had some difficult weeks when she felt very low: She knew that, normally, she would spiral downward again. On one such occasion, she was in the doctor's office with one of the children. She felt pressured because she had had to take time off work to be there, thinking not only "What will the boss say?" but also "Why shouldn't I be here? I'm entitled to it," and so on and on.

She noticed what was happening, but not in the old way, when she dealt with it by telling herself not to be so stupid. Instead, she took a moment. She acknowledged what she was feeling: angry, tired, confused, and very worried about her child. Then she felt her perspective broaden and found herself able to say, "It's OK to feel like this; it's OK." She allowed the feelings just to be there, without struggling to chase them away. They dissipated in a way that she later called "miraculous." She had never before experienced anything like that in her life.

So both cognitive therapy and MBCT emphasize that thoughts are best seen as events in the mind, events to which we are ordinarily so close that it is often difficult to realize they are mental events. Mindfulness gives this different relationship to thoughts a more explicit focus. It does not emphasize gathering evidence for or against them, nor answering them back as a first step in gaining distance from them. Instead, it encourages people to bring a different mind, a different quality of attention to bear upon them; to observe them as part of a whole package that, although we do not know where it has come from, now needs to be acknowledged and treated with an attitude of gentleness and acceptance.

Notice the emphasis here on thoughts as part of a "package." If we refer back to Figure 14.1, we can see how thoughts and feelings give rise to body sensations and impulses to act in certain ways, but the figure is incomplete without realizing (1) that that there is often a *context* for the situation—something that happened recently that has affected our mood (discussed later), and (2) that there are important feedback loops *from* body sensations and impulses to act *back* to our feelings.

According to this view, what we experience as "emotions" is a *package* of thoughts, feelings, body sensations, and impulses. The elements of the package are so closely entangled that it is sometimes very difficult to distinguish them—yet by learning to approach them, then to explore them, we can see how the separate elements reinforce each other, magnifying and exacerbating our distress, and our efforts to repair the damage the distress is causing. Once we see this clearly, we can more easily reduce some of the effort we have expended in dealing with them, as if they are telling the truth about the world or ourselves, the past, or the future. We also stop allowing ourselves to be controlled by them or, at least, we begin to see that tendency emerge in the present moment. Once we see negative thoughts from this perspective, from behind the cascading waterfall, our emotional response to them will be different in subtle but important ways.

Mindfulness training encourages people to observe thoughts as part of a whole package that, although we do not know where it has come from, now needs to be acknowledged and treated with an attitude of gentleness and acceptance.

SEEING THE "TAPE IN THE MIND" FOR WHAT IT IS

The meditation teacher Larry Rosenberg[95] points out that when we get to the point where we've watched the mind a great deal and seen the same old thoughts come up again and again, we don't rise to the bait anymore: "It's like seeing *Gone with the Wind* for the fifth time or the twelfth, however many it takes you. The first eleven were great, but the twelfth doesn't work anymore. You just don't care. The same thing happens with the movie in your mind, if you really start to watch it" (p. 142).

Naming our familiar thought patterns is one way that helps us to recognize them when they start up. It allows us to say, "Ah, I know this tape. This is my 'I can't stand my boss' tape or my 'No one recognizes how hard I work' tape." This will not necessarily switch it off, or even if it appears to, it will almost certainly return soon, like a children's movie at holiday season. The difference is in the way we relate to it: on one hand as "fact" that should be addressed seriously, for example, by phoning the boss and complaining to him or her; or on the other as a tape running in the head that will continue to affect us until the "batteries run down" and it ceases of its own accord. Acknowledging the familiar patterns, and the hurt they can cause, may allow us to realize that it's OK not to like or to want these mind states around. Such acknowledging can free us from the adhesive quality that comes, ironically, from our very aversion to them.

Such a stance toward our own thoughts does not come naturally, and for people who have been depressed, certain thoughts can be so powerful that seeing them "simply as thoughts" can be a huge challenge in itself. Furthermore, many people do not experience their minds as having "thoughts" as such. They may "think" in images or pictures. For example, if they feel rejected by their friends, they may not have the thought "My friends are sick of me." They may simply see, in their mind's eye, a picture of their friends huddled in a corner, laughing and talking among themselves.

Many participants notice that body sensations often seem to be magnets for thoughts. Thoughts may arise as a reaction to an awareness of sensations: "Why am I feeling this way?"; "It's my age. I'll never have the energy I used to have"; "If this headache doesn't go away, I will have to cancel my plans for tonight." To approach these thoughts mindfully does not require that we do anything different from what we have been doing up to now for sensations and feelings. We can imagine we are in a cinema or theater and simply decide to watch the film or theater of the mind as thoughts come and go on the screen or stage. We can also look out for those thoughts that seem to "come from behind" in the theater—like a whisper in the ear from the seat behind (e.g., "This is not going so well"; "There's no point in doing this"; "It's not going to work, so why bother?"; "This pain is killing me"; "I wish this practice would end"; "This is so hard, I'm never going to be any good at it, and things will never change"). These are difficult to see as mental events, for they do not appear "on the stage" we are watching.

So the instructor may point out that some thoughts come from other "places," and that these (to change the analogy) can get "under the radar" of our practice of "observing thoughts." We may invite participants to think of their theater as having surround sound—or if they imagine themselves sitting on the banks of a river, that part of the river may be running behind them, easily missed, but also carrying some leaves in its stream. However, we also point out that this is not easy to do, and it should be practiced for only 3 or 4 minutes at a time in the early stages.

REPORTING ON HOME PRACTICE

In the week preceding this session, participants have been invited to try formal practice without using recordings on certain days. This proves difficult for some, who find that they simply cannot concentrate. A range of negative thoughts and images arises, many of which are often very self-critical and reactive.

In this example, notice how this difficulty was compounded by thoughts for one participant. First, in contrast, previous weeks were so good that now there is great disappointment; second, if she could not do it "well," it was useless to do it at all:

P: I had a dreadful week, a really dreadful week. I didn't do any meditation, and I didn't get around to reading any of the book. The weeks before were so good, I was really getting into it. I just can't concentrate on anything at all at the moment.

I: What do you think was going on?

P: I really don't know. I think it is just loneliness. I have been busy, but I was making time before. I was consciously making time because I enjoyed it. It was my time.

I: Right, but when you needed it most, you lost it?

P: Yes. There were a couple of times in the week when I tried to do it at work, and I just couldn't do it. My mind wouldn't concentrate. It was constantly running.

In this case, a *fact* (that her mind was constantly running) was mixed with an *interpretation* (this means "I couldn't do it"). There is a choice here for the instructor. He could have pointed out the fact–interpretation issue or addressed what the practice actually demands. He decided to do the latter first.

"That's OK. I think what is really important, particularly at times like this, is not to assume that you have got to sit down and be able to 'do it properly.' Simply sitting down for the allotted time and watching your mind race is much better than not doing it at all, even though it is not so easy to bring yourself to practice in such circumstances. But these are some of the best times to practice. The truth is, if you look back with the benefit of hindsight, you can see that the times you just sat with all that stuff raining down on you have actually been as or more valuable than the times when you have been peaceful and calm."

Later, the instructor found the opportunity to come back to the way that thoughts get mixed up with facts.

"Often when we are practicing and the mind is all over the place, we find ourselves getting angry and frustrated. The thoughts and feelings seem like a huge waterfall, and we feel as if we are being hurled down with the force of the water. At these times, as best you can, see if you are able to stand behind the waterfall. Watch the thoughts and feelings, including the understandable frustration you feel. The thoughts and feelings cascade past you. They are very close. You can feel the force of them, but they are not you."

All of these points may arise out of discussion of both the sitting meditation practice at the start of the session and the home practice. Recall that participants have practiced using the 3-minute breathing space regularly during the day and taking a breathing space whenever difficult things come up. This will become an increasingly important "scaffold" for dealing with difficulties, including negative thoughts, and we return to it later. For now, we wish to explore another way of illustrating the core theme of this session: the alternative ways to relate to thoughts.

WHEN CONTEXT, MOODS, AND THOUGHTS CONSPIRE AGAINST SEEING ALTERNATIVE VIEWPOINTS

Our colleague Isabel Hargreaves devised the following moods and thoughts exercise, which demonstrates to participants some of the ways in which feelings can determine how we think about a particular situation (it is adapted here by permission of Isabel Hargreaves). The instructor gives each person a piece of paper with a scenario written on it: Version 1 on the front of the paper, and Version 2 on the back. Participants write down what they would think, first using Version 1, then Version 2.

Version 1 says:

"You are feeling down because you've just had a quarrel with a colleague at work. Shortly afterward, you see another colleague in the General Office, and he or she rushes off quickly, saying he or she couldn't stop. What would you think?"

Version 2 says:

> "You are feeling happy because you and a work colleague have just been praised for good work. Shortly afterward, you see another colleague in the General Office, and he or she rushes off quickly, saying he or she couldn't stop. What would you think?"

In the discussion that follows, class members compare the thoughts and feelings brought up by each description. Note that this is not simply about exclusively positive interpretations in one scenario versus negative interpretations in the other. While it's not unusual to hear that the first situation is associated with thoughts of being rejected or hurt by the colleague hurrying away, in the second scenario, the colleague rushing off may draw out the thought that he or she might be jealous, or curious or concerned for his or her welfare. For example:

P: In the first case, it would keep going over in my mind, why my colleague hadn't spoken to me, whereas in the other one, I would just accept it without another thought.

I: So we have got exactly the same objective situation [the actual evidence is that the person said he or she couldn't stop and rushed off], but at least to some of us, the frame of mind we bring to it creates a radically different interpretation, a different set of feelings. This makes the very obvious point that just because we think something doesn't make it so.

FRAMES OF MIND

Thoughts carry credibility. We believe them. But recall that a thought is a mental event containing a seed of reality surrounded by a shell of inference. We have this capacity to make many different interpretations of the same situation. If these interpretations are going to be determined by the frame of mind that we bring to it, and we are in a negative frame of mind, we are in danger of getting trapped in the shell of interpretations that frame of mind produces, our mood gets worse, and then down we go.

So the first stage is really to get thoroughly aware of this difference between thoughts and facts. Part of the point of meditation is to perceive this distinction; we note our thoughts as passing events in the field of awareness; we note their content and their "emotional charge," and then we bring our attention back to the breath. As best we can, we do not get caught in the thought stream. We just say, "Oh, there's another thought"; then, we go gently but firmly back to the breath.

The important point here is that interpretation of events reflects what we bring to it as much or more than what is actually there. We have already seen how what we think can influence how we feel, but the new element here is that what we think is also determined by our background mood or "context" at the time we are thinking.

> Feelings "give birth" to thoughts. What we think is determined by our mood at the time we are thinking.

The idea that *thoughts are not facts* is as relevant to people who have recovered from depression as to those who are still depressed. Discussing how the same event can be interpreted differently, depending on what happened immediately beforehand, suggests that there is no single truth that our thoughts are telling us. This exercise suggests thoughts are interpretations that reflect a number of different influences, including learning from our past and current mood states. Just because our thoughts are compelling does not make them true.

The message of this session builds on the message of Sessions 2 and 4 concerning the connection between thoughts–interpretations and our moods. What does this session add? First, just as we saw in the "John was on his way to school" example, interpretations come so quickly, as part of our moment-by-moment processing of what's going on in the world, that we do not see them coloring our reaction to situations. Second, this session focuses on the way mood can give birth to thoughts: Feelings (often created by something that happened recently, or a reminder of a past event) can determine a whole frame of mind that then determines which thoughts and interpretations come to mind. Third, this session homes in on why we find it so difficult to see thoughts as mental events. *Because*

thoughts are born out of context and feelings, they seem real to us: They are so
well camouflaged by the context that they are difficult to see.

SO WHAT IS THE NEXT STEP?

Participants need to feel that there is something they can do immediately,
when they feel their thoughts getting the better of them. We therefore
emphasize that taking a breathing space (no matter how briefly) is always
the first step. Stepping out of autopilot and bringing awareness to the
whole "package" of thoughts–feelings–body sensations that arise before
shifting attention to the breath, a person has a greater chance of acknowledging what is going on with him- or herself at this moment, without
taking it personally. With this awareness often comes the sense of a greater
choice about how to respond.

> When thoughts threaten to overwhelm, taking a breathing space
> (no matter how briefly) is always the first step.

One picture we have in mind is that the breathing space is like a door.
Opening the door reveals a number of different corridors down which we
might decide to go. In Session 5 we explored how to add to the breathing space an invitation to see what effects any difficult thoughts have
on the *body*, to open to physical sensations that accompany repetitive
thoughts and feelings. In the next session, we'll consider how people can
choose to take *action* following a breathing space. Here, we focus on how
best to deal with thoughts. The critical thing is to become aware that
there is a choice. But the message remains: Take a breathing space as a
first step.

So, if negative thoughts are around, after taking a breathing space,
there are a number of options as to what to do next if participants wish
to focus on thoughts themselves. First, participants might use some of
the tools developed by cognitive therapists for people who become aware
of trains of thought that have a strong emotional charge.[96] These are
included in the participant handouts for people to try on their own:

1. Simply to simply watch your thoughts come and go in the field of awareness, without feeling that you have to follow them.
2. To view all your thoughts, and particularly negative thoughts, as mental events rather than facts. It may be true that a particular thought "event" is often associated with strong feelings. It is therefore tempting to think of it as being true. But it is still up to you to decide to what degree it is true, if at all, and how you want to deal with it.
3. To write your thoughts down on paper. This lets you see them in a way that is less emotional and overwhelming. Also, the pause between having the thought and writing it down can give you a moment to take a wider perspective.
4. To focus, with a sense of compassion, on the feelings that may be giving birth to the thought, by asking: "What feelings are here right now?"; "What feelings are giving rise to these thoughts: What is this? Is it fear? Loneliness? Anger? Sadness?"; "What physical sensations in the body are here?"; "How can I best look after myself right now?"

With time, participants may begin to see thinking *as an activity*, and just note when it is happening. This reveals the process of thinking as it unfolds, but without getting lost in its content or what the thoughts are trying to say. If participants can relate to their experience of thinking in this way, it may enable them to choose between those thoughts they wish to act on and those they can simply let be.

A fundamental point is that if we are able to recognize our self-talk in this way, we place ourselves in a better position to *choose* what we want to do about it. If, when we notice an avalanche of thinking, we take a breathing space, there are a number of things we can do next, if need be. These include not only observing our self-talk, or writing it down, but also bringing our awareness to the feelings behind it, as best we can, with an attitude of gentleness: "There may be other ways to see what's happening to me right now."

Finally, paying such careful attention to our sensations and thoughts can give us a moment to take a different view of our difficulties, so that they become less stressful. For example, if we are criticized by our boss at work, instead of letting it snowball into insecurity or defensiveness, with mindfulness, we can watch our initial reactions go by before we speak, then speak more consciously and therefore more effectively.

The important point is that *all thoughts are mental events (including the thoughts that say they are not!).*

A "DIFFERENT RELATIONSHIP TO THOUGHTS" IS NOT JUST ANSWERING THEM BACK

Many people report that using the breathing space as a first step in dealing with negative thinking proves very helpful. But we must be cautious. There is a subtle but important difference between attempting to use the breathing space to strengthen us to fight against the thoughts and standing in a different relationship to them. In the first case, simply trying to find more and more clever answers to negative thoughts may leave us with a greater sense of hopelessness.

Note, in the transcript that follows, how this person moves from simply trying to "answer back" her negative thoughts in the first part, to simply seeing them as thoughts in the second. In particular, notice the dangers of the "answering back" mode; it too easily lapses back into self-criticism, while the "seeing thoughts as thoughts" mode brings a different tone.

P: I know from the start when I'm having a bad day.

I: It starts the moment you wake up?

P: Yeah, well, I can have a good start and it can deteriorate throughout the day, but sometimes, first thing in the morning, it's one of those days. Sometimes I get increasingly frustrated with myself for not being able to do what I think I should be able to do. That's when reminding myself that it's not my fault and it will be better in the next day or in the next couple of hours is helpful.

I: So you challenge some of your thoughts with those thoughts?

P: Yeah, and I use the breathing space for that sort of thing . . . and for things that have happened in the past that are of no consequence, or shouldn't be of any consequence. Things somebody said that weren't meant to hurt suddenly hurt, you know. They had no intentions to hurt and I shouldn't take them to heart, you know. I'll suddenly think of something that somebody said 2 weeks ago—"I bet she meant such and such," "Why did she say that?"—and my mind just races and races.

I: It can pick up on small things?

P: Really and, you know, it's stupid. There is no sense whatsoever in having that thought and keeping it going round and round in your head. It just does it.

Notice that, at this point, it looks as though this person is using the breathing space as a sort of tool to "pull herself together." The struggle to keep on terms with her negative thinking is very evident, and a tendency to use self-criticism is clear from comments such as "It's stupid" and "There's no sense whatever in having that thought." But later, it becomes clearer that the breathing space does connect her to other aspects of the classes:

P: I also think of that saying—"Thoughts aren't facts," was it? That one really clicked with me. "Thoughts are not facts" and the other bit that said " . . . even the ones that tell you they are." I thought that was really good (*laughs*)—"Thoughts are not facts, even the ones that tell you they are"—because if you've got that sort of thing going around in your head, you can say, "Now come on. That is not real. This is real. You're here in this room and look at all the good things that are around you." And then the other thought would come back in. "But she really did say that. That really did happen." And then I was able to pick up on the next phrase, " . . . even the ones that say they are" (*laughs*). Then I do the breathing space and I usually find that it's gone.

IDENTIFYING RELAPSE SIGNATURES

The research we reviewed in Chapter 3 showed that when people have been depressed many times, the process of becoming depressed can become more and more autonomous. The depression gathers at a very fast pace and seems to escalate without external triggers. This means that it is important to identify in advance, and while mood is stable, those changes (in mind and body) that might signal that depression is developing. By being able to recognize these signs early, participants will be in a better position to use the skills that they have been practicing. These signs of relapse, referred to as "relapse signatures," are unique for each individual.

Note that this assumes an acceptance that depression will occur again, but we are working with how to handle or deal with it when it occurs. It would be a mistake to think that taking a mindfulness class means that you might never feel sadness again. It is rather a question of learning better how to take care of ourselves when it happens, charting the territory of depression, so that we can navigate through it with less fear.

In the first edition of this book, we had left the identification of warning signs until Session 7. Further experience of teaching the program has led us to the conclusion that it is sometimes better to introduce it earlier, and that the Session 6 discussion of thoughts and how to recognize them as "mental events" leads naturally to discussion of how we might use negative thoughts (and how adhesive they seem) as an important warning sign of depression. They may signal a tendency to get drawn back into old and unhelpful patterns of thinking that might escalate into a relapse.

We examine relapse signatures by setting an exercise for the class that is best started in pairs or small groups. The task is to make a list of the specific warning signals that depression might be trying to take hold again. Once finished, the instructor writes some of the signals on the blackboard. Here are some examples from one class.

- Seeing negative thoughts and feelings taking hold—finding them adhesive, difficult to dismiss
- Becoming irritable with self and others
- Withdrawal from social participation—just "not wanting to see people"
- Changing sleep habits
- Changing eating habits
- Getting easily exhausted
- Giving up on exercise
- Not wanting to deal with business (opening mail, paying bills, etc.)
- Postponing deadlines

Each person's particular combination of signs of the worsening mood that might have once signaled impending relapse or recurrence is unique—that is why it is called a "signature." Becoming aware without becoming hypervigilant for these signs is an important balance to discover. But just noticing these changes isn't enough. It is easy to list them when we are feeling good, but when our mood starts to worsen, we may no longer believe that it is useful to heed these warnings at all. Recall that part of the "territory" of depression is hopelessness, and hopelessness tends to make us feel that none of these practices is worth doing, that "I am back to square one." That is why participants are encouraged to take advantage of their present intention to look after themselves and include others in their plans. They need to ask themselves two questions: "What, in the past, has prevented me from noticing and attending to these feelings (e.g., pushing away, denial, distraction, self-medication with alcohol; arguments, blaming family members or colleagues)?" and "How can I include other family members in my early warning system for detecting the signs of a relapse?" We use the Working Wisely with Unhappiness and Depression–I worksheet (Session 6–Handout 4). Participants can start it in class, then finish it at home.

PREPARING FOR THE FUTURE

At the end of this session, there are only two classes left. At this point, therefore, we allow time for participants to explore their own way of making the practice part of their daily lives. To help them, the instructor provides audio of mindfulness meditation practices, 10-minute and 20-minute sitting meditation practices, as well as audio of only the sound of bells at intervals to provide minimal structure for a person's own practice. Participants are asked to choose their own selection from these and earlier meditations, and practice for a minimum of 40 minutes per day.

The implicit message here is that by offering the opportunity to explore these different means, we invite participants to settle into long-term practice. Mindfulness is a way of life rather than a short-term therapy that will "cure" whatever has "gone wrong" with the person. The more people can incorporate formal practice into their lives, and make it as routine as brushing their teeth or taking a bath or shower, the more likely the change that has begun during the 8-week program will continue.[97] Ultimately, it is the "everydayness" of the practice that is important, not exactly which practice is used or for how long. Some people will hear the message, "Unless I continue for 40 minutes a day, I will not stay well." This is not what we wish to imply. But we are more and more convinced that it is important to be clear about the future: Putting time aside on a daily basis to sample the "being" rather than "doing" mode is one of the most helpful gifts that people can give to themselves. If we wish to be mindful *all* moments of the day, it is useful to find some moments of the day when we practice *only* being mindful—moments when we can allow ourselves to meet and then to nourish what is deepest and best in us.

Summary of Session 6:
Thoughts Are Not Facts

It is amazing to observe how much power we give unknowingly to uninvited thoughts: "Do this, say that, remember, plan, obsess, judge." They have the potential to drive us quite crazy, and they often do!

—JOSEPH GOLDSTEIN[89]

Our thoughts can have very powerful effects on how we feel and what we do. Often those thoughts are triggered and run off quite automatically. By becoming aware, over and over again, of the thoughts and images passing through the mind and letting go of them as we return our attention to the breath and the moment, it is possible to get some distance and perspective on them. This can allow us to see that there may be other ways to think about situations, freeing us from the tyranny of the old thought patterns that automatically "pop into mind." Most important, we may eventually come to realize "deep in our bones" that *all thoughts are only mental events* (including the thoughts that say they are not), that *thoughts are not facts*, and that *we are not our thoughts*.

Thoughts and images can often provide us with an indication of what is going on deeper in the mind; we can "get hold of them," so that we can look them over from a number of different perspectives, and by becoming very familiar with our own "top 10" habitual, automatic, unhelpful thinking patterns, we can more easily become aware of (and change) the processes that may lead us into downward mood spirals.

It is particularly important to become aware of thoughts that may block or undermine practice, such as "There's no point in doing this" or "It's not going to work, so why bother?" Such a pessimistic, hopeless thought pattern is one of the most characteristic features of depressed mood states, and one of the main factors that stop us from taking actions that would help us get out of those states. It follows that it is particularly important to recognize such thoughts as "negative thinking" and not automatically give up on efforts to apply skillful means to change the way we feel.

From thoughts come actions. From actions come all sorts of consequences. In which thoughts will we invest? Our great task is to see them clearly, so that we can choose which ones to act on and which simply to let be.

—JOSEPH GOLDSTEIN[89]

Ways You Can See Your Thoughts Differently

Here are some of the things you can do with your thoughts:

1. Just watch them come in and leave, without feeling that you have to follow them.

2. See if it is possible to notice the feelings that give rise to the thoughts: the "context" in which your thoughts are but one link in a chain of events.

3. View your thought as a mental event rather than a fact. It may be true that this event often occurs with other feelings. It is tempting to think of it as being true, but it is still up to you to decide whether it is true and how you want to deal with it.

4. Write your thoughts down on paper. This lets you see them in a way that is less emotional and overwhelming. Also, the pause between having the thought and writing it down can give you a moment to respond to it differently.

5. For particularly difficult thoughts, it may be helpful to take another look at them intentionally, in a balanced, open state of mind, as part of your sitting practice. Let your "wise mind" give its perspective, perhaps labeling the feeling out of which, it arises, and holding a sense of curiosity, as best you can: "Ah, here is sadness"; "Here is the voice of depression"; "Here is the familiar harsh and critical voice." *The keynote attitude to take with your thoughts is gentle interest and curiosity.*

Based in part on Fennell.[96]

Relapse Prevention

What are your warning signals that depression might be trying to take hold again (e.g., becoming irritable; decreased social contact—just "not wanting to see people"; changes in sleeping habits; changes in eating habits; getting easily exhausted; giving up on exercise; not wanting to deal with business, such as opening mail, paying bills; postponing deadlines)?

Set up an Early Warning System—write down on the next worksheet the changes that you should look out for (if it feels comfortable, include *those with whom you share your life* in a collaborative effort to *notice* and then to *respond* rather than to *react* to these signs).

Working Wisely with Unhappiness and Depression–I

SEEING CLEARLY (NOTICING THE FIRST SIGNS OF DEPRESSION)

This worksheet offers an opportunity to increase your awareness of what happens for you when depression appears. The aim is, carefully and with curiosity, to investigate the thoughts, feelings, body sensations, and patterns of behavior that tell you that your mood is starting to drop.

What triggers depression for you?

- Triggers can be external (things that happen to you) or internal (e.g., thoughts, feelings, memories, concerns).

- Look out for small triggers as well as large ones—sometimes something that appears quite trivial can spark a downward mood spiral.

What sort of thoughts run through your mind when you first feel your mood dropping?

What emotions arise?

(cont.)

What happens in your body?

What do you do, or feel like doing?

Are there any old habits of thinking or behavior that might unwittingly keep you stuck in depression (e.g., ruminating, trying to suppress or turn away from painful thoughts and feelings, struggling with it instead of accepting and exploring it)?

Home Practice for the Week Following Session 6

1. Practice with your own selection from the new meditations and previous ones (audio tracks 4, 10, and 13) for a minimum of 40 minutes a day (e.g., 20 + 20). Record your reactions on the Home Practice Record Form.

2. 3-Minute Breathing Space—Regular (audio track 8): Practice three times a day at times you have determined in advance. Record each time by circling an R on the Home Practice Record Form; note any comments/difficulties.

3. 3-Minute Breathing Space—Responsive (audio track 9), if you choose (see Session 5–Handout 2): Practice *whenever you notice unpleasant feelings*. Record each time by circling an X for the appropriate day on the Home Practice Record Form; note any comments/difficulties. If negative thoughts are still around after the breathing space, you might like to use some of the ideas in Session 6–Handout 2 to get a different perspective on these thoughts.

4. Complete the Working Wisely with Unhappiness and Depression Worksheet–I you started in class. Please include family members and friends, if you like. They may also notice early warning signs if your mood is low.

Home Practice Record Form—Session 6

Name: _____

Record on the Home Practice Record Form each time you practice. Also, make a note of anything that comes up in the home practice, so that we can talk about it at the next meeting.

Day/date	Practice (Yes/No)	Comments
Wednesday Date: _____	Which formal practice chosen? R R R X X X X X X X X X X	
Thursday Date: _____	Which formal practice chosen? R R R X X X X X X X X X X	
Friday Date: _____	Which formal practice chosen? R R R X X X X X X X X X X	
Saturday Date: _____	Which formal practice chosen? R R R X X X X X X X X X X	

R, 3-Minute Breathing Space—Regular Version; X, 3-Minute Breathing Space—Responsive Version.

(cont.)

Day/date	Practice (Yes/No)	Comments
Sunday Date: _____	Which formal practice chosen? R R R X X X X X X X X X X	
Monday Date: _____	Which formal practice chosen? R R R X X X X X X X X X X	
Tuesday Date: _____	Which formal practice chosen? R R R X X X X X X X X X X	
Wednesday Date: _____	Which formal practice chosen? R R R X X X X X X X X X X	

Stepping Back from Thought

It is remarkable how liberating it feels to be able to see that your thoughts are just thoughts and not "you" or "reality." For instance, if you have the thought that you must get a certain number of things done today and you don't recognize it as a thought but act as if it's "the truth," then you have created in that moment a reality in which you really believe that those things must all be done today.

One patient, Peter, who'd had a heart attack and wanted to prevent another one, came to a dramatic realization of this one night, when he found himself washing his car at 10 o'clock at night with the floodlights on in the driveway. It struck him that he didn't have to be doing this. It was just the inevitable result of a whole day spent trying to fit everything in that he thought needed doing today. As he saw what he was doing to himself, he also saw that he had been unable to question the truth of his original conviction that everything had to get done today because he was already so completely caught up in believing it.

If you find yourself behaving in similar ways, it is likely that you will also feel driven, tense, and anxious without even knowing why, just as Peter did. So if the thought of how much you have to get done today comes up while you are meditating, you will have to be very attentive to it as a thought or you may be up and doing things before you know it, without any awareness that you decided to stop sitting simply because a thought came through your mind.

On the other hand, when such a thought comes up, if you are able to step back from it and see it clearly, then you will be able to prioritize things and make sensible decisions about what really does need doing. You will know when to call it quits during the day. So the simple act of recognizing your thoughts as thoughts can free you from the distorted reality they often create and allow for more clear-sightedness and a greater sense of manageability in your life.

This liberation from the tyranny of the thinking mind comes directly out of the meditation practice itself. When we spend some time each day in a state of nondoing, observing the flow of the breath and the activity of our mind and body, without getting caught up in that activity, we are cultivating calmness and mindfulness hand in hand. As the mind develops stability and is less caught up in the content of thinking, we strengthen the mind's ability to concentrate and to be calm. And if each time we recognize a thought as a thought when it arises and register its content, and discern the strength of its hold on us and the accuracy of its content, then each time we let go of it and come back to our breathing and a sense of our body, we are strengthening mindfulness. We come to know ourselves better and become more accepting of ourselves, not as we would like to be, but as we actually are.

The Train of Associations

The thinking level of mind pervades our lives; consciously or unconsciously, we all spend much or most of our lives there. But meditation is a different process that does not involve discursive thought or reflection. Because meditation is not thought, through the continuous process of silent observation, new kinds of understanding emerge.

We do not need to fight with thoughts, struggle against them, or judge them. Rather, we can simply choose not to follow the thoughts once we are aware that they have arisen.

When we lose ourselves in thought, identification is strong. Thought sweeps the mind and carries it away, and, in a very short time, we can be carried far indeed. We hop on a train of association, not knowing that we have done so, and certainly not knowing the destination. Somewhere down the line, we may wake up and realize that we have been thinking, that we have been taken for a ride. And when we step down from the train, it may be in a very different mental environment from where we jumped aboard.

Take a few moments right now to look directly at the thoughts arising in your mind. As an exercise, you might close your eyes and imagine yourself sitting in a cinema watching an empty screen. Simply wait for thoughts to arise. Because you are not doing anything except waiting for thoughts to appear, you may become aware of them very quickly. What exactly are they? What happens to them? Thoughts are like magic displays that seem real when we are lost in them but then vanish upon inspection.

But what about the strong thoughts that affect us? We are watching, watching, watching, and then, all of a sudden—whoosh! We are gone, lost in a thought. What is that about? What are the mind states or the particular kinds of thoughts that catch us again and again, so that we forget that they are just empty phenomena passing on?

It is amazing to observe how much power we unknowingly give to uninvited thoughts: "Do this, say that, remember, plan, obsess, judge." They have the potential to drive us quite crazy, and they often do!

The kinds of thoughts we have, and their impact on our lives, depend on our understanding of things. If we are in the clear, powerful space of just seeing thoughts arise and pass, then it does not really matter what kind of thinking appears in the mind; we can see our thoughts as the passing show that they are.

From thoughts come actions. From actions come all sorts of consequences. In which thoughts will we invest? Our great task is to see them clearly, so that we can choose which ones to act on and which simply to let be.

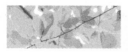 CHAPTER 15

A Day of Mindful Practice

When we started our project in 1993 to see how the 8-week MBSR program might be adapted for the prevention of recurrent depression, we were aware of an important component that we, at that time, could not include: the day of mindfulness between Sessions 6 and 7 that provides patients with an opportunity to practice under conditions of silence and simplicity. The randomized trial we were asking our funders to support required us to look closely at the issue of health economics (the direct costs and the "opportunity costs" of the additional time it would take for participants and for instructors, compared to other therapies). This meant we would need to minimize the cost and time devoted to the program, and for that reason we didn't include it. Over the past decade, however, having taught the MBCT program with and without an all-day, we have seen evidence of its benefit. In addition, the health economic argument is helped by the fact that the day is open to all those who have been through the program in previous classes. In this way it presents attendees with an opportunity to maintain wellness and strengthen their practice, both of which lead to lower health care costs if relapse is kept at bay. (Note, however, in clinical trials with an active control group, the all-day may still not be used, since the comparability of number of hours of contact time may have to be controlled in some trial designs.)

The all-day is usually scheduled, as in MBSR, between Sessions 6 and 7, since by the end of the sixth session patients will have been exposed to all the formal mindfulness practices. In the all-day they can now see what it is like to experience these familiar practices back to back, much as is done on a silent retreat (see Figure 15.1). This resemblance is accurate in

9:45–10:00	Arrival
10:00–10:05	Sit for 5 minutes in silence
10:05–10:20	Welcome, introductions, ground rules
10:20–10:50	Sitting meditation: Breath, body, sounds, thoughts, and choiceless awareness
10:50–11:30	Mindful stretching
11:30–12:00	Body scan
12:00–12:05	Instructions for lunchtime: Bringing focus of awareness to eating, tasting, chewing, swallowing, slowing down
12:05–1:05	Lunch: On one's own either outside or inside, followed by going for a mindful walk
1:05–1:20	Brief sitting
1:20–1:50	Walking meditation
1:50–2:20	Mountain meditation
2:20–2:40	Mindful stretching
2:40–3:00	Silent sitting or extended breathing space
3:00–3:30	Feeding back experiences of day in pairs
3:30–4:30	Large-group discussion

FIGURE 15.1. Example schedule for a day of mindful practice.

another sense as well. Because the Day of Mindfulness usually takes place on the weekend, it can represent a conscious setting aside of the usual running around and getting things done, in favor of paying attention from one moment to the next from midmorning to late afternoon. Patients are encouraged to wear comfortable clothes and layers, so that they can take off or put on clothes to warm up or cool down throughout the day. They bring their own lunch, including a beverage, and rainwear or a warm jacket in case they would like to do walking meditation outdoors and it is rainy or chilly. As in the class, mats, cushions, and chairs are provided, but patients bring whatever else they might need to be comfortable during extended periods of practice. These might include a pillow, a blanket, or a yoga mat.

Once people have arrived the instructor rings the bells and invites them to sit in silence for a few minutes. People may briefly introduce themselves to each other, then the instructor welcomes the group and discusses some of the ground rules for the day. These ground rules are intended to simplify the time spent together by removing the need for external interaction and allowing participants to deepen their exploration of the mindfulness practices. At a practical level, the instructor asks participants to refrain from talking or making deliberate eye contact throughout the day. Because it is not unusual for a variety of physical or emotional reactions to arise during a day of practice, these rules make it easier for participants to use their energy to observe whatever is present. The instructor then explains that a bell will ring to indicate when a practice starts and when it ends (so people may take off their watches if they choose), and that if anyone is having a difficult time or needs to speak to the instructor about anything else they should not hesitate to do so.

The choice and sequence of practices can vary from setting to setting. Here is a schedule that we have used. The first practice may be a 30-minute sitting meditation with a focus on breath, body, sounds, thoughts, and choiceless awareness. Patients move from focusing their attention on a specific object of awareness, such as the breath, to a more receptive awareness in which whatever is in moment-to-moment experience can become the object and focus of awareness. This is followed by 40 minutes of mindful movement that is guided slowly and gently, always leaving room for people to listen to their bodies. The body scan, the last practice before lunch, is positioned so it offers participants the opportunity to notice the contrast between mindfulness of the body at rest compared to the active stretching and exertion that come from the mindful movement.

In discussing the lunch period, the instructor emphasizes that patients are on their own for this period and they are asked to continue to maintain silence. They are invited to explore what happens to their experience of food when eating takes places more slowly, leaving time for curiosity, chewing, tasting, and swallowing. Depending on the setting, participants may have the option of eating in the classroom or going outside, and when they finish, perhaps taking a mindful walk around the neighborhood until it is time to return. If they go out, then they may wish to put their watches back on and take responsibility for the time for this period.

Because it is easy for participants' energy to dip after lunch, the next practice we introduce, after a brief sitting, may be a walking meditation in which patients are asked to find a track of 10 or so paces that they can walk along unhindered, back and forth (see Session 4–Handout 2). Once again, slowing down the act of walking can heighten the sensations that come from shifting the weight from one leg to the other, lifting the toes, placing the heel, and feeling the body in motion. Walking becomes just walking, and participants may notice that no thinking is required to keep it going; it is an opportunity to cultivate moment-to-moment awareness of something that we usually take for granted.

The mountain meditation[66] may be the last new formal meditation of the day. It draws on the image of a mountain to help people embody sitting with a posture that feels grounded, connected to the earth yet lifted skyward. It also embodies a sense that we can remain grounded regardless of the "weather systems" that might come and go as we watch our minds, be they painful sensations or disturbing thoughts and feelings. Following the mountain meditation, the group continues with more mindful stretching and then takes time to sit in silence (or a minimally guided extended breathing space) as a way to pause between the end of silent practice and discussion.

To start the discussion, we ask participants to break into pairs and share in turn their reactions about the day with each other: one as speaker, the other as listener, before changing roles. In order to keep the energy in the room from peaking too quickly, participants speak softly and whisper as they take turns to listen and to speak, and have a period of speaking more naturally as a transition to when the group members come back as a whole and share their experience of the day, and how their practice is going more generally in their life.

THE LARGER QUESTION OF FOLLOW-UP ONCE MBCT HAS ENDED

As with any short-term treatment, the end of the MBCT program comes too quickly for some patients, and instructors are often faced with requests for follow-up groups or meetings. In part, this is an understandable reaction to letting go of the general support of the group and the sense of shared journey over the 8 weeks. But it also reflects another reality—there are few venues available for former MBCT participants who want to practice with others. This is one of the main reasons that when a Day of Mindfulness is held, graduates of previous classes are invited to attend along with participants in an active MBCT group. The idea of welcoming others who have been through the program sends a message of community and connection through sharing a few hours of joint practice.

Another option for follow-up has been to offer between two and four additional classes spaced over a year after the MBCT group's end date. This has most commonly been done in the randomized trials that have been conducted and less so in community practice. These sessions resemble a typical MBCT class, and patients divide their time between practicing mindfulness and discussing the challenges and discoveries they have had in keeping depression at bay since the course ended. Many patients find this combination of refreshing their skills and sharing with others very helpful (see Figure 15.2). Note that it will be important to define from the outset how many follow-up sessions will be offered. Of course, since these follow-up classes are usually offered only to the original class members, it may not be a solution for the larger number of former MBCT participants.

A third option that is less limited in scope is to offer a regular (weekly or monthly) sitting group that places more emphasis on practice and less on discussion or review. One format employs a 1 hour duration for these meetings, divided into 20 minutes for mindful movement, 25 minutes for sitting meditation, then 15 minutes for discussion. Another format, used in the Oxford Mindfulness Centre once a week, is an early evening (6:15 P.M.) group, starting with a 30- to 40-minute period of practice guided by an instructor, then a refreshment break for "catching up," followed by a 40 minute period of silent practice. Some come for the whole time; others drop in for either the first or second part only. This type of group can be open to all "graduates" of previous MBCT programs and has the advantage of running continuously throughout the year and being organized by the participants themselves. In addition participants are often grateful for information about other centers that hold retreat days or sitting groups.

Finally, in some programs, at the end of Session 8, the instructors give to each participant a copy of the book *The Mindful Way through Depression*[76] as "food for the journey." It has meditations narrated by

0:00	Welcome
	Practice
	Sitting: breath, body, sounds, thoughts. Option of reading a poem at the end of the sitting
0:35	Brief practice review
0:45	Home practice review
	Pairs → large group
	What are your experiences with the practice since the course finished?
	What have you noticed?
1:05	Action plan review (contemplation → refresh, review)
	Pairs → large group
	Have there been difficult situations, times of feeling low?
	How have you responded?
	What did you learn?
	What would you like to incorporate into your action plan?
1:25	Informal chat and refreshments
1:45	Sitting and close

FIGURE 15.2. Example schedule for follow-up meeting after MBCT.

Jon Kabat-Zinn, so participants can experience a different voice to guide them; and, by the end of eight classes, they will recognize a common pattern or familiar teaching whatever page they turn to in the book. The classes have shown participants that they are not alone, that what they thought of as their own peculiar and unique imperfections, are so common in many sufferers, and such a book speaks to this as well. This can be an enormously liberating insight in itself. The classes and the book do not stop there: They link such insight and understanding with practice, a practice that invites us again and again to have the courage to turn toward our deepest distress, to see clearly the patterns of the mind that can exacerbate it, and to bring to our experience a quality of warm attentiveness and compassion that allows us to inhabit our lives more fully.

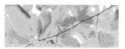 CHAPTER 16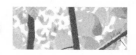

"How Can I Best
Take Care of Myself?"

Session 7

Take a moment to bring to mind what you do during a typical working day. If you spend much of your day apparently doing the same thing, try breaking the activities down into smaller parts: talking to colleagues, e-mailing, making coffee, filing, word processing, eating lunch. And what about evenings and weekends? What sort of things do you find yourself doing then? Make a list in your mind's eye or on paper. What things on the list lift your mood, give you energy, nourish you? And what things on your list dampen your mood or drain your energy?

This exercise helps us to discern the close connection between our activity and our mood. Skillful use of activity is a central aspect of cognitive and behavioral approaches to depression. It is now time to weave it into MBCT.

THE IMPORTANCE OF TAKING ACTION
IN DEALING WITH DEPRESSION

When we started this project to develop a program to help people prevent depression from coming back, our first thought had been to develop a maintenance version of CBT. Prominent in our plans for such an approach was to focus on teaching people how to notice early signs of impending relapse, then take action to avoid the escalation of negative mood. As you can now see, the program we eventually adopted contained less CBT and instead became embedded within a mindfulness-based approach.

But from the outset, we were also concerned that we not lose sight of the fact that cognitive therapy contains many important elements that, together, reduce the chances of relapse. CBT is an empirical, action-oriented approach, and recent research on behavioral activation (BA)[98] shows how the action element is a vital part of CBT. Scheduled homework in these approaches encourages patients to become more aware of the pattern of not only their thinking but also the activities in their lives (what they are doing that maintains their depression, what they are not doing that might allow mood to improve). Learning to monitor such daily activities allows patients to notice when their lives begin to get out of control.

> In monitoring our actions, we become more aware of the pattern of our lives—what we are doing that maintains a mood state, what we are not doing that might allow things to improve.

But CBT and BA do not stop at monitoring activities: They schedule activities. The theme of "taking action" is all-pervasive, as a way of counteracting a period of fatigue or negative mood, or, in CBT, of testing the reality of a negative thought, attitude, or belief. We thought it important that MBCT include this element. From time to time, and especially when depression threatens to overwhelm a person, there is a need to explore how activity may help.[99] Such exploration may simply reveal that the amount of activity needs to be increased, or that the quality of activity needs to change.

TAKING CARE OF YOURSELF

It is important to be aware of a major stumbling block for participants in noticing warning signs and taking action. No amount of awareness of the signs of relapse and planning to take action is likely to affect what actually happens to participants unless they are able to learn gradually to take care of themselves. (Relatedly, we may read a poem such as Mary Oliver's "The Summer Day" during this session; see Box 16.2.) Participants

BOX 16.1

Theme and Curriculum for Session 7

THEME

Using skillful action to take care of ourselves in the face of lowering mood. We can lift depressed mood by intentional skillful action. We can respond more promptly and effectively to lowering mood by learning to recognize our personal pattern of warning signs. After taking a breathing space, we kindly take care of ourselves by acts that give pleasure or a sense of mastery, or provide a clear focus for mindfulness.

AGENDA

- 30- to 40-minute sitting meditation—awareness of breath and body; noticing how we relate to our experiences through the reactions we have to whatever thoughts, feelings, or body sensations arise; especially when difficulties arise within the practice, noting their effects and reactions to them, on the body.
- Practice review.
- Home practice review (including shorter meditations and breathing spaces).
- Exercise to explore links between activity and mood (see Session 7–Handout 3).
- Plan how best to schedule activities for when mood threatens to overwhelm
  - o Rebalancing nourishing and depleting activities
  - o Generating list of pleasure and mastery activities
- 3-minute breathing space as the "first step" before choosing whether to take mindful action.
- Identifying actions to deal with threat of relapse/recurrence (Session 7–Handout 4).
- 3-minute breathing space or mindful walking.
- Distribute Session 7 participant handouts.

|*(cont.)*

- Home practice assignment:
  o Select, from all the different forms of practice, a pattern you intend to use on a regular basis.
  o 3-Minute Breathing Space–Regular (three times a day).
  o 3-Minute Breathing Space–Responsive (whenever you notice unpleasant feelings).
  o Develop action plan to be used in the face of lowered moods.

PREPARATION AND PLANNING

In addition to your personal preparation, remember to bring a black- or whiteboard and writing materials to class for the activity and mood links, and Action Plan exercises. You are also invited to read Mary Oliver's poem "The Summer Day."

PARTICIPANT HANDOUTS FOR SESSION 7

Session 7–Handout 1. Summary of Session 7: "How Can I Best Take Care of Myself?"

Session 7–Handout 2. When Depression Is Overwhelming

Session 7–Handout 3. The Exhaustion Funnel

Session 7–Handout 4. Working Wisely with Unhappiness and Depression–II

Session 7–Handout 5. Home Practice for the Week Following Session 7

Session 7–Handout 6. Home Practice Record Form—Session 7

may discover 101 reasons why they do not deserve to take a rest or do things they enjoy, especially when they are feeling down. Recall the CBT approach to this situation. What is imaginative about CBT is that it does not wait until the person feels like doing something before scheduling it to occur. Instead, CBT identifies those actions and activities associated, for each patient, with being nondepressed, and then works collaboratively with the person to build these into the daily routine.

BOX 16.2

"The Summer Day"

Who made the world?
Who made the swan, and the black bear?
Who made the grasshopper?
This grasshopper, I mean—
the one who has flung herself out of the grass,
the one who is eating sugar out of my hand,
who is moving her jaws back and forth instead of up and down—
who is gazing around with her enormous and complicated eyes.
Now she lifts her pale forearms and thoroughly washes her face.
Now she snaps her wings open, and floats away.
I don't know exactly what a prayer is.
I do know how to pay attention, how to fall down
into the grass, how to kneel down in the grass,
how to be idle and blessed, how to stroll through the fields,
which is what I have been doing all day.
Tell me, what else should I have done?
Doesn't everything die at last, and too soon?
Tell me, what is it you plan to do
with your one wild and precious life?

From *House of Light* by Mary Oliver.[100] Published by Beacon Press, Boston. Copyright © 1990 by Mary Oliver. Reprinted by permission of The Charlotte Sheedy Literary Agency, Inc.

Normally, we can wait until we want to do something before we actually do it. In depression, we have to do something *before* we are able to want to do it.

It is important not to wait until we *feel* like doing something before actually doing it. Instead, we do it anyway—as an experiment to see what we discover.

Importantly, cognitive therapists realize that depression reverses the motivation process. Normally, we can wait until we want to do something before we actually do it; in depression, we have to do something *before* we are able to want to do it. Furthermore, the tiredness and fatigue that occur in depression can be misleading. When we are not depressed, tiredness means that we need to rest. In this case, rest refreshes us. When depressed, however, resting can actually increase tiredness. The fatigue of depression is not normal tiredness; it calls not for rest but for increased activity, if only for a short while. Part of "taking care" of yourself in those moments is to "stay in the game" or keep participating in activities, even if your mood and thoughts seem to say that there is no use.

> The fatigue of depression is not normal tiredness;
> it calls not for rest but for increased activity,
> if only for a short while.

Because MBCT was designed for people who were between episodes of depression, it was likely that participants would be able to appreciate the message about "taking care of yourself," if only because they might see the difference between their attitude when depressed and their present attitude, when their mood allowed them to be more evenhanded. Nevertheless, participants felt reluctant to take time for themselves. Actually, this is true for many of us.

ANNA'S STORY

Anna worked as a secretary during the day, but she took an avid interest in ice skating and attended many classes at night. She especially enjoyed going to competitions with her classmates, and she had one coming up on the weekend. Anna was also under a lot of stress at work and had been telling herself that she was capable of doing a better job. As she dressed for a skating session, she became aware of thinking that she was not a very good skater and had little chance of scoring well in the competition.

In the past these thoughts would have overwhelmed her. Many times over the past few years, she had given up enjoyable activities because she thought that taking time for herself was self-indulgent. Especially when there was pressure at work, Anna felt that she ought to spend all her available time doing extra tasks for the firm.

This time, Anna became aware of her low mood and decided to take a breathing space. She described becoming aware of and acknowledging what was on her mind, then bringing her attention to her breathing. Finally, she expanded her attention to the body as a whole and noticed its effect on her thoughts or feelings. Anna said that by doing this, she was able to step back and see that there was a bigger picture to what she was experiencing. She saw that her view of the competition was narrow and focused only on having to do well. She also became aware that some of her doubts came from conflicted feelings about her job and were not necessarily about skating, which she enjoyed.

The breathing space enabled Anna to take an alternative view of some of her more critical thinking, and to devise a plan to take action despite its messages of despair. She acknowledged that although the doubtful thoughts might still be with her, she could go out and compete anyway. Anna said that by taking this wider view of what was happening to her, she could see more clearly that her task at this moment was to be at this event and do her best. This allowed her to participate with more enthusiasm and commitment.

Afterward, it became clear that the breathing space had not just given Anna a pause. It had connected her to the regular formal meditation practice that had become an important aspect of her new daily routine. It was as if, during that short breathing space, Anna had been able to bring to the situation the "wider perspective" she had discovered during her longer, more formal sittings and her work in the classes. She had found particularly helpful the way that formal sitting meditation mixed focusing on the breath with "choiceless awareness" of whatever came up, which meant that whatever was in moment-to-moment experience could become the object and focus of attention as if it were the breath. The task was to observe anything that arose and allow it to remain in awareness without judging it, or taking it personally. Anna had been surprised at how much meaning could be attached to this moment-by-moment experience, for example, hearing a simple sound. Most of the time, she did not expect sound to carry any emotional overtones whatsoever. Yet for her, listening in this way brought greater awareness of emotions, especially anger and tension. She had also become more aware of how, when tense, her tendency, almost a reflex, was to brace or tighten different parts of her body that had previously escaped her awareness.

The instruction to "open" to such feelings, to "soften" in response to them, allowed Anna to stay with such sensations longer than she might previously have done. The attitude of the instructor had also been important, encouraging Anna's curiosity about such observations, and allowing her to take a wider perspective on experience. She found the instructor's questions became her own. Was this thought or feeling pulling for her attention? What did she notice about this experience? How long did it last? Did it change or stay the same? Was she aware of any thoughts alongside what she was experiencing? How did it fade, if at all? All of this formal practice was now available to her, made present in each situation by her greater awareness of what was going on. Anna's experience when preparing for her competition was that the breathing space was helpful because it was continuous with the rest of her practice rather than an isolated "quick fix" and a substitute for regular formal practice.

Anna's experience raises an important issue: that the sense of "opening" to difficult thoughts, feelings, and sensations allowed her to see more clearly when she was vulnerable to thinking in old and unproductive ways. She was beginning to identify her own relapse signature. But more than all this, Anna learned that feeling down really affected her ability to engage in activities that would nourish her. Notice the description at the start of her story: "Many times over the past few years, she had given up enjoyable activities because she thought that taking time for herself was self-indulgent. Especially when there was pressure at work, Anna felt that she ought to spend all her available time doing extra tasks for the firm."

Anna is not alone. Depression depletes us. It drains us of the vital energy we need that normally get us up in the morning and keeps us going during the day. Even worse, it takes away any anticipation of pleasure from things we normally enjoy. Even *thinking* of such pleasures is aversive. Anna took a breathing space, but after it, she knew that there were times that taking action was the most important thing: Simply having the courage to do something she did not feel like doing was what her body and mind needed.

NOTICING THE LINKS BETWEEN ACTIVITY AND MOOD

In order to introduce this theme, after the sitting meditation at the beginning of the session, and the inquiry into the practice and the home practice, we ask participants to do the exercise with which this chapter started: to reflect in silence on, then to write down, some of the typical things they do in a day.

When the list is complete, participants categorize the activities into *N*, the activities in daily life that *nourish*, and *D*, the activities in life from day to day that deplete, that drain one of energy.

Each participant may then look at the *balance* between N and D activities. Sometimes, participants feel that whether an activity is nourishing or depleting *depends*—for instance on their mood or on other external circumstances. In these cases the instructor encourages them to ask "What does it depend on?" and become curious about what are the factors that change the same activity from "nourishing" into "depleting" and vice versa.

Then, in pairs or small groups, participants ask the following questions:

> "Of the nourishing activities: How might I change things so that I make more time to do these things more often or become more aware of them when I do?"
>
> "Of the depleting or draining activities: How might these best be done less often or handled more skillfully?"

When doing this exercise in class, one theme that often emerges is a greater awareness of the activities that deplete rather than those that nourish.

> "I always feel half-dead when I awake. It's dreadful just dragging myself out of bed."
>
> "I rush so much to get the kids out to school, it feels so bad—so depleting. But sometimes, when I don't have an early appointment at work, I can take more time, then we get to talk more and it's really great—much more nourishing."

Another way of illustrating this that we sometimes use in the class is to talk about the exhaustion funnel (see Session 7–Handout 3).

ACTION TO TAKE WHEN MOOD IS SLIDING

The next step is to encourage participants to discover how they might best deal with periods of low mood that may lead to depression by knowing, from direct experience, which activities are likely to be most helpful, then to cultivate such activities as tools to cope with periods of worsening mood. Having these tools already available means that participants will be more likely to persist with them in the face of the negative thoughts—such as "Why bother with anything?"—that are simply part of the territory of depressed mood. Working by themselves or in pairs, and having already seen the connection between actions and mood, participants move on to consider ways in which they might change *what* they do or *how* they do things, in order to deal with low mood. Let's start with the *how*, then move to the *what*.

Dealing Skillfully with Day-to-Day Life

A common theme in depression is a sense of hopelessness, coupled with guilt when people seek to make changes in their favor, for instance, taking more time for themselves.

> "There are things in life over which you don't have a choice, like going to work."
>
> "Most of us are not raised to take time for ourselves."
>
> "You can only do something nice for yourself once your obligations to others, or to your work, have been satisfied."
>
> "I am balancing being a mom, a career woman, a wife, and a housekeeper. Where do I find the time for myself?"
>
> "My parents are elderly and need caring for. It would be wrong for me to put myself first."

These comments describe how we are all pulled in many directions much of the time. Yet there is another aspect we would do well to notice: These comments seem to be very general, and to imply that there is no room for things to be different than they are. We can see the impasse here. If we want things to be different but our thoughts tell us things won't change, then we are stuck. But what if, by becoming more aware of what is happening, we start to "taste the raisin"—to pay more attention even in the midst of the busy-ness? Is there a possibility of "looking for the spaces" even when things are hectic, so that looking after yourself is not an optional extra? Taking action starts with simply noticing what is going on around you.

Take the case of Jackie, a nurse on a busy hospital ward, always, as she said, "being knocked off her feet" with one thing after another. There simply seemed to be no time for her to relax, far less to sit and meditate. But she started to pay more attention within the busy-ness. She noticed that little spaces opened up even at the most hectic times. She said, for example, that she had needed to phone someone in another part of the hospital to get some test results on a patient. She phoned several times but got no reply. This was one of the most frustrating aspects of her job, waiting for someone in another department to answer the phone, when she had so much to do. She started to get angry.

Then, she stopped. Here was 30 seconds in which she could not rush around; here was a moment of potential silence in the noise of the day. She started to use the lack of an answer as an opportunity to take a breathing space, to step back. Gradually, she started to notice many other times when she could step back, for example, pushing a drugs trolley, whose speed limited the pace of movement along the corridor, or walking to the other end of the ward to see a patient's family. Prior to this, she had thought that meditation practice might best be done when taking a lunch break or going to the restroom. Now, she found she could look for the "in-between" spaces throughout the day, spaces that transformed her thoughts, feelings, and behavior for the rest of the activities of the day.

In a way, she had found a way of "turning toward" rather than escaping or avoiding her experience. This is exactly what we ask of participants: to hold the difficult aspects of their daily lives, as well as their beliefs or expectations about them, and to move closer to them. After all, it is what they have been doing in the practice for the past 6 weeks with body sensations, feelings, and thoughts. Having mapped the territory, seeing more clearly what is going on by using the breathing space, it may be time to consider taking action.

Changing Actions: Focusing on Mastery and Pleasure

When people feel sad, there are two types of activities that can lift their mood, but that depression tends to undermine. The first type of helpful activity is one that gives pleasure. Once people are depressed, it is harder to enjoy the things they once found enjoyable (e.g., going out for a meal with a friend; taking a nice, long bath; eating dessert; or buying something simply because it would be fun to have).

The second type of helpful activity that depression undermines is one that gives a sense of mastery. These kinds of activities nourish participants by contributing to a sense of accomplishment, or a feeling that they are "taking care of business." Some of these include writing a letter, filling out an income tax form, shopping for groceries, or mowing the lawn. Notice that these may not be inherently pleasurable, but something in the world is different after doing them.

Expanding the List

So in considering what action might be taken to deal with low mood, participants look at their list of daily activities and consider which give a sense of pleasure, which give a sense of mastery, and how to add further activities that might increase both. It is interesting to see what examples participants can generate from their own experience. Many may seem trivial (e.g., watching a video, phoning a friend). They may have seemed too unimportant to put on the earlier list of things that either nourish or drain energy. The instruction is to expand the list of "nourishing" activities and put a *P* next to those that give pleasure and an *M* next to those that give a sense of mastery, no matter how trivial.

How Can This Be Used in Day-to-Day Life?

The next step is for participants to select those activities that might be scheduled in the future (including breaking them down into small steps), so that they are not omitted by default.

THE BREATHING SPACE: ADDING THE ACTION STEP

The core of the breathing space has involved three steps: (1) acknowledging what is going on in the mind and the body, (2) bringing attention to the breath, then (3) expanding attention to the body. When feeling down, the first step is always to take a breathing space.

Then, we choose what to do next: this might be to focus on the body (see Session 5, Chapter 13) or thoughts (see Session 6, Chapter 14), or after Session 7, to take mindful action.

There are both general messages and a specific one here. The general message is that by actually being present in more of our moments, and making mindful decisions about what we really need at each of those moments, we can use activity to become more aware and alert, and to regulate mood. The specific message is that depressed mood cannot be overlooked. We must always make a choice about what (specifically) to do next. The nature of depression demands such specificity.

We include some hints (Session 7–Handout 3) as to how participants, after reconnecting with an expanded awareness in the breathing space, can move to take some skillful action. As we have seen in dealing with depressed feelings, activities that are pleasurable or give a sense of mastery may be particularly helpful. However, doing things that give pleasure or increase mastery is particularly difficult when mood is low, and the handouts include additional material that participants can read and share with partners or family members outside the class. Whatever action is taken, the idea is to act mindfully, to ask "What do I need for myself right now? How can I best take care of myself right now?", and to answer these questions in the knowledge that they may not *feel* like doing anything at all—but that doing something, no matter how small a step it seems, can be a large step toward health and well-being.

SOME TIPS ABOUT TAKING ACTION WHEN MOOD IS LOW

Some people have found the following "tips" are useful in keeping perspective on what activity can or cannot do for them:

- As best you can, perform your action as an experiment, without prejudging how you will feel after it is completed. Keep an open mind about whether doing this will be helpful in any way.
- Break an activity down into smaller, more manageable steps, either by time (doing something for only a few minutes, then giving yourself permission to stop) or by activity (doing only one aspect of a larger activity; e.g., such as clearing one part of a desk rather than the whole desk).
- Consider a range of activities, and don't limit yourself to a favorite few. Sometimes, trying new behaviors can be interesting in itself. "Exploring" and "inquiring" often work to diminish "withdrawal" and "retreat" reactions.
- Don't expect miracles. Carry out what you have planned as best you can. Putting extra pressure on yourself by expecting your new approach to alter things dramatically may be unrealistic. Rather, activities are helpful in building your overall sense of control in the face of shifts in your mood. They are also helpful in allowing you to see how the practice of mindfulness can influence your behavior.
- Remember not to wait until you *feel* like doing it.

ACTION PLAN TO DEAL WITH THREAT OF RELAPSE/RECURRENCE

The aim of this session is for participants to arrive at the point where they have some specific plans for how to deal with periods of heightened vulnerability. The groundwork for this has been done. Now, participants work with the worksheet (see Session 7–Handout 3), and then return to their pairs or small groups to check in with each other and discuss their action plans. They examine what sort of specific strategies they might actually adopt and—very importantly—to consider *what obstacles* might stop them from taking such action and how they might deal with them:

- The first step always is to take a breathing space.
- The second step is for participants to make a choice, using other practices that they have found helpful in the past to gather

themselves as best they can (e.g., listening to a mindfulness practice audio track; reminding themselves what they learned in the class; determining what they found helpful then; going back to something they read or heard during class that captured the essential message of the program; reminding themselves that the feelings are very intense right now, but what they need now is no different from what they practiced then).

- The third step is to take some action, especially action that in the past would have given a sense of *pleasure* or *mastery*, even if it seems futile to do so right now (see Session 7–Handout 1). Break activities down into smaller parts (e.g., doing only part of a task, or restricting yourself to doing it for only a short and easily manageable period of time).

The important thing is to let the past experience of relapse be the teacher. Some participants decide to write themselves a letter, including a list of actions to take, with an instruction to choose at least one, even if they expect not to feel like doing it at the time. Then, they seal the letter and open it only when they start to feel depressed. This, they decide, is the best way to give themselves the benefit of the hard-earned wisdom that might not be available to them at that time.

Participants report that the worst times are often when depression comes out of the blue. For example, waking up in the morning is a very vulnerable period for many. Even people who have not been depressed in the past can find the period immediately after wakening to be difficult, as the body may take time to wake up, and plans for the day can besiege the mind, bringing a sense of anticipated exhaustion. For those who have been depressed, such early morning periods can mimic the symptoms of an episode and evoke huge fears that it is all coming back.

At these times, we encourage them to start by taking a breathing space. Afterward it may be possible to ask themselves: "How can I best be kind to myself right now? What is the best gift I can give to myself at this moment?" Asking specific questions is helpful: "I do not know how long this mood will last; how can I best look after myself until it passes?" Given that the negative thinking can be quite overwhelming in such situations, participants have the chance to observe the tendency of the mind at these moments to be drawn into rumination ("Why am I feeling like this?";

"What's wrong with me?"; "I should be better than this"; "A good parent would feel more energetic about getting their children ready for school, which means I am a bad parent").

Most participants say that it is very helpful to shift attention deliberately into the body and spend some time observing—with gentleness and curiosity—how and where the mood is affecting physical sensations, in order to "open" and "soften." Then they find it easier to make an intentional choice about what to do next.

What we are saying here is that when things are tough, the task is really to focus on each moment, to "handle each moment as best you can." If the quality with which a person handles a difficult moment shifts even by 1%, then that is an important shift because it affects the next moment, and the next, and so on; so one small change can have a large impact in the end.

USING HOME PRACTICE TO PREPARE FOR THE END OF THE CLASSES

Given that this will be the last home practice to be assigned, it is important for participants to continue to develop routines for practicing on their own (we return to this theme again in Session 8, to remind people of the importance of regular practice). We ask them to spend some quality time between now and the next session making concrete plans for relapse prevention.

We ask them to choose—from among all the different types of formal mindfulness practice they have experienced—a form of practice on which they intend to settle on a regular, daily basis for the next few weeks (or until the first follow-up meeting of the class), no matter how long or short. Having chosen, their instructions are to use this practice on a daily basis this week and record reactions on the Home Practice Record Form.

In addition to the 3-minute breathing space, participants are given instructions about how to add an action step to it, whenever they notice unpleasant thoughts or feelings (see Session 7–Handout 1 for details).

Finally, there are instructions for how to involve family members in the task of detecting relapse and working wisely with dealing with such vulnerable moments. The task we give participants is to write down suggestions for an Action Plan that might be used as a framework for coping action, once they or their friends or family notice early warning signs. They are reminded to address their frame of mind at the time (e.g., "I know you probably will not be keen on this idea but I think that, nonetheless, it is very important that you . . . "). For example, they might do some mindful walking, put on a mindful movement, body scan, or mindfulness practice; remind themselves what they learned during the class, what was helpful then; take breathing spaces leading into bodily focus, thought review, or considered action (appropriately broken down into simple steps, if necessary); read something that would "reconnect" with their "wiser" mind; and so on. It is important that instructors review these ideas during the next, final class.

Summary of Session 7:
"How Can I Best Take Care of Myself?"

What we actually *do* with our time from moment to moment, from hour to hour, from one year to the next, can be a very powerful influence affecting our general well-being and our ability to deal skillfully with depression.

You might like to try asking yourself these questions:

1. Of the things that I do, what nourishes me, what increases my sense of actually being alive and present rather than merely existing? (*N* activities—for nourishing)

2. Of the things that I do, what drains me, what decreases my sense of actually being alive and present, what makes me feel I am merely existing, or worse? (*D* activities—for depleting)

3. Accepting that there are some aspects of my life I simply cannot change, am I consciously choosing to increase the time and effort I give to nourishing activities, and to decrease the time and effort I give to depleting activities?

By being actually present in more of our moments and making mindful decisions about what we really need in each of those moments, we can use activity to become more aware and alert, and to regulate mood.

This is true for dealing with both the regular pattern of our daily lives and periods of low mood that may lead to depression—we can use our day-by-day experience to discover and cultivate activities we can use as tools to cope with periods of worsening mood. Having these tools already available means that we will be more likely to persist with them in the face of negative thoughts (e.g., "Why bother with anything?") that are simply part of the territory of depressed mood.

For example, one of the simplest ways to take care of your physical and mental well-being is to take daily physical exercise—as a minimum, aim for at least one brisk, 10-minute walk a day; also, if at all possible, engage in other types of exercise, such as mindful stretching, yoga, swimming, jogging, and so on. Once exercise is in your daily routine, it is a readily available response to depressed moods as they arise.

The breathing space provides a way to remind us to use activity to deal with unpleasant feelings as they arise.

(cont.)

USING THE BREATHING SPACE: THE ACTION STEP

After reconnecting with an expanded awareness in the breathing space, it may feel appropriate to take some *considered action*. In dealing with depressed feelings, the following activities may be particularly helpful:

1. Do something pleasurable.
2. Do something that will give you a sense of satisfaction or mastery.
3. Act mindfully.

Ask yourself: What do I need for myself right now? How can I best take care of myself right now?
Try some of the following:

1. **Do something pleasurable.**

   Be kind to your body: Have a nice hot bath; have a nap; treat yourself to your favorite food without feeling guilty; have your favorite hot drink; give yourself a facial or manicure.

   Engage in enjoyable activities: Go for a walk (maybe with the dog or a friend); visit a friend; do your favorite hobby; do some gardening; take some exercise; phone a friend; spend time with someone you like; cook a meal; go shopping; watch something funny or uplifting on TV; read something that gives you pleasure; listen to music that makes you feel good.

2. **Do something that gives you a sense of mastery, satisfaction, achievement, or control.**

   Clean the house; clear out a cupboard or drawer; catch up with letter writing; do some work; pay a bill; do something that you have been putting off doing; take some exercise. (*Note*. It's especially important to congratulate yourself whenever you complete a task or part of a task, *and to break tasks down into smaller steps and only tackle one step at a time.*)

3. **Act mindfully** (read Staying Present, Session 4–Handout 5).

   Focus your entire attention on just what you are doing right now; keep yourself in the very moment you are in; put your mind in the present (e.g., "Now I am walking down the stairs . . . now I can feel the banister beneath my hand . . . now I'm walking into the kitchen . . . now I'm turning on the light . . . "); be aware of your breathing as you do other things; be aware of the contact of your feet with the floor as you walk.

(cont.)

REMEMBER

1. Try to perform your action as an experiment. Try not to prejudge how you will feel after it is completed. Keep an open mind about whether doing this will be helpful in any way.

2. Consider a range of activities and don't limit yourself to a favorite few. Sometimes, trying new behaviors can be interesting in itself. "Exploring" and "inquiring" often work against "withdrawal" and "retreat."

3. Don't expect miracles. Carry out what you have planned as best you can. Putting extra pressure on yourself by expecting this to alter things dramatically may be unrealistic. Rather, activities are helpful in building your overall sense of control in the face of shifts in your mood.

When Depression Is Overwhelming

Sometimes you may find that depression comes out of the blue. For example, you may wake up feeling very tired and listless, with hopeless thoughts going through your mind.

When this happens, it may be useful for you to tell yourself, "Just because I am depressed now does not mean that I have to stay depressed."

When things come out of the blue like this, they set off negative ways of thinking in everyone.

If you have been depressed in the past, it will tend to trigger old habits of thought that may be particularly damaging: full of overgeneralizations, predictions that this will go on forever, and "back to square one" thinking. All of these ways of making sense of what is happening to you tend to undermine your taking any action.

Having these symptoms does not mean that the depression needs to go on for a long time or that you are already in a full-blown episode of depression.

Ask yourself, "What can I do to look after myself to get me through this low period?"

Take a breathing space to help gather yourself. This may help you see your situation from a wider perspective. This wider perspective allows you to become aware of both the pull of the old habits of thinking and what skillful action you might take.

The Exhaustion Funnel

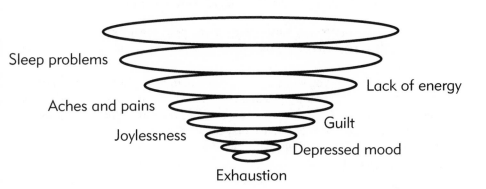

Sleep problems

Lack of energy

Aches and pains

Guilt

Joylessness

Depressed mood

Exhaustion

The narrowing area of the circles illustrates the narrowing of our lives as we give up the things that we enjoy but that seem "optional." The result is that we stop doing activities that would nourish us, leaving only work or other stressors that often deplete our resources. Professor Marie Asberg suggests that those of us who continue downward are likely to be those who are the most conscientious workers, those whose level of self-confidence is closely dependent on our performance at work (i.e., those who are often seen as the best workers, not the lazy ones). The diagram also shows the sequence of accumulating "symptoms" experienced by one participant as the funnel narrowed and he became more and more exhausted.

Working Wisely
with Unhappiness and Depression–II

**RESPONDING WISELY (CARING FOR YOURSELF
WHEN YOU NOTICE THE FIRST SIGNS OF DEPRESSION)**

In Session 6–Handout 4, you wrote down what triggers downward spirals in mood for you, and what you notice as the signs that your mood is dropping (e.g., thoughts, feelings, body sensations). On this sheet, we consider how you might skillfully respond when you find yourself in this position. It may be helpful to look back over your course handouts, to remind yourself of what you have done and see whether you have discovered anything that might help.

In the past, what have you noticed that helped when you were becoming depressed?

What might be a skilful response to the pain of depression? How could you respond to the turmoil of thoughts and feelings without adding to it (including what you have learned in the classes)?

(cont.)

How can you best care for yourself at this difficult and painful time (e.g., things that would soothe you, activities that might nourish you, people you might contact, small things you could do to respond wisely to distress)?

YOUR ACTION PLAN

Now write down suggestions to yourself for an Action Plan that you can use as a framework for coping, once you or your friends/family have noticed early warning signs (remember to address the frame of mind that you might be in at the time; e.g., "I know you probably will not be keen on this idea but I think that, nonetheless, it is very important that you . . . "). For example, you might put on a mindful movement, body scan, or sitting meditation recording; remind yourself of what you learned during the class that was helpful then; take frequent breathing spaces leading into thought review or considered action; read something that will "reconnect" you with your "wiser" mind; and so on.

It may be helpful to remind yourself that what you need at times of difficulty is no different from what you have already practiced many times throughout this course.

Home Practice for the Week Following Session 7

1. From all the different forms of formal mindfulness practice you have experienced, settle on a form of practice that you intend to use on a regular, daily basis until our first follow-up class. Use this practice on a daily basis this week, and record your reactions on the Home Practice Record Form.

2. Complete the Action Plan (Working Wisely with Unhappiness and Depression–II, Session 7–Handout 4) to prepare for times when mood threatens to overwhelm you. Feel free to include others—family or friends—in this planning.

3. 3-Minute Breathing Space—Regular (audio track 8): Practice three times a day at times that you have decided in advance. Record each time you do it by circling an R for the appropriate day on the Home Practice Record Form; note any comments/difficulties.

4. 3-Minute Breathing Space—Responsive plus action (audio track 9): Practice *whenever you notice unpleasant thoughts or feelings*. Record each time you do the coping breathing space by circling an X for the appropriate day on the Home Practice Record Form; note any comments/difficulties.

Home Practice Record Form—Session 7

Name: _____

Record on the Home Practice Record Form each time you practice. Also, make a note of anything that comes up in the home practice, so that we can talk about it at the next meeting.

Day/date	Practice (Yes/No)	Comments
Wednesday Date: _____	Which formal practice chosen? Planned—R R R Responsive— X X X X X X X X X X	
Thursday Date: _____	Which formal practice chosen? R R R X X X X X X X X X X	
Friday Date: _____	Which formal practice chosen? R R R X X X X X X X X X X	
Saturday Date: _____	Which formal practice chosen? R R R X X X X X X X X X X	

R, 3-Minute Breathing Space—Regular Version; X, 3-Minute Breathing Space—Responsive Version.

(cont.)

Day/date	Practice (Yes/No)	Comments
Sunday Date: _____	Which formal practice chosen? R R R X X X X X X X X X X	
Monday Date: _____	Which formal practice chosen? R R R X X X X X X X X X X	
Tuesday Date: _____	Which formal practice chosen? R R R X X X X X X X X X X	
Wednesday Date: _____	Which formal practice chosen? R R R X X X X X X X X X X	

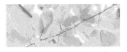 CHAPTER 17

Maintaining and Extending New Learning

Session 8

If there were a way to pull together the central ideas covered in the program, what would it be? Perhaps it is this: that when relapse-related automatic thought patterns are triggered, there are ways of seeing this happening earlier, and then skillful ways of responding. These ways do not deny that there is a problem with which people must deal. But they remind us that there are choices, one of which is to face whatever is causing the depression, and the depression itself, in a radically different way. Instead of ruminating about the problem; instead of asking unanswerable questions such as "Why me?" and "What is it about me that causes this?", instead of the thoughts of failure that just go around in circles, there exists another possibility.

The task becomes that of holding whatever we become aware of—thoughts, feelings, impulses, or sensations—in a more spacious awareness, anchored in the present moment by the breath. As we have seen before, we never know what we might find! In due course, people may come to understand, and to experience at a very deep level, that the mind has a way of processing the "stuff of everyday life" that is wiser than they might have imagined. Learning to trust that this process will occur without interference from other, more problem-solving modes of mind is difficult.

> The mind has a way of processing the "stuff of everyday life" that is wiser than any of us might have imagined.

Using a computer analogy may help. Many people buy computers to do relatively simple tasks such as word processing or tracking accounts. We are now told that much of the computing power on an average desktop PC is never called upon to perform. Now, imagine that the situation with our minds and bodies is something similar: that we have a "processor" in our mind–body system (the "Great Computer Within") that can, if allowed to do so, help to process the difficulties and problems that accumulate during our lifetimes; that the reason for allowing it to do so is because it is able to handle things in a much wiser and gentler way than we ever could do normally; that this different mode of mind is always available to us, though the busy-ness of our lives often obscures it.

Whether or not we find this analogy helpful, it remains true that not all situations call for action or efforts to make changes. In the realm of emotions, things often don't follow logically. It might be that in some areas of our lives, the harder we try, the more we can achieve. But this rule seldom applies when we are dealing with feelings that we don't want to have or aspects of ourselves of which we are critical.

It may be a paradox, but if we cope with our unpleasant feelings by pushing them away or trying to control them, we actually end up maintaining them. This is the last thing we would expect; yet it remains true. In avoiding or "pushing away" our experience, we remain limited in understanding its wider context. Yet as soon as we accept that we feel sad or anxious, in that moment, it is already different. Accepting that we feel a certain way doesn't mean that we have to approve of it, nor does it mean that we are finally defeated by it and might just as well give up. Quite the contrary: by accepting how we feel, we are just telling ourselves that this is our starting point. We are actually in a better position to decide what to do.

> If we cope with our unpleasant feelings by pushing them away or trying to control them, we actually end up maintaining them.

Of course, the ability to decide which course to take—whether to act to bring about change or to accept how things are for now—will depend on many things, not least of which is our momentary awareness of what is called for in any situation. *Sometimes wisdom means not to act.*

It might be that our situation is genuinely difficult or chaotic. If so, we may need simply to "be with" the sense of difficulty or chaos. "Being with" is not about gritting our teeth and putting up with things. Rather, it implies that we allow ourselves to see it clearly, to explore the difficulty itself and our reactions to it with gentleness and compassion. This seeing might bring up a sense of uncertainty, and if so, some anxiety. But if we can be willing to experience such "not knowing," resisting the temptation to act just because we cannot stand the uncertainty, then there is a much greater chance that we will see things clearly.

> By *allowing* ourselves to see how we feel, we are reminding ourselves that *this is our starting point.* We are in a better position to decide what to do.

If we can experience the chaos and uncertainty consciously, the chaos itself can take us to the clarity. And if we need a brake on the mind's tendency to want to act impulsively, its tendency to prefer any course of action to the anguish that accompanies confusion, then we can always come back to the breath.

COMING FULL CIRCLE

We start this last session by first using the body scan as the formal practice, to give a sense of coming full circle. Second, we make time for participants to look at the relapse prevention action plans they started to work on in Session 7 and the home practice during the week. Third, participants recall their experiences over the course of the program, in a scheduled exercise that allows people to think back. While the last class together naturally brings to mind thoughts of endings and partings, there is a way in which Session 8 is more like the end of the beginning rather than the beginning of the end. Because what is being asked is not bounded by time limits or deadlines, "the real Session 8," as Jon Kabat-Zinn has said, "is the rest of our lives."

We set aside a little time for participants to tell of their experience with the body scan but do not conduct a full inquiry. It is interesting to

BOX 17.1

Theme and Curriculum for Session 8

THEME

Planning for a new way of living. Maintaining and extending a more mindful and caring way of being requires clear intention and planning. It is helpful to link intentions for regular mindfulness practice to a personally significant value or positive reason for taking care of oneself.

AGENDA

- Body scan practice.
- Brief practice review.
- Home practice review (including early warnings and relapse prevention action plans).
- Review whole course: what has been learned—in pairs, then go around whole group.
- Give out questionnaire for participants to give personal reflections on the program.
- Discuss how best to keep up momentum developed over the past 7 weeks in both formal and informal practice.
- Check and discuss plans, and link them to positive reasons for maintaining the practice.
- Distribute Session 8 participant handouts and book (e.g., *The Mindful Way through Depression*[76]).
- End the classes with a concluding meditation (marble, stone, or bead) or with participants wishing each other well.

PREPARATION AND PLANNING

In addition to your personal preparation, remember to bring the Session 8 questionnaire. A black- or whiteboard may be helpful to record participants' choices for maintaining practice and relapse prevention plans. Also, remember to bring a memento or a book for each participant, to mark the end of the program, depending on your practice.

(cont.)

hear how people respond to the practice now that they have come to the end of the classes. With a greater sense of how attention can be trained and reclaimed, the body scan is viewed by most in a different way than it was 8 weeks earlier. This does not mean that participants have all fallen in love with it. In fact, those who found parts of it boring or tedious still often say that this was the case. What is new, however, is that when people find it boring, it bothers them less. They have learned to relate differently to their own mind states. They are better able to recognize that even this "negative" experience can teach them about being with boredom or tedium, if that is what they are experiencing. Others in the class remember the body scan as very helpful to them and, when the home practice has given them the opportunity, have returned to it in some form. For them, the opportunity to do the body scan again in the class is an affirmation of their practice with it over the past 7 weeks.

RELAPSE PREVENTION ACTION PLANS

And what of participants' relapse prevention action plans discussed in Session 7? Participants were to continue to develop such plans during the week as home practice. The idea was that if people had an early warning system in place and had written down some helpful things to do, they could draw on these in times of need. Participants discussed a number of these ideas, many of which were based on their experience of *not* having a plan like this available the last time they became depressed.

Jennifer, a woman in her mid-40s, pointed to the classes providing her with a better understanding of the "territory of depression," especially how her moods could shift day to day. To be well prepared to respond to her changing moods, Jennifer drew from the activities that gave her pleasure or contributed to a sense of mastery, and came up with what she called "My Antidepressant Activity List." She filed it away until she needed to consult it. For her, this list would include material from the participant handouts, with the instruction to herself, "Jenn, although you may not feel like doing any of these, select at least one and do it anyway":

- Do something today just because you enjoy it.
  - o Phone a friend.
  - o Rent a DVD or download a film you enjoy.
  - o Have a nice, hot bath.
  - o Have a nap.
  - o Treat yourself to your favorite food, without feeling guilty.
  - o Have your favorite hot drink.
  - o Go for a walk (maybe with the dog or a friend).
  - o Visit a friend.
  - o Do your favorite hobby.
  - o Spend time with someone you like.
  - o Cook a meal.
  - o Go shopping.
  - o Watch something funny or uplifting on television.
  - o Read something that gives you pleasure.
  - o Listen to music that makes you feel good.
- Do something that gives you a sense of mastery, satisfaction, achievement, or control.
  - o Clean one part of the house (for no more than 20 minutes).
  - o Clear out a cupboard or drawer.
  - o Catch up with letter writing.
  - o Pay a bill.
  - o Do some gardening.
  - o Do something that you have been putting off doing.
  - o Take some exercise.
- Remember to take that big task and break it down into smaller steps (e.g., just do 10 minutes of it) and to congratulate yourself afterward.

There can be many such ideas. The important thing to emphasize is that any of these might be used in tandem with an early warning system, so long as people decide to do something early enough in the process. Remember that *having the idea is not enough*: Translating the idea into action (no matter how small) is critical.

LOOKING BACK

Following the feedback on the practice and the home practice, we set time aside for people to look back. The instruction is to spend some time, alone or in pairs, reflecting on a number of questions:

"Think back to why you came originally—what were your expectations and why did you stay?"

"What did you want/hope for?"

"What did you get out of coming, if anything? What did you learn?"

"What were the costs to you?"

"What are your biggest blocks/obstacles to continuing?"

"What strategies might help you not get stuck?"

In addition to this exercise, participants spend a few minutes writing down their personal reflections about the program. We use a simple questionnaire that asks people to rate, on a scale from 1 to 10 (1, *not at all important*, and 10, *extremely important*), how important the program has been to them. We then leave the page blank and say to them, "Please say why you have given it this rating."

Reading these comments after the program is over, it is impossible not to be struck by the commonalities in the participants' experience: It has usually been hard, but again and again they say that it has been a challenge worth accepting.

"It has given me the opportunity to learn how to give myself space for slowing down and *being*—especially being in the moment. I know that I have a safe place—an inner, safe place that allows me to be me, without any hassles, criticisms, and so on, from other people—and learning to give it priority (the space, that is) on a regular basis helps defuse negative mental thoughts before they cause any more damage."

"This program has confirmed and repeated some things I already knew about depression—but it has been more effective to be able to go through it with other people who know what it's like."

"The good and the not so good—it is a tremendous beginning for me to learn about myself and accept all thoughts and feelings. The breath has been unexpectedly rewarding."

"I have discovered an inner strength."

"I now have tactics when I sense a low mood/depression starting."

"It has removed my sense of shame about having been depressed and anxious in the past, therefore giving me greater self-acceptance."

"I have discovered a way of moving into an inner place of calm/centeredness."

"My depression and associated anxiety had made me very unhappy. . . . I have been able to actually enjoy and be in the present moment . . . realizing this is the only time I have to live . . . so instead of constantly worrying about the future and my past failures, I can more evenly and calmly embrace the present moment. This has allowed me to realize what it is that makes me depressed . . . and how I can recognize these factors to hopefully alleviate any relapse."

"The meditation brought up a lot of strange emotions that worried me at first, but now I realize that they were just emotions I had been repressing for years and that to really live my life, I had to feel them. Although I may get down again at times, my whole perspective on life has changed."

These statements are representative of the immediate responses given during Session 8 of the program and written down when the instructor was nearby. It is always possible that, under these circumstances, participants might wish to speak more about the benefits and less about any difficulties. It is interesting, therefore, to see what participants said some months later, when interviewed. Listen to participants interviewed by researcher Oliver Mason as they look back over the MBCT classes.

We pick up a first interview as the participant is discussing with Oliver his early experience with the formal practice.

P: I did the body scan every day, and like everybody else, found it relaxing, perhaps too relaxing. But that had its benefits, too, because one of the things when you are depressed is this difficulty in relaxing and finding sleep, finding recuperation. You seem to have this motor that's overrunning all the time inside you. So something that gives you that deep relaxation was and is quite valuable. But in the rest of the practices, I did what I was supposed to do.

I: So you went through the course as it was presented to you. Any discoveries or surprises that stick out?

P: The key thing overall has been that often what goes through your mind are just mental phenomena. They are just thoughts, they are just that, they are just thoughts, not necessarily truths. And you do have some choice about which ones to follow. I mean, I am not saying it's necessarily easy to do that. But that idea I found very, very helpful: that you are not a victim of thoughts going on in your mind, a sort of helpless victim just bobbing along with them. You can choose to disregard some and look at others more closely, and look at why those are cropping up more often and with more insistence.

The participant goes on to describe how he is now more able to bring a wider, decentered view to his thoughts and feelings.

I: And you are not quite so close to the problem, either? It's there but you are not it?

P: Yes, exactly. It's not just happening to you; you can see it happening to you. There is a very very big difference there, I think. And I've always felt the biggest challenge comes when you are feeling pretty low. Because at those times, it is less easy to meditate. I find there's less motivation to do it, but the need to do it is greater. I suppose at good times I tend not to do so much formal meditation, but when things are bad, it's important to do it, I think, because it reconnects you to the whole program and the whole ethos behind it, which you can easily forget, you know, if you just start to go down.

This raises the issues that were discussed in Session 7: How do people recognize their relapse signatures?

I: So how do you spot that, when you start to go down?

P: For me, I think the triggers are sluggishness, disturbed sleep, waking up at all times of the night, futility, and hopelessness about things. Not dramatic, but a lowering of your morale and a sort of physical slowness or weakness pervading things.

I: So does that bring you back to meditating straightaway?

P: Not straightaway, at least not always. It's a prompt to do something, certainly. I don't always honor that. I don't always respond to that prompt. But before the program, I would have simply been dragged along, dragged down by it, and I would have felt more hopeless, like there were no kinds of support or props, there was no way other than taking pills.

I: So it's a sense that there is at least something you can do?

P: Yes, it doesn't promise to cure depression, but it's a strategy for dealing with it, which gives you some control over what is happening to you. I suppose that is the key of it, really.

This participant appears to feel differently about his depression. By knowing what the signs of impending depression are for him, and seeing them as prompts, he is able to talk about having choices. He admits how easy it is to forget the program when he feels his mood lowering, but he is able to use the practice to "reconnect to the whole program." Fundamentally, his relationship to his thoughts has altered: " . . . what goes through your mind are just mental phenomena. They are just thoughts, they are just that, they are just thoughts, not necessarily truths. And you do have some choice about which ones to follow." He appears to have a spirit of discovery about his moods and his thoughts. Finally, he has no illusions about the future, nor about a "cure" for his depression.

His experience was that, even months after the classes had finished, he felt able to deal with upsetting events in a way that did not trigger the severe depression that, he felt, would have occurred before. For him, the program appeared to have prevented recurrence of major depression. His experience raises important issues: first, how to keep the practice alive once the classes have ended; and second, how to deal effectively and skillfully with future downturns in mood.

LOOKING FORWARD

Finding a way to set up and maintain practice in the absence of weekly classes is a challenge faced by all participants. It is important to set time aside to hear what type of practice people have decided they will settle on. Because there are a number of choices, the plans are quite varied. Sometimes we find it helpful to list them on the blackboard. Some participants say that they will continue to practice for 30 minutes on a regular basis. Others report that they will alternate between a regular sitting practice and yoga. Usually, participants say that they do not know whether they can sustain the same level of practice they achieved during the course. Instead, they aim to use the breathing space throughout the day, then practice more formally on the weekend or when they feel the need to "refresh" their practice. Others have found one of the guided meditations from the variety of meditations distributed in Session 6 particularly helpful. For others, the track that simply contains the sound of bells gives them sufficient structure to sit without instructions. Whatever the proposed plan, the important thing is that it should be realistic.

Occasionally, the question arises: Is it OK just to sit on the weekends, if one sits long enough? It is important for instructors to be sensitive about giving choices and instruction. Of course, the choice is up to participants, but experience shows that regular, daily, brief practice is preferable to longer but infrequent practice. There is something about the "everydayness" of the practice (no matter how short) that is important. Continuity builds and sustains motivation and momentum. Because relating to our experience mindfully is not part of the territory of the depressed mind, we need all the help we can get in connecting back to it. People need whatever support they can give themselves, whether it is a favorite CD, special quotations, or any other reminders. It is like learning a foreign language: It is better to keep speaking it at every opportunity and on a regular basis.

One of the main reasons instructors devote so much time to this topic has to do with the fact that stress is unpredictable. Nobody knows when and where depression will hit. Yet we also know from studies of both cognitive therapy and MBCT/MBSR that the people who benefit most from the treatment are those who do the home practice.[101] If people can manage to keep the practice fresh, to keep it there each day, each week, then it is much more available than if they let it go. We need to keep our tools oiled, so that they are ready for use when we actually need them. This means, for example, that if participants have decided to use the breathing space as their regular practice, it is best to find time to do one or two breathing spaces each day at regular times, in order to support its use when it is needed to respond to difficulties and stress during the day.

To support this ongoing work, most centers at which mindfulness is taught run a range of follow-up classes and day retreats for those who have participated in 8-week classes. There will be some reunion meetings of each class itself, and even if some cannot arrange to be there, it is an opportunity for the teacher to be in touch to see how things are going. Many MBCT programs now have a silent practice day between Sessions 6 and 7 (see pp. 332–337), and all those who have been through a previous program are invited. Other centers have a regular sitting group (see p. 336).

GIVING ONESELF A REASON
FOR SUSTAINING THE PRACTICE

Our experience has shown that no matter how good these resolutions are, unless they are linked to a positive reason to do them, they are very difficult to adopt. We find it helpful, therefore, to ask each participant to think of one positive reason for sustaining the practice and having relapse prevention strategies in place. The idea is to link the everyday practice with something about which they care deeply.

So as a short meditation/contemplation practice, we ask participants to allow the following question to drop into the mind as a small stone might fall down a deep well:

"What is most important to me in my life (what do I most value) that this practice might help with?"

After a period of silence an answer may come, and the stone can be allowed to drop some more, until it settles on the bottom of the well. What answers come now?

Following this short (2- or 3-minute) practice, participants write whatever came up on cards we have given them. This is for them. There is no need to share it with anyone else, though some participants wish to say what came up.

One participant, Joanne, found that during the classes she seemed to have more time for her children, that she felt more "available" to them and enjoyed them more. This, she felt, was ironic, given that earlier on in the program she had been very concerned that the formal practice was taking time away from her children and her husband. She was able to link the plan to maintain some form of everyday practice with her wish to remain available for her children.

At its base there is, in a sense, one core reason for ensuring that the practice is nourished and sustained and having relapse prevention strategies in place: "Because I care for myself." Of course, taking care of oneself is *the* problem in depression. What was it that Joanne was discovering?

In the Welsh language, there is a word, *trugaredd*, which comes from the root word *caru*, meaning "to love." But because it includes a sense of kindness and unfailing affection, it is often translated as "mercy" or "lovingkindness" and is closely linked to a sense of compassion for self and others. It refers precisely to the qualities we have said are an essential feature of all mindfulness classes, embodied by instructors and "caught" by participants (Chapter 8).

Depression brings with it the opposite of *trugaredd*. Instead we experience attitudes of self-criticism, self-denigration, and even self-loathing. Depression undermines the motivation to be kind to oneself and, with it, the capacity to be available to others. The mindfulness approach invites people to explore a different way in which they may relate to themselves and their world, with a quality of attention that has something of *trugaredd* about it. *Trugaredd,* lovingkindness, never works in one direction only. What Joanne found, to her surprise, was that if she took care of herself, she became more available to others: Greater compassion toward herself brought about greater compassion for others—and not just experiences of participants bear witness to this change; research findings bear it out as well.

These may seem like impossible goals, but we are not talking about striving for goals. Instead, we are speaking of having an intention: to continue exploring how to become more aware of "where we are" from moment to moment; to explore how to step into "being" mode rather than remain in "doing" mode. This involves practicing mindfulness throughout the day. Here are Larry Rosenberg's tips for how this is done:

1. When possible, do just one thing at a time.
2. Pay full attention to what you are doing.
3. When the mind wanders from what you are doing, bring it back.
4. Repeat Step 3 several billion times.
5. Investigate your distractions.[95] (pp. 168–170)

UNPLANNED BENEFITS

What we have found remarkable is that the program can have profound effects on participants, without these ever being part of the explicit "agenda" of the sessions. In particular, the mindfulness practice seems to allow the wider perspective, which has been learned in relation to ordinary daily events, to generalize in unexpected ways. Listen to the following account of someone looking back on the difference it made to practice mindfulness, first in dealing with the humdrum routine of each day, then in coping at a very difficult period of his life, when his father died.

P: This morning, for instance, is a case in point. I had a lot of things to do this morning as usual. It's Monday morning, the dustbin had to go out, and I only had about half an hour to do these things, and I found myself, oh God, I reached the point when I stopped and I couldn't go in any direction. It's as if I had gone totally into mind overload. And I thought, "Oh, hang on." And it's as if there is a switch in the mind now that goes: "Hang on, stop. Be mindful, and we will start with this bit first." It's like an automatic correction. Instead of getting bogged down with the mind, trying to do a whole lot of stuff up front, as it were, and overload me . . . it's the ability to step back from that and hold the mind there. Just sort it out, as it were, just do one thing. I think that is the thing that it does. It gives focus all the time. Because it is easy to be swamped by whatever's on the mind.

I: And that ability remains even in periods of lowness?

P: It does, yes. I don't know what it does. It's so powerful, yet it is so simple. . . . And I can go to that point through mindfulness or meditation and hold or be with whatever happens. If I get low, for instance, or like I lost my father last year, so there was a lot of grief. And I was able to meditate with that grief and actually see it or feel it come up and allow it to come out. Because one of the problems I had was bottling things up. So I feel myself getting unhappy about losing my father, so I'm able to sit quietly, allow it come up and have a good cry. Before, I wouldn't have been able to cry, it was just a pain here. So that's just being able to sit and just to watch the thing come up, so that's one of the things it does. . . . It's been a very valuable grief, and a very honest and pure one, and I find now, when I think of my father, there is less of a sense of loss and grief, and more of a sense of honoring him, so its been good in that respect. Though I still miss him, it is a different thing.

Notice what happened here. At no point in the program had we dealt with his responses to loss or bereavement in the past, or the vulnerable attitudes he might have had that made it difficult for him to cope with strong emotions. Yet his experience was that something fundamental had changed for him. Recall that, at the outset, we had wanted to develop an approach that might be used with people who were vulnerable to depression, but who were OK at the moment. We had chosen to explore mindfulness because, among other things, it seemed to provide a way in which people might use the moment-by-moment events of everyday life to learn things that would help them respond to the more difficult events and more severe moods. This participant's experience suggests that, for him, this approach had done just that. Like the participant whose comments we read earlier, MBCT appeared to help him deal with events in his life in a way that helped to prevent a recurrence of major depression. The question remained whether this "preventive" effect would occur in enough participants for us to be confident that these comments were not just isolated incidents. It was a question we would not be able to answer until we had done the necessary statistical evaluation of the whole program, and we come to this issue in Chapter 19.

ENDING THE CLASS

How should the last class end? Simply saying "good-bye and good luck" seems rather weak. People naturally feel they want to remember each other, to wish each other well. Originally, we would arrange to give each participant a small object (e.g., a marble, stone, or bead) and would lead the class in a short meditation in which the class examined the object as we examined the raisin in the first session. The object was a reminder to participants that they have been in the class, a reminder of the hard work they have done over the past 8 weeks, and of the people who shared this experience with them. There are many other ways of ending.* Some classes finish with participants looking around the class, starting with the person on their left, and moving their gaze from one participant to the next, breath by breath, and silently wishing each person well.

There are many ways to end, but all contain something that reminds participants to continue the process they started, to discover a way of living alongside the parts of themselves they feel are broken, and holds before them the possibility of responding to their own fragility in an ever more gentle and more caring way.

---

*In Oxford, in addition, we give participants a copy of the book *The Mindful Way through Depression*[76] as a gift at this last session, so that everyone has something to sustain him or her into the future—a new voice guiding, and new forms of words to explain each practice to add to the handouts given out during the MBCT course.

Summary of Session 8:
Maintaining and Extending New Learning

The advantages of awareness, acceptance, and mindfully *responding* to situations rather than immediately running off preprogrammed, "automatic" *reactions* have been a recurring theme throughout this course.

Acceptance may often be the springboard to some form of skillful action directed at changing your inner or outer worlds. However, there are also situations and feelings that it may be very difficult, or actually impossible, to change. In this situation, there is the danger that by carrying on, trying to solve an insoluble problem, or by refusing to accept the reality of the situation one is in, one may end up "banging one's head on a brick wall," exhausting oneself, and actually increasing one's sense of helplessness and depression. In these situations, *you can still retain some sense of dignity and control by making a conscious, mindful decision not to attempt to exert control and to accept the situation as it is, if possible, with a kindly attitude to the situation and your reactions to it. Choosing* not to act is much less likely to increase depression than being forced to give up attempts at control after repeated failures.

In the so-called "Serenity Prayer," we ask for the *grace to accept with serenity the things that cannot be changed, the courage to change the things that should be changed, and the wisdom to distinguish one from the other.*

Where do we find this grace, this courage, this wisdom? At some level, we *already* have all of these qualities—our task is to realize them (make them real), and our way is none other than moment-by-moment mindful awareness.

THE FUTURE

Decide, right now, what your regular pattern of practice will be over the next weeks, until we meet again, and stick to it as best you can throughout this period. Note any difficulties you have, so that we can discuss them next time.

Also, remember that the regular breathing space practice provides a way of "checking in with yourself" a few times a day. Let it also be your first response in times of difficulty, stress, or unhappiness—KEEP BREATHING!

Daily Mindfulness

- When you first wake up in the morning, before you get out of bed, bring your attention to your breathing. Observe five mindful breaths.

- Notice changes in your posture. Be aware of how your body and mind feel when you move from lying down to sitting, to standing, to walking. Notice each time you make a transition from one posture to the next.

- Whenever you hear a phone ring, a bird sing, a train pass by, laughter, a car horn, the wind, the sound of a door closing—use any sound as the bell of mindfulness. Really listen and be present and awake.

- Throughout the day, take a few moments to bring your attention to your breathing. Observe five mindful breaths.

- Whenever you eat or drink something, take a minute and breathe. Look at your food and realize that the food was connected to something that nourished its growth. Can you see the sunlight, the rain, the earth, the farmer, the trucker in your food? Pay attention as you eat, consciously consuming this food for your physical health. Bring awareness to seeing your food, smelling your food, tasting your food, chewing your food, and swallowing your food.

- Notice your body while you walk or stand. Take a moment to notice your posture. Pay attention to the contact of the ground under your feet. Feel the air on your face, arms, and legs as you walk. Are you rushing?

- Bring awareness to listening and talking. Can you listen without agreeing or disagreeing, liking or disliking, or planning what you will say when it is your turn? When talking, can you just say what you need to say without overstating or understating? Can you notice how your mind and body feel?

- Whenever you wait in a line, use this time to notice standing and breathing. Feel the contact of your feet on the floor and how your body feels. Bring attention to the rise and fall of your abdomen. Are you feeling impatient?

- Be aware of any points of tightness in your body throughout the day. See if you can breathe into them and, as you exhale, let go of excess tension. Is there tension stored anywhere in your body? For example, your neck, shoulders, stomach, jaw, or lower back? If possible, stretch or do yoga once a day.

- Focus attention on daily activities such as brushing your teeth, washing up, brushing your hair, putting on your shoes, or doing your job. Bring mindfulness to each activity.

- Before you go to sleep at night, take a few minutes and bring your attention to your breathing. Observe five mindful breaths.

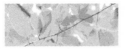 CHAPTER 18

Reprise

The 3-Minute Breathing Space as the Spine of the Program

In the early 1990s, when MBCT was first being developed, a great deal of attention was paid to protecting the integrity of the mindfulness practices featured in the program and being clear about the rationale for their inclusion. We were, after all, about to ask participants to do things that would fall well outside the standard menu of ingredients for building a brief, cognitively focused prevention treatment. We wanted to include exercises from CBT, for not only the strong evidence of their benefit in depression but also because the emphasis on continued practice outside the therapeutic hour was entirely consistent with the approach in our new treatment. As central as the formal mindfulness practices were in MBCT, we did not see them as an endpoint, but rather as the training ground for the types of skills in attention deployment, curiosity, kindness, and grounding that would help participants respond to real challenges in their everyday lives. Cognitive therapies had always stressed the need for new learning to be practiced repeatedly, especially in affectively challenging situations. This was how new therapeutic learning was consolidated, and there is a great deal of evidence from the cognitive therapy (CT) literature that participation in homework between sessions is associated with better outcomes.[102] In order to provide MBCT group members with the same opportunity, we developed the 3-Minute Breathing Space (3MBS). Now that you have encountered the 3MBS in its different formats, let's pause and reflect on this brief practice and its larger role in the overall program. In doing so, we remind ourselves of the many general themes and strategies of the whole MBCT program.

A GENERAL SCHEMATIC
FOR THE 3-MINUTE BREATHING SPACE

The 3MBS is a mini-meditation that was designed to bring the perspective of the longer formal sittings into participants' everyday lives. It is to be used as the first step in dealing with difficult situations and feelings. In many ways, it forms the spine of MBCT because its varied use provides for participants a quick and effective way to switch into being mode when they most need to do so, and, session by session, incorporates the learning that is taking place from the longer formal sittings and educational components at each stage of the program.

The skill being taught in the 3MBS is the intentional and flexible engagement of two types of attention: one that is open and wide-angle, and another that is focused or narrow-angle. To prepare for the practice, the invitation is to notice and adjust posture so as to embody a sense of "waking up" from autopilot, and a willingness to turn toward what is arising from moment to moment. The practice then follows a set sequence of three steps. Step 1, the emphasis is on awareness, especially recognizing and acknowledging one's current experience. Step 2 emphasizes gathering, particularly by bringing the attention to the sensations of the breath in a particular place in the body. Step 3 is about expanding the awareness into the body as a whole, using the particular sensations of the breath as an anchor, while opening to the range of experience that is present. A useful teaching metaphor is to consider the movement of attention in the 3MBS as following the path of an hourglass—starting with a wide opening, moving to a narrow neck, and expanding once again at a wide base. The instructions given as guidance are relatively spare, allowing participants to spend some time at each step. New instructors may find themselves unwittingly adding extra instructions borrowed from other, longer practices, but the point of the breathing space is its directness and simplicity. In preparing participants to integrate the 3MBS into their day, it can be helpful to allow some time during the class to discuss when participants will actually do it. One idea is to anchor the practice to a specific activity in one's day (e.g., morning coffee, before or after meals, taking children to school, or sitting at the computer).

Such a "directive" yet simple three-step structure for presenting a practice in which openness and curiosity are paramount is no accident. The risk with such brief practices is that they are seen as providing a time-out in the midst of an ongoing crisis, and not the important shift in mode of mind—from doing to being—that is needed. When guiding the 3MBS it is helpful if the instructions carefully target what is intended—a deliberate change of stance toward what is occurring in any moment. In the early stages of introducing the 3MBS, the instructor should be clear and precise in guiding the three steps, even labeling them (Step 1, Step 2, Step 3), so that participants know very explicitly where they are in the process.

More concretely, although the term "breathing space" implies that the primary focus of attention is on the breath, breathing is not featured until the middle of the practice. As we have mentioned, the practice does not start until there has been an intentional shift in body posture—especially an awareness of one's posture and the invitation to sit in a way that embodies alertness and wakefulness. The effect of a simple alteration in body position in standing or sitting can be profound in terms of the inner message it communicates about our stance toward our experience. Only then does Step 1 begin, and this is an invitation to acknowledge what is arising in thoughts, feelings, and body sensations, allowing them to be just as they are. It is Step 2 that narrows attention to the sensations of breathing. So even in this brief practice there is a sense of pausing and preparing, opening and acknowledging, before the more focused awareness on the breath—a sequence that echoes the program as a whole, which starts by teaching participants how to step out of automatic pilot.

In addition to discussing implementation, it is also important to be clear about the intention behind the 3MBS. Especially since it requires a certain amount of effort, it may seem natural to look for a payoff. However, as with all meditation practices, if we become too goal-oriented about it, we'll revert from being mode back into doing mode, thereby reducing our chances for new learning. One of the more powerful demonstrations of this intention can come out of the instructor taking a 3MBS in the middle of a class. For example, the instructor may wish to introduce another mode or perspective, especially when the class finds itself in a lengthy discussion or when strong feelings or reactions surface. Seeing how the 3MBS can be flexibly integrated into the teaching, without a specific therapeutic outcome being required, can be a very useful model for participants' use of the 3MBS in their own lives.

Finally, it is helpful to encourage participants not to worry about the exact amount of time involved. Although it is initially practiced for 3 minutes, there may be later occasions when there is time for only a few breaths. Soon one may be using it in varying degrees in many situations when unpleasant feelings or sensations are present.

THE 3-MINUTE BREATHING SPACE AS THE SPINE OF THE MINDFULNESS-BASED COGNITIVE THERAPY PROGRAM

The way the 3MBS is used gets refined across the 8-week program:

- Preprogrammed times, three times a day (after Session 3).

This pattern of preprogrammed breathing spaces continues throughout the remainder of the 8-week program, and is supplemented with the following:

- "Responsive" breathing space whenever unpleasant feelings are noticed (after Session 4—reentry).
- "Responsive" breathing space whenever unpleasant feelings are noticed, adding a sense of "opening to the difficult" through the body (after Session 5—the body door).
- "Responsive" breathing space as the "first step" before taking a wider view of thoughts (after Session 6—the thought door).
- "Responsive" breathing space as the "first step" before taking mindful action whenever unpleasant feelings or thoughts are noticed (after Session 7—the action door).

Throughout the program, participants are invited to think of the 3MBS as a natural first step in a more mindful response to unpleasant feelings. A helpful image is to see it as a door through which we can pass from "the hot, murky, cramped, 'driven' places in our minds to a lighter, cooler, more accommodating space."[76] Because the nature of the mind in one moment affects thoughts, emotions, and behavior in the next moment, the 3MBS facilitates approaching the next moment in a new way. Once we have opened the door and connected with a different space in our minds, a number of other doors are visible. Each door offers a different option for further mindful responding when it comes to being stuck in automatic tendencies, carried away by difficult thoughts, or deciding how best to look after oneself. Let's take a closer look at the "doors" available.

Reentry

Sometimes the simplest option after having completed the third step of the breathing space is to consider it done. This allows us mentally to reenter the original situation that prompted taking the breathing space, but with a new mode of mind in place. It may be that the unpleasant feelings, thoughts, or sensations are still there, but encountering them in being mode through a more spacious perspective can make all the difference. Reentry allows us to approach these experiences directly, and by avoiding the types of tunnel vision and automatic reactions that may only add fuel to the fire allows us to clarify what our next step might be. While the concept of reentry suggests a distinct chronology of before and after an event, instructors can also tell participants that it is never too late to do a 3MBS, even if, paradoxically, it is after the fact! Reentry in this case may refer to what happens when the event is over and, even then, taking a 3MBS may make sense. This is because what is being trained is an orientation and a willingness to practice that can strengthen the likelihood that the next time present moment awareness is needed, the 3MBS will present itself as a skillful option.

The Body Door

Since the difficulties we often face are associated with negative feelings, once the initial breathing space has ended, we may wish to work further on emotions that are still present. As we have learned all along, when we have strong emotions, our aversion or resistance to them is often registered as physical sensations such as tension, tightness, or pressure. To work wisely with these phenomena, we can direct our attention to what we are feeling in the body. We begin by taking an open and friendly attention to the part of the body where these sensations are making themselves known, and returning to the framework learned in the body scan, we can use the inbreath to carry attention and breathe into the area, and we breathe out from the area on the outbreath. Sometimes simply bringing awareness to the resistance (the "not wanting") itself may change the intensity of these sensations. Another option for turning toward our feelings is to choose to move our attention more directly into the area of discomfort and spend some time investigating the qualities of the sensations themselves, perhaps lightly noting whether they are continuous or intermittent, strong or subtle, sharp or dull, and so on. If the feelings become too intense, then switching to a strategy of "working the edge" may be possible, moving the attention up toward the edge of a strong sensation but not right into it, getting a sense of its size and shape, moving away from and up to the sensation as we choose. This allows us to remain in a stance of being "turned toward" the experience, but without having to "dive in" all at once. At any time, if our feelings become overwhelming, we can always compassionately shift our attention to some other grounding and neutral focus, such as the breath or the soles of the feet. Whichever approach is used, working through the body door allows us to cultivate a more "allowing" relationship to intensely unpleasant experiences.

The Thought Door

As our awareness expands in the first step of the 3MBS, we may notice that judgmental or critical thoughts are the most salient feature of our experience, ways of speaking to ourselves that, although painful, have become familiar or repetitive. If these thinking patterns are still present when we have completed the 3MBS, there is the option of working with them through the thought door by making a conscious choice to relate differently to thinking. Some ways of doing this might involve recording the thoughts on paper; observing their coming and going in the mind; seeing if we can watch them as mental events instead of facts; seeing if they are arising from a particular mood state (e.g., anxiety, sadness, loneliness or exhaustion); and looking to see if they are one of the patterns of mind we recognize as familiar, even if they come "camouflaged." It is also possible to ask ourselves gently whether these thoughts popped into our minds when we were fatigued and run down, whether we are jumping to conclusions or possibly thinking in black-and-white terms.

By using the thought door, we quickly start to appreciate that there are a number of approaches for relating differently and creatively to disturbing thoughts. Many of these strategies will have come directly from participants' previous exposure to mindfulness practice, and all reinforce the core message that we are not our thoughts, and that thoughts are not facts. Over time, this perspective will help lessen the command element of thinking and allow negative thoughts to move more freely through the mind, rather than drawing on our mental energy to keep them in place.

The Door of Skillful Action

A final option that is available is to open the door of skillful action following 3MBS completion. Becoming active is an important complement to the attitudes of openness and acceptance that may have been brought to unpleasant experiences in Step 3. Working through this door also suggests that sometimes "acknowledgment" is only the first step in looking after ourselves. But what type of action is called for? Thankfully, the wider perspective that is available following the 3MBS can help participants make this decision based on a greater awareness, rather than a narrower view, of the problem at hand. Most often, activities that allow us to take care of or show kindness to ourselves are what are called for.

Because low moods can diminish our ability to enjoy what we do or to keep up with the demands in our lives, two types of activities are well suited to help us look after ourselves. After the breathing space, we may choose to do something that once would have given us pleasure and enjoyment, such as buying a special coffee on the way home, sharing a meal with a friend, or listening to music that makes us feel good. Alternatively, we could do something that supports our sense of mastery or satisfaction and makes us feel like we are taking care of business. No action is too small to count, and in the case of mastery, paying bills, driving in a carpool, picking up dry cleaning, and washing the car are among the numerous ways we can begin to feel that our actions are having an effect in the world. Instructors also come to realize that one of the advantages of skillful action is that it needn't wait until we want to do it. Indeed, it cannot wait until we want to do it. Simply doing it as an experiment takes the emotional dimension out of the equation just at that time when a participant's emotional state may be unmotivated or dismissive.

By placing the emphasis on engagement over the size of the activity, and the intention for self-care over the magnitude of outcome, the door of skillful action sums up the intention for the breathing space practice whenever it is used during or after the program: an important opportunity for the embodiment of self-compassion and choice when we come face-to-face with old patterns of thinking and feeling.

PART III
EVALUATION
AND DISSEMINATION

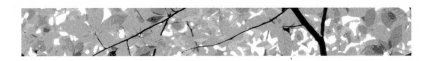

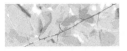

CHAPTER 19

Does Mindfulness-Based
Cognitive Therapy Work?

Mulla Nasrudin, the wise fool of many teaching stories in the Middle East, was throwing handfuls of crumbs around his house when a bemused onlooker asked him what he was doing. "Keeping the tigers away," the Mulla replied. "But surely there are no tigers in these parts," the onlooker responded. The Mulla beamed knowingly: "That's right. Effective, isn't it?"

As the story indicates, we can never be sure that actions intended to prevent some unwanted event are effective simply because the event does not occur—it might never have happened anyway. So, having developed the MBCT program to prevent future relapse to depression, how were we to find out whether our program delivered the desired effects? It was clear that simply running groups of recovered depressed patients through the program and counting how many relapsed in the following year, for example, would not tell us much—if there were few relapses, perhaps that is exactly what would have happened anyway; if there were many relapses, there might still have been fewer than if patients had not been through the program.

As you might expect, we were not the first to face such questions. Fortunately, a sophisticated methodology has been developed to address these issues, both in the evaluation of psychological treatments and in the assessment of the usefulness of clinical interventions more generally. At the heart of this methodology lies a process as random as tossing a coin.

393

THE POWER OF RANDOMIZATION

The randomized controlled trial (RCT) as a way to evaluate the effectiveness of clinical interventions was one of the most important developments in clinical and community medicine in the 20th century. In an RCT comparing the effectiveness of two treatments, the particular treatment, A or B, that any patient receives will be decided by a toss of a coin (or equivalently, by a computer-generated random sequence)—tails, the patient gets treatment A; heads, the patient gets treatment B. Patients then receive the treatment to which they have been allocated (having agreed in advance to their treatment being decided in this way). All patients are then assessed to determine the state of their clinical condition, and a score reflecting how well they are or how much improvement they have made is recorded. The numbers that have improved with treatment A and treatment B are then evaluated. Knowing the kind of differences that might be expected by chance alone, it is then possible to say, with a known level of confidence, that A is better than B, that B is better than A, or that the difference between A and B is not greater than would be expected by chance. The more patients in such a study, the more confident we can be in knowing that a difference of any given size between A and B is not simply due to chance. Equally, the greater the number of patients studied, the more confident we can be that we have not missed the possibility of small, but possibly important, differences between treatments that might be attributed to chance with smaller numbers of patients.

In medicine, in evaluating a new drug, the two treatments compared in an RCT are commonly the new drug and a placebo pill that looks and tastes the same as the new drug but lacks its chemically active ingredients. If the RCT shows that patients who took the new drug improved more than those who took the placebo, then we can have some confidence that the active chemical ingredients of the drug contributed to those effects. It is, of course, essential in such trials that the person assessing the extent to which patients have improved does not know what kind of treatment (A or B) any given patient has received. Otherwise, his or her assessments might be biased by beliefs, conscious or unconscious, about the effectiveness of the two treatments—this is obviously likely to be a problem if the assessor has a financial or personal investment in the effectiveness of one treatment; for example, if he or she has invested many years in its development. For such reasons, in RCTs, assessments have to be made by assessors blind to treatment condition; that is, strenuous efforts have to be made to prevent assessors knowing or discovering the kind of treatment patients have actually received.

RANDOMIZED CONTROLLED TRIALS AND MINDFULNESS-BASED COGNITIVE THERAPY

In the simple but powerful RCT method, we had a way to overcome Nasrudin's error, the false belief that an action is effective in preventing an unwanted outcome, simply because the outcome does not occur. By randomly allocating recovered depressed patients to receive either the MBCT program or some comparison condition, and following up to see how many people relapsed in the two groups, we would discover whether our efforts had paid off in producing an effective program.

But what should the comparison condition be? In fact, the choice of an appropriate comparison condition in an RCT often is determined by the state of knowledge in a particular field at a particular time. At the time we planned our first RCT of MBCT, there was no published evidence that any psychological intervention offered to patients after recovery from depression could reduce future rates of relapse. This made our choice of a comparison condition easier, as the first and most important step was to see whether MBCT could produce better outcomes than the treatments patients would normally receive. So we settled on a design for an RCT in which patients would be randomly allocated either simply to continue with the treatment they would normally receive, or, in addition, be offered participation in the MBCT program.

Having worked out our general strategy for evaluating MBCT, what did we actually do, and what did we find?

The First Clinical Trial of Mindfulness-Based Cognitive Therapy

The aim of our trial (reported in detail in Teasdale and associates[103]) was to answer the question: Does MBCT reduce rates of relapse and recurrence in patients who have recovered from major depression, compared to the treatment that such patients would normally receive? Our initial calculations suggested that if we were to have a reasonable chance of coming up with a definite answer to this question, one way or the other, we would have to study a lot of patients. Specifically, considerations of statistical power told us that if MBCT could, in reality, reduce relapse rates from 50 to 28%, we needed to have at least 120 patients completing both treatments if we wanted to have even an 80% chance of being sure of showing that difference, if it existed, in our trial. Given the inevitability of a proportion of patients dropping out before completing treatment, we knew that we would actually need to include a larger number than that in our trial. The only way we were going to get such numbers was by each of us offering MBCT to suitable patients at each of our three workplaces—Toronto, Bangor (North Wales), and Cambridge—and pooling the results.

What Did We Do?

In our three-center clinical trial to evaluate MBCT, we recruited 145 patients who had recovered from major depression, that is, patients who had previously experienced episodes of major depression but had been well for the last 3 months, with no more symptoms of depression than one might expect of anyone in the normal population. These patients were randomly assigned to one of two conditions. In the first condition, treatment as usual (TAU), patients continued with the treatment they would normally receive, including seeking help, as they needed it, from other sources, such as their family doctor. In the second condition, patients were allowed to seek their usual treatment, but in addition, they took part in the eight sessions of the MBCT program. To enter the trial, patients had to have had at least two previous episodes of major depression (in fact, 77% had experienced three or more episodes). All patients had previously been treated with antidepressant medication but had been off medication for at least 3 months before entering the trial.

Before describing our results, we need to say a little more about one aspect of clinical trial methodology. In clinical trials such as the one we conducted, it is conventional to categorize each patient on certain baseline variables that might be related to the primary clinical outcome of interest before randomly assigning him or her to one treatment or another. The reason for using this procedure, known as "stratification," is to make sure that patients in the two treatment groups have comparable personal characteristics that are known to be associated with good or poor outcomes, regardless of the treatment they may receive. We were aware that the scientific literature on depression had identified two such factors, and so we decided to stratify based on (1) how recently the last episode of depression had occurred and (2) how many previous episodes of major depression patients had experienced (two vs. three or more).

What Did We Find?

The outcome that most interested us was whether patients experienced a relapse or recurrence of their depression in the 60 weeks after their baseline assessment. As is conventional, before conducting the main statistical analyses of such a trial, we first checked that the effects of the treatments being compared were the same in patients in the different groups (strata) that stratification creates. When we did this, we found that, compared to TAU, MBCT was not as effective in patients with only two previous episodes as in patients with three or more previous episodes of depression; there was a statistically significant difference between these two groups in the extent to which MBCT reduced relapse compared to TAU. In patients with three or more episodes (77% of the total sample), MBCT significantly reduced relapse compared to TAU. In patients with only two episodes (23% of the total sample), there was no difference in relapse rates between patients receiving MBCT and TAU. In other words, the beneficial effects of MBCT were shown only in the patients with more extensive histories of depression. We had not expected this result, though the fact that we had stratified on this variable before randomization was very important: It meant that the pattern of results could be reported as part of the primary analysis rather than as a secondary post hoc test. We consider possible explanations for this interesting finding below. For now, let us focus on the patients with three or more episodes, the considerable majority in the sample we studied (see Figure 19.1).

Of these, patients who simply continued with the treatment that they would normally have received showed a 66% relapse rate over the total 60-week study period, whereas those who received MBCT showed a relapse rate of 37%. The probability that we would get a difference this large by chance (if there were no real difference) was less than 1 in 200.

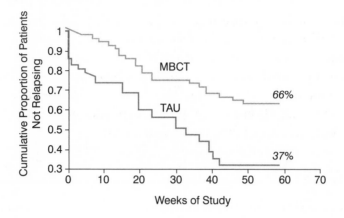

FIGURE 19.1. Survival curves comparing relapse–nonrelapse to major depression for treatment as usual (TAU) or MBCT in patients with three or more past episodes of depression.

Adding MBCT to the treatment that patients would normally receive had the effect of reducing risk of relapse almost by half. Furthermore, differences in the use of antidepressants by patients in the MBCT group did not account for benefits of MBCT; the proportion of patients using antidepressants at any time during the study period was actually less in MBCT than in TAU patients.

These findings were very heartening. In considering their implications, it is important to remember that MBCT was specifically designed for patients who had been depressed in the past but were relatively well at the time that they started the MBCT program. In particular, we felt that it was important to caution against interpreting our findings to support the use of MBCT with patients who are acutely depressed. At that time, there was no evidence to suggest that MBCT would be useful with this group (although see below the interesting work with treatment-resistant or partially remitted patients). Indeed, our best guess was that MBCT was unlikely to be effective in the treatment of acute depression, where factors such as difficulties in concentration and the intensity of negative thinking might make it very difficult for patients to develop the attentional skills central to the program.

In summary, it appeared that for patients with three or more previous episodes of depression, we had achieved our aim of developing a new, cost-efficient way to reduce risk of relapse/recurrence of depression. But why was MBCT not helping patients with only two previous episodes of depression?

In 1998 Helen Ma came to the Cognition and Brain Sciences Unit in Cambridge to work with John Teasdale. This gave the Cambridge team a wonderful opportunity to take the research further. But what should the next step be? They could do a dismantling study to examine what component of the MBCT was essential. They could offer MBCT with or without the home practice to answer the pragmatic question of how much the outcomes depended on participants' own work by themselves.

In the end, they decided to do something very simple, and hugely important—to carry out a "procedural replication" of the Teasdale and colleagues study in 2000.[104] Resisting the temptation to hurry on, their study of 75 patients who met the same study entry criteria as those in the 2000 study would become a landmark study in its own right. Why? Because its results exactly replicated the 2000 study. This time, those patients who had three or more episodes of depression prior to entry into the trial relapsed without MBCT (i.e., with TAU alone) at a rate of 78%. By contrast only 36% of those who had MBCT relapsed.[104]

Once again, however, no such effects were observed for those with only two prior episodes, and, taken together with the results of the first trial, it looked as if mindfulness might even be *harmful* for patients with only two prior episodes. The question that this new trial could now help to answer was therefore very pressing indeed: Why were there very different outcomes for those with three or more prior episodes and those with only two? Is it really a question of how many episodes one has had, or are these data hiding another, more important, variable?

Why Did Mindfulness-Based Cognitive Therapy Not Help Patients with Only Two Previous Episodes of Depression?

In the first trial, we had not expected the benefits of MBCT to be restricted to patients with three or more previous episodes. At that time, we were able to come up with some plausible explanations for these findings, but we had to admit that these ideas were just that—unverified hunches that awaited further demonstrations and explorations of the pattern of results that we observed. And since only one trial had found this pattern anyway, it was unclear whether the pattern was a "one-off" that sometimes happens in any research; something that never happens again. So the first important outcome of the second trial was the fact that it exactly replicated the finding that those with the longest histories of depression benefited the most, and those with only two episodes were no better for having done MBCT and may have been slightly worse.

The findings are of particular interest with respect to the theoretical background of MBCT.[54,57] As we described in Chapter 2, the MBCT program was specifically designed to reduce the extent to which patterns of depressive thinking reactivated by sad moods could feed the factors responsible for relapse/recurrence. Such sadness-linked thinking, we assumed, resulted from repeated associations between the depressed state and characteristic negative thinking patterns within each depressive episode. Perhaps the strengthening of these associations with repeated episodes contributed to making relapse increasingly autonomous or automatic, so that it took less and less to actually trigger the return of symptoms. This view is supported by the observations of Post and by Kendler and colleagues that environmental stress appears to play a progressively less important role in bringing on relapse/recurrence with increasing number of episodes experienced.[34,105]

Such findings suggested the possibility that in these trials of MBCT, (1) the greater risk of relapse in patients with three or more past episodes was to a large extent due to autonomous relapse processes involving reactivation of depressive thinking patterns by sad moods, and (2) the preventive effects of MBCT arose, specifically, from disruption of those processes at times of potential relapse/recurrence.

Within this analysis, it is possible that relapse in patients with only two previous episodes of depression may have been substantially related not to the reactivation of more autonomous, relapse-related processes (recurrence of old habits of dysfunctional patterns of thinking) but rather to the occurrence of major life events, such as unemployment, deaths or serious illness in the family, or breakdowns in relationships. This relationship between life events and relapse in patients could now be carefully measured, and that is what Ma and Teasdale did.[104] First, they found that patients with three or more episodes of depression reported a greater number of adverse *early* life experiences than patients with two episodes and those who had never been depressed. By contrast, the rates of reported negative early experiences did not differ between patients with only two episodes and never-depressed controls. Furthermore, although those with only two previous episodes had a childhood and adolescence that was free of serious stressors, when they relapsed during the study, the relapse was far more likely to follow a serious life event. By contrast, relapses in those with three or more prior episodes were more autonomous: They "came out of the blue."

This strongly suggested that the reason for the difference between those with two versus three or more prior episodes is that these patients come from two different "base populations": that is, they are suffering from different types of depression. Importantly, it implies that the number of episodes is a marker of another, more significant variable: whether a depression is autonomous or follows a major upsetting event. In other words, the "two only" versus "three or more" does not simply reflect patients who are at different points in the same "trajectory" of depression.

Why is this so important? First, it cautions us against offering MBCT as a first approach to helping those whose depression follows immediately after a serious life event. Of course, it remains possible that patients who have been meditating for years may find the practice helpful in the midst of a tragedy, for they will more likely know when it is helping and when to ease off. But our patients had not done meditation before, and how best to help those whose depression emerges in reaction to such severe life events in later life remains an important question.

Second, the findings are important because of their implications for those with three or more depression episodes prior to coming for MBCT who turn out to have a 20-year history of depression that started in adolescence or early adulthood. It raises the possibility that MBCT might be useful for people with *early* onset of depression or for adolescents who show signs of belonging to this very vulnerable group, even before they have accumulated three episodes. This is an important priority for future research.

Subsequent Clinical Trials of Mindfulness-Based Cognitive Therapy

Up to this point in time, we had what appeared to be a reliable finding on the effectiveness of MBCT and for whom it was most effective.

But there was another problem. These findings were generated solely by us—the treatment's developers. According to U.S. criteria, we had a treatment approach that was "probably effective," but it would not meet the highest criteria for efficacy until we knew how the treatment would fare in someone else's hands. Findings from one controlled trial in Switzerland[106] seemed to give ambiguous results. It recruited only patients with three or more prior depression episodes but showed little overall difference between the 12-month outcome of MBCT versus TAU, though MBCT significantly delayed relapse by 19 weeks compared to TAU, which in other respects did unusually well compared to other trials. Another trial conducted in Ghent, Belgium,[107] was unambiguous. It also recruited only those with three or more previous episodes and found that MBCT reduced relapse from 68 to 30% over 12 months. Now there were four trials, two of which had been conducted independent of the treatment developers. MBCT could be seen as a robust approach for those with the most recurrent history of depression.

The Belgian trial was interesting in another respect. For the first time, patients were allowed to enter the trial while still taking antidepressants, and three-fourths of the patients in each group were on such medication at the outset of the trial. Yet the outcome replicated the previous results shown for those who were not taking medication. This is important, showing that patients do not have to choose between MBCT and medication: Both can be used at the same time. But the study was not designed to examine how MBCT would fare against antidepressants alone. This requires different research designs, and fortunately, two studies, one in the United Kingdom and one in Canada, were researching just this question. Research was now at a point where we needed to evaluate our MBCT approach against a more active and powerful comparison group—maintenance antidepressant pharmacotherapy.

HOW PROTECTIVE IS MINDFULNESS-BASED COGNITIVE THERAPY COMPARED TO ANTIDEPRESSANT MEDICATION?

Just as in the early 1980s, cognitive-behavioral therapy's credibility as a treatment for depression was established via head-to-head comparisons with antidepressant medication, establishing MBCT's true clinical value requires knowing how it fares against the current standard of care offered to patients in remission. Preventing relapse by continuing antidepressant treatment well into the period of recovery reduces the chances of relapse to between 30 and 40%,[22] and, along with being highly endorsed by clinical practice guidelines, is also the strategy most widely used by physicians. Willem Kuyken and his colleagues[108] at the University of Exeter were the first to compare these two treatments in their study of 123 recurrently depressed patients, all of whom had been treated with antidepressants for at least 6 months and were now in remission or partial remission. In order to study what happened to patients once their medication was removed, they randomly assigned one group to receive MBCT, with the understanding that they would discontinue their medication within 6 months of starting the MBCT course, while they asked another group to continue taking their medicine for 15 months. Rates of relapse over the 15-month follow-up did not differ significantly between medication (60%) and MBCT (47%), even though 75% of those in the MBCT group completely stopped taking an antidepressant. This important finding suggests that MBCT can be just as effective as the current treatment of choice for preventing depressive relapse. Even more impressive, MBCT was significantly *more* effective than medication in reducing residual depressive symptoms and psychiatric comorbidity, and in improving quality of life. There was no difference in average annual cost between the two groups.

Another approach to this question involves studying what happens when antidepressants and MBCT are used sequentially, so that patients get the benefit of medication for acute depressive symptoms but then stop taking their pills and receive MBCT to prevent relapse. Asking patients to discontinue their medication once they are well actually mimics what tends to happen in the most doctors' offices—up to 40% of patients stop treatment far too soon, either because of the burden of side effects or a growing unwillingness to take medicine for years.[36] Could MBCT fill this gap and provide such patients with further protection? Segal and colleagues[109] addressed the issue directly by first treating 160 depressed patients with drugs alone and, only then, randomly assigning the 84 patients who achieved remission to one of three experimental arms. In the first group, patients came off their medication and received MBCT; patients in the second group also discontinued their medication and received a placebo pill—identical to the medication they received in the acute phase but chemically inert; patients in a third group continued to take medication for 18 months. What was new is that this study allowed the investigators to compare the effectiveness of sequencing pharmacological and psychological treatments versus keeping the same treatment—antidepressants—in place over the long term.

Because Segal and colleagues[109] recruited and treated acutely depressed patients within the study itself, it was also possible to examine whether the quality of their improvement—how well the medication was able to bring depressive symptoms under control—interacted with the type of prevention treatment patients went on to receive.[110] In other words, we could see whether what happened during the first stage of treatment sequence had an impact on the second. This, in fact, is what was found. For patients who experienced periodic flurries of symptoms (those with unstable remission) during the acute depression but still got well, discontinuing their medication and receiving MBCT significantly lowered their risk for relapse or recurrence risk (28%)—no different from the group that continued with medication alone (27%). By contrast, those unstable remitters who discontinued the active medication and went onto a placebo were highly significantly more likely to relapse (71%; see Figure 19.2).

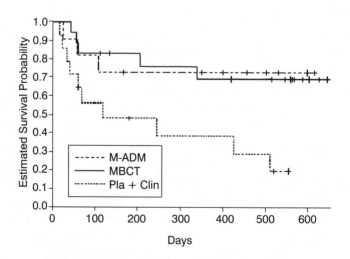

FIGURE 19.2. Cumulative proportion of unstable remitters who survived without relapse during maintenance/follow-up. M-ADM, maintenance antidepressant monotherapy; Pla + Clin, placebo plus clinical management.

For patients who responded well and whose remission was stable—not marked by transient elevations in depressive symptoms—all three groups showed similar prevention outcomes (40–50% range).

The real-world implications of these findings are hugely important, as sizable numbers of patients are unwilling or unable to tolerate maintenance antidepressant treatment. For them, we now know that MBCT offers equal protection from relapse. While the idea that sequencing pharmacological and psychological interventions is still novel, the fact that it may help to keep more patients in treatment and protect them for a longer period of time suggests that it warrants wider adoption.

META-ANALYSIS, MINDFULNESS-BASED COGNITIVE THERAPY, AND RELAPSE PREVENTION

Depressed patients looking to stay well often face having to make a dichotomous decision about whether to continue or to refrain from following a certain course of treatment. Consulting individual randomized trials for guidance may not be the most informative route because these studies are frequently designed to address a wider scope of concerns. One solution to this dilemma has been to rely on statistics to boil down the results of multiple studies into a single number that reflects the benefits of a particular treatment. Such calculations are made easier if investigators report similar clinical outcomes, for example, depression scores from the same questionnaire or ratings of clinical improvement from an interview.

The problem we faced when we wrote the first edition of this book was that there were simply too few studies to enable this type of broad overview. As the number of MBCT studies has grown, this is now feasible. "Meta-analysis" is the name given to the statistical procedure that generates a weighted average of the outcomes from multiple clinical trials. This indicator, called an "effect size," is scaled in such a way that small effect sizes suggest little benefit from receiving treatment, while larger effect sizes indicate increasing benefits from receiving an intervention. Because a meta-analysis provides a numerical indicator of a treatment's impact, it is increasingly preferred over other types of evaluations of clinical evidence in which an author's conclusions are based largely on subjective appraisals.

Drawing on six randomized trials of 593 patients, a meta-analysis by a group in Aarhus, Denmark, reported that in comparisons between MBCT and inactive control groups, MBCT significantly reduced the risk of relapse, relative to staying with usual care, by 35%, and for patients with three or more past episodes, the reduction was 44%.[111] They also reported that both MBCT and antidepressant medication reduced relapse risk to a similar degree. In a second meta-analysis, Hoffman and colleagues[112] approached the issue from a different angle. They scrutinized 1,140 patients receiving mindfulness-based interventions for a variety of mental health conditions and examined reductions in symptoms of anxiety and depression, rather than whether a person relapsed or not. Treatments featuring mindfulness training, of which MBCT is a prominent example, were each associated with large effect sizes of 0.97 for anxious and 0.95 for depressive symptoms. They also found, as might be expected for a framework that encourages the practice of mindfulness as a general life skill, that these benefits were maintained past the point at which patients were no longer receiving treatment.[97]

Perhaps the most compelling endorsement for MBCT comes from the United Kingdom's National Institute for Health and Clinical Excellence (NICE), an independent national body that provides clinical guidelines for evidence-based care to patients using the National Health Service. Guidelines are formulated through a stringent review of empirical and clinical studies for a particular medical or psychiatric condition, and recommendations reflect a ranking of the most to the least supported treatment options. The NICE guidelines for unipolar depression have, since 2004, consistently endorsed MBCT as an effective means for prevention of relapse and recurrence, which in turn has provided patients with an additional resource at their disposal for comprehensive depression care.[9]

EXTENDING THE REACH OF MINDFULNESS-BASED COGNITIVE THERAPY BEYOND DEPRESSIVE RELAPSE

Finally, robust support for MBCT in preventing depressive relapse has encouraged adaptations of the framework for other difficulties. As we would expect, in many of these approaches, elements of MBCT's eight-session framework were modified to make room for material relating to the particular disorder being treated. Promising examples are MBCT for children[113,114]; mindfulness-based relapse prevention for substance abuse[115]; MBCT for pregnant women at risk for depression[116]; MBCT for hypochondriasis,[117] chronic fatigue syndrome,[118] tinnitus,[119] auditory hallucinations,[120] insomnia,[121] social phobia,[122] generalized anxiety disorder,[123] panic disorder,[124] and depression in primary care[125]; and MBCT for cancer patients.[126,127] More generally, MBCT has been shown to increase positive and reduce negative emotions,[128,129] to help in the clarification of life goals,[130] and to increase adaptive regulation of experimentally induced fear and anxiety.[131]

Coming back to the area of mood disorders, there is also growing interest in finding out whether MBCT can be used with treatment-resistant or chronic depression. Positive findings from two uncontrolled studies[132,133] and two RCTs[134,135] suggest that this is an area deserving of further study. In a similar vein, there is the possibility that MBCT, through its effects on reducing anxiety and improving executive functioning, may benefit patients with bipolar disorder who are taking mood stabilizers.[136–139] In time, we should have sufficient new data to determine the staying power of all these promising trends.

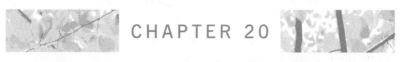

CHAPTER 20

How Does Mindfulness-Based Cognitive Therapy Achieve Its Effects?

That the MBCT program can produce marked reductions in rates of depressive relapse/recurrence supports its clinical adoption and dissemination. However, what do we know about the active ingredients behind its effectiveness? What are people actually saying has helped them? One indication might come from the most straightforward of sources—patients' own comments collected at the last MBCT class, in which they say what has helped them. Two patients wrote, "I am now better capable of recognizing when I am about to enter the 'train wreck' thought zone and detach myself from it," and "I have learned strategies to become more aware of my thoughts and physical reactions. Even though I may not be able to stop an automatic reaction, I can be aware of it and bring myself back or 'reset.'" Working with difficult emotions was another theme that emerged in patients' feedback: "Now I can distinguish how feeling good and feeling bad feel like . . . and I'm not afraid of the bad to come because I found the confidence of knowing that I can figure out ways to deal with it." Patients also pointed out that MBCT allowed them to develop a kinder way of relating to their experiences: "The qualities of acceptance and compassion for things within and situations outside my life are behaviors that this program helps me to develop. . . . I had none of these before coming in."

How much can we take from these comments? Although, as clinicians, it is pleasing to see them, they were all collected from people at the end of the program, when they might possibly have been saying something to please the instructor. A systematic approach that gathers this

408

information independently of the teacher might be preferred. One study to have done so was by Allen and colleagues,[140] who interviewed patients who had taken part in the clinical trial of Kuyken and colleagues[108] a year after the program ended, and whose findings provide a rare, long-term view of MBCT's utility. Looking back, patients reported they were better able to detect relapse triggers, to activate themselves if depressive symptoms threatened, and to improve the quality of their relationships. For example, patients noted a heightened awareness of the bodily and cognitive signs of low-level depressive symptoms, and if low mood was present, they would deliberately engage in neutral or positive activities such as gardening, walking the dog, or taking a 3-minute breathing space. Interpersonally, patients felt closer to friends and family, and had increased empathy for other people's struggles. What is especially relevant to the rationale for MBCT is that patients described being better able to objectify depression, specifically by shifting over time to (1) seeing thoughts as thoughts and (2) depression as "not me." The opportunity during MBCT to get to know others who had had depression and hear them talk about their experiences made it easier for patients to accept symptoms as part and parcel of an emotional disorder ("I just thought it was me going mad. . . . It's surprising how many other people are out there thinking the same thing"), and not as a judgment of who they were ("It is really important to realize that your thoughts aren't a reflection of who you really are"). Approaching depressive phenomena from this new perspective also made it easier not to judge or engage with the content of the thoughts themselves: "It's almost like you've got an awareness, that you've got this aspect of yourself, . . . and we call them our thoughts . . . and I think that's really helped."

While the range of changes reported from this study is impressive, we also note that such qualitative accounts would not convince our more hard-nosed colleagues, who would say that relying on these reports to answer the question "What is the critical thing(s) learned in MBCT?" is insufficient. After all, these data are uncontrolled and can never be collected from participants who are unaware or blind to what is being assessed. How could one know whether the feedback reflects only those elements of MBCT about which the patient felt enthusiastic or worked hard at, rather than the critical ingredients? The challenge for constructing a scientific account of the mechanisms behind MBCT is to judge which of these changes are reliable and accompany treatment.

WHAT IS THE PROCESS OF CHANGE
IN MINDFULNESS-BASED COGNITIVE THERAPY?

Both the individual accounts of participants and studies using more formal self-report questionnaires have now shown that important changes in psychological functioning occur across the eight weekly classes. Self-reported changes include decreases in depression, anxiety, rumination, insomnia, and tension, and increases in mindfulness, compassion, concentration, resilience, optimism, and quality of life.[141] Cognitive changes also occur: Overgeneral memory is reduced in MBCT subjects compared to controls. This is potentially important, in that such overgeneral memory has been linked to increased vulnerability to onset of depression and increased persistence of depressive symptoms.[142-144] However, the question remains: Which—of all the things that change when people do MBCT—are the critical variables that underlie and explain its relapse-reducing effects?

Trying to understand *which* of these factors helps to keep relapse at bay is a complex issue—especially if many variables change. Why is this a problem? One reason is that not being able to distinguish the critical ingredients from all the changes that occur limits our ability to improve MBCT, sharpen how it is taught, and adapt it to new populations. To better understand how a treatment operates, investigators have turned to a statistical approach known as "mediation analysis."

Let's take, for example, the finding that MBCT reduces rumination. It is known that high levels of rumination make depression's return more likely, but reduction in this variable may or may not be the *critical* change that accounts for MBCT's preventive effects. Perhaps reductions in rumination are a proxy for patients becoming more mindful, and it is this change that actually protects them. In terms of its technical definition, in order for a variable to be considered as a mediator, two conditions must be met: It needs to show greater change in MBCT than in a control condition, and it needs to explain the majority of a treatment's effects on outcome. Going back to rumination, we would want to test whether reductions in rumination were greater for MBCT patients compared to controls, then examine what happens to the relapse rates when these reductions are statistically removed from the comparison between the MBCT and control groups. If MBCT patients' protective effects were diminished or no longer different from those of the control group, we would be on firm ground saying that MBCT works through reducing rumination in recovered depressed patients. If MBCT's outcomes remained unchanged, then we could conclude that rumination may still change after MBCT, but it does not play a critical mediating role.

The first comprehensive examination of MBCT treatment mediation was carried out by Kuyken and colleagues,[145] who drew on the findings from their 2008 study to examine whether changes on a number of distinct, theory-driven variables mediated MBCT's reduction of depressive symptoms over 15 months of follow-up. Two measures in particular stand out. First, the Kentucky Inventory of Mindfulness Skills[146] was used to assess four facets of mindfulness: observing—"I notice the smells and aromas of things"; describing—"Even when I'm terribly upset, I can find a way to put it into words"; acting with awareness—"When I'm doing something, I'm only focused on what I'm doing, nothing else"; and accepting without judgment—"I pay attention to how my emotions affect my thoughts and behavior." Second, Kuyken and colleagues assessed self-compassion using a scale developed by Kristen Neff,[147] including items such as "I try to be loving toward myself when I'm feeling emotional pain" and "I'm tolerant of my own flaws and inadequacies."

Kuyken and colleagues'[145] results showed larger increases in both mindfulness and self-compassion over the 8 weeks in the MBCT group compared to changes seen over a similar interval in the control group, whose members were on maintenance antidepressant medication. Furthermore, increased mindfulness and self-compassion significantly predicted depression levels 13 months later, even after the effects of treatment and background symptoms were taken into account. The strength of these findings lies in their a priori status: They were predicted by the theoretical model underlying MBCT's development and were statistically robust. The fact that patients who did not acquire mindfulness or the capacity for self-compassion had higher rates of depressive symptoms is strong evidence of the essential role played by mindfulness and self-compassion in the benefits derived from the 8-week program. In addition, the findings have direct implications for instructors: MBCT's overarching aim of cultivating the mindful, being mode of mind, the "what" of teaching, now has a solid empirical basis, and, most important, the embodiment of compassion as a crucial aspect of the "how" of mindfulness teaching is also supported by quantitative data.

But there was an even more remarkable aspect to Kuyken and colleagues' [145] results. They had asked their patients to participate in a mood challenge experiment similar to that used in the early research on vulnerability to depression by Zindel Segal and colleagues in 1999 and 2006 (reported in Chapter 2).[53,54] They assessed the MBCT group after completing the MBCT course and the medication group at an equivalent point in time. All received the sad mood induction, which involved listening to a sad piece of music and recalling a sad personal event from the past. Before and after the mood induction, their levels of dysfunctional attitudes were assessed. Recall that Segal and colleagues (in 1999 and 2006) had found that the larger the increase in scores on this questionnaire after a mood challenge (i.e., the more patients endorsed things such as "I should be happy all the time"), the more likely a patient would experience a recurrence of depression in the future.

Kuyken and colleagues' results were fascinating. They showed that those patients in the continued medication group who reacted "badly" to this experiment (showing large increases in dysfunctional attitudes) were much more likely to become depressed again over the following year. By contrast, in the MBCT group, equivalent (or even higher) levels of reactivity did not have any predictive power at all. It was as if the MBCT patients had learned something that, while not reducing their primary reactivity, did reduce the impact of that reactivity on whether it escalated into a full-blown relapse. What might have been learned that might have this effect? The data were clear, as shown in Figure 20.1. The more change in self-compassion, the greater the prophylactic effect.

Those who had learned to be compassionate toward themselves, although they might experience equivalent or even greater levels of reactivity in the mood challenge experiment, were those who were likely to be most protected from future episodes of depression.

A second mediation analysis by Beiling and colleagues[148] tested a similar group of variables in those depressed patients who were initially treated with an antidepressant, then, once well, were assigned to receive MBCT, maintenance pharmacotherapy, or a placebo pill as part of the Segal and colleagues[109] trial. In addition to measuring mindfulness, they completed the Experiences Questionnaire.[149] This is a measure of "metacognitive awareness," that is, a person's ability to observe thoughts and feelings without being pulled into their story. Sample items on this

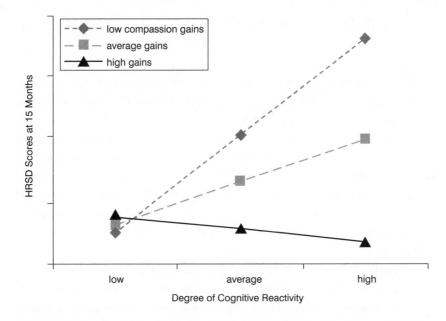

FIGURE 20.1. Changes in compassion during MBCT reduce the effects of cognitive reactivity on depression. *Note.* HRSD, Hamilton Rating Scale for Depression.

scale include "I can observe unpleasant feelings without being drawn into them" and "I can actually see that I am not my thoughts." Results indicated that patients in MBCT showed increased mindfulness and metacognitive skills over the 8 weeks of the program, whereas those taking an antidepressant or placebo did not. Consistent with the analysis of mediation, these changes were also associated with lower depression scores 6 months later.

What is interesting about both sets of findings is the picture they paint about two equally effective approaches to depressive relapse prevention. Whereas the mechanisms underlying antidepressant treatment are largely pharmacological, increases in mindfulness, self-compassion, and the acknowledgment of negative affect without becoming overwhelmed by it[150,151] are skills more likely to be employed by patients in MBCT and are important drivers of its protective benefits. When considered alongside the qualitative descriptions of enhanced emotional and cognitive processing acquired during MBCT, it seems that people's own sense of what changed for them psychologically resonates with what the research shows.

HOW DOES THE PRACTICE OF MINDFULNESS AFFECT THE BRAIN?

A few decades ago, the dominant view in brain science held that our subjective experience is the product of activity in brain regions or networks that are specialized for discrete functions. This relationship was seen as a one-way street—the amygdala fires and we are suddenly gripped with fear. To ask whether the opposite could be true, that mental training could lead to rewiring of brain circuits, was often seen as a fundamental misunderstanding of the workings of the brain. These days, however, the concept of "neuroplasticity," the idea that specific forms of sustained mental training can alter brain activity, has taken firm hold in neuroscience. Researchers are now asking how, not whether, this occurs.

One of the first studies to examine neural changes associated with the practice of mindfulness meditation was by Davidson and colleagues,[152] using electroencephalography (EEG) to assess brain wave patterns before and after an 8-week MBSR course. The background to this work is that greater activity in the left, relative to the right, frontal brain regions is associated with a positive affective style—a personal set-point for emotional responses that favors approach, or positive emotion, over avoidance, or negative emotion. The opposite pattern is a marker of negative affect. Would the practice of mindfulness, which has been shown to aid emotion regulation and even increase the capacity for happiness, have any impact on this biological measure of affective style? Participants in the study were not referred for clinical problems, but were part of a wellness program at a midsize biotechnology corporation. The findings revealed that over 8 weeks, mindfulness practitioners, compared to nonpracticing control participants, showed increased levels of left-sided asymmetrical activation, a pattern indicating a shift toward more positive emotions that persisted 6 months later, and, importantly, remained in place even when participants underwent a mood challenge procedure. That is, following MBSR, participants were able to experience just as much sadness, but to do so while remaining "open" in a way that suggests sadness would be far more likely to be transient.

In a clinical replication of this work by Barnhofer and colleagues,[153] 22 previously depressed patients with a history of suicidal ideation were randomized to receive either MBCT or usual care. All patients were well at the outset of the study but at high risk of relapse. EEG results indicated that both groups showed equal degrees of relative left- and right-sided frontal activation at pretreatment, but over an 8-week span, the usual care group showed a significant decline on this index, while MBCT patients maintained their pretreatment levels. The authors suggest that for patients with an affective disorder, the practice of mindfulness may not increase, as much as maintain, a balanced activation in brain areas that direct the regulation of positive emotion.

The findings from both these studies show that not only does mental training have the capacity to change the brain, but also its reach can extend to those very processes that are intimately related to the regulation of emotion. In patients with a mood disorder, the possibility of new neural learning in these domains may be invaluable.

TRAIN YOUR MIND AND CHANGE YOUR BRAIN

Measuring brain wave activity provides important clues to which neural regions may be involved in the practice of mindfulness, but this approach is limited because its level of resolution is too broad. EEG recordings can pinpoint effects on the left, the right, the front, or the back of the brain, but details about specific brain structures are harder to come by. With the advent of neuroimaging, the neural changes associated with mindfulness practice can be detected in different ways, such as measuring increases in the size of brain structures, or which brain areas are more or less active during the performance of specific tasks. Sara Lazar and her colleagues took advantage of the high-quality brain images available from magnetic resonance imaging (MRI), to examine this very question.

Lazar and colleagues[154] reported that brain regions controlling the attentional and sensory processing functions harnessed by meditation practice, particularly the prefrontal cortex and right anterior insula, were significantly thicker in meditators than in nonmeditators. This startling finding suggested that regular practice was associated with increases in the size of those brain regions that meditation recruited. Whether this was due to the growth of new brain cells, increased synaptic connections, or dendritic lengthening has yet to be determined, but the principle had been established. They also found that the degree of thickening in these regions was associated with greater amounts of meditation experience, and not just the simple dichotomy of whether someone practiced or not. This is further strong evidence for a training effect.

A further important demonstration of the neural effects of mindfulness training was reported by Hölzel and colleagues,[155] who tested patients with no meditation experience, before and after an 8-week MBSR program and compared them to a wait-list control group. She found that even over this relatively brief period of time, cortical thickening was found in the left hippocampus, posterior cingulate, and temporoparietal junction, brain regions that direct self-related processing, emotional learning, and memory. This is some of the strongest evidence to date that through the types of mindfulness practices offered in MBCT and MBSR, people are being taught skills that change the structure of their brains.

The prospect of being able to rewire neural connections or increase the size of brain regions through the practice of mindfulness is an exciting development and was certainly not even considered by the field when the first edition of this book was published. Looking ahead, we need to ask how these findings can help us optimize MBCT, so that patients can learn how to work with negative emotion in ways that prime neural reorganization and effectively reduce relapse risk. To address this possibility we need to know what happens in the brain when people feel sad and practice mindfulness.

MINDFULNESS AND THE NEURAL EXPRESSION OF SADNESS

A recurring point of emphasis in MBCT is that mindfulness training helps patients separate the momentary subjective experience of sadness from the conceptual analysis of what it means to feel sad. Since helping patients experience this for themselves is one of MBCT's central teachings, being able to characterize this in neural terms could identify specific brain regions that serve as markers of one or the other mode being more active. But how does one set about investigating these two modes in the scanner?

Norman Farb and his colleagues,[156] using functional MRI (an MRI that measures brain activity while the person is engaged in mental tasks), trained participants to ask themselves a number of questions about self-descriptive adjectives while being scanned. Drawing on previous work by Watkins and Teasdale,[157] the questions reflected either a narrative/analytic mode ("What does this say about me," "Is this good or bad?") or an experiential/concrete mode ("What is occurring from one moment to the next" or "What am I aware of in my body"). Once participants were trained, it was possible to examine how mindfulness training interacted with these two modes, and to see whether each had a unique neural signature. Two groups were tested, the first just before enrolling in an MBSR program and the second after completing the program.

Results indicated that for participants trained in mindfulness, there were marked reductions in the medial prefrontal cortex (often linked to analysis of self-related material—thinking *about*) and increased activation in a right lateralized network comprising the lateral prefrontal cortex and viscerosomatic areas, such as the insula (linked to direct, moment-by-moment sensory experience), secondary somatosensory cortex, and inferior parietal lobule. Analyses of the strength of connectivity among these brain regions suggested that the strong coupling between the right insula and the medial prefrontal cortex in those who had not undergone mindfulness training was "uncoupled" in those who had completed a mindfulness program. The fact that these regions are coupled together prior to learning meditation suggests that it is usually very difficult for a person to focus on momentary bodily experience without this experience starting off thoughts *about* the self. After mindfulness training, the uncoupling suggests that the person is now able to maintain attention on body experience, without it automatically activating "stories" about the self. These data are hugely important. They are the first to support the notion of a fundamental neural dissociation between two distinct forms of self-awareness—narrative and experiential modes—that are habitually integrated but can be uncoupled through mindfulness training.

Having shown that training in mindfulness sharpens the contrast between the narrative and experiential modes of processing, and cognizant of the associated reductions in reactivity this can produce, the question most relevant to a prevention treatment such as MBCT is whether patients can learn to do this when they are feeling sad.

Farb and colleagues[158] examined this directly by having patients who were about to start or had recently completed MBSR watch sad and neutral film clips while being scanned. For all participants, sadness provocation was associated with activation along the back and front regions of the middle of the frontal cortex, as well as in language and conceptual processing centers. These areas direct the type of analytic thinking and self-focus that is characteristic of reappraisal. Lower levels of activity were also found in the somatosensory cortex and right insula, areas that convey information about body sensations associated with emotion. However, when the effects of mindfulness training were examined, the group that completed the 8-week program demonstrated less neural reactivity to sadness provocation than those who had not undergone training. The pattern changed: The frontal regions that direct self-focus showed less activation, and there was now far more activity in the insula.

As we have seen, accessing information about what is occurring in the body during the experience of sadness and being able to watch emotions as they arise—without getting caught up in thinking about them—is a core skill practiced during MBSR and MBCT. It may also be one path through which mindfulness helps to restore the balance between neural networks that support both analytic (ruminative) and body-based representations of emotion, when they are tipped too strongly toward the former by a stressor or setback in our everyday lives.

To summarize, it is important to stress that while we don't want to overestimate what can be learned from brain science, there is an astonishing coherence to the story unfolding thus far. Taking what people said was effective about MBCT as our starting point, we found that the themes of mindful awareness and compassionate action were equally valid when examined through qualitative interviews and quantitative methods. Changes have been indicated in just those elements that theory says are important. Building on this, the brain imaging data show that a key attentional shift taught in the program—from narrative to experiential mode—is neurally discernable, and that training in mindfulness enables this shift even in the presence of sad thoughts and feelings. It may well be that future researchers will discover other important mechanisms of MBCT, but the convergence found in the accounts to date offer striking support for the higher-order teaching points embedded and embodied in the program.

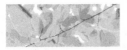 CHAPTER 21

Moving the Program Off the Page and into the Clinic

Supports for Mindfulness-Based Cognitive Therapy Instructors and Their Patients

If you are intrigued by the possibility of integrating mindfulness training with aspects of cognitive therapy as a way to reduce suffering and promote well-being, there are a variety of resources at your disposal. While this was certainly not the case when the first edition of this book was published, the broader exposure that mindfulness has recently received should make it easier for you to engage with the topic. Here, we offer some suggestions to guide your further exploration.

STARTING YOUR OWN PRACTICE OF MINDFULNESS

A central message in MBCT is that in order to do this work, therapists should practice mindfulness themselves. This principle, while foundational, has nonetheless sparked some controversy in psychotherapy circles, perhaps because training in meditation is not in the standard curriculum for psychotherapists.

If you would like to dip your toe in the water and simply find out more about mindfulness before committing to a personal practice, there are a number of excellent sources of further information available. *Wherever You Go, There You Are*, written by Jon Kabat-Zinn,[66] is a wonderful book that conveys the spirit of bringing mindfulness to everyday experience, together with suggestions for practice. Another excellent source for a more detailed description of insight meditation, the tradition from which clinical applications of mindfulness are most directly derived, is *Seeking the Heart of Wisdom: The Path of Insight Meditation* by Joseph Goldstein and Jack Kornfeld.[159]

On the other hand, perhaps you are ready to dive right in and directly experience the practice of mindfulness training. The best way is to be taught face-to-face by an experienced meditation teacher (see later details of how to find one). However, you might first like to "do it yourself" using the guided meditation instructions that are available for download at *www.guilford.com/MBCT_materials*. These will not only help you establish a regular practice but also provide a direct sampling of the exercises used by patients in the program (for other materials, see *http://oxfordmindfulness.org/learn/resources*).

Ideally, one learns meditation from personal contact with an experienced meditation teacher. There are many different forms of meditation. Therefore, from the perspective of preparing oneself as a potential instructor of MBCT, it is important to choose a tradition and teacher that are compatible in spirit and form with the MBCT program. In practice, this likely means exploring the teachings offered by centers related to the Westernized insight meditation tradition. Information about these centers can be obtained from the following: in North America, the Insight Meditation Society in Barre, Massachusetts (*www.dharma.org*), or Spirit Rock in Woodacre, California (*www.spiritrock.org*); in Europe, Gaia House in Devon, England (*www.gaiahouse.co.uk*); and in Australia, the Australian insight meditation network (*www.dharma.org.au*).

TRAINING GUIDELINES FOR MINDFULNESS-BASED COGNITIVE THERAPY INSTRUCTORS

If you are a therapist or counselor who is interested in applying mindfulness clinically, then the best way to characterize the current training opportunities in MBCT is to say that capacity is germinal but growing. Postgraduate training leading to a master's degree in MBCT is available at Oxford University and the University of Exeter, while Bangor University offers a master's in mindfulness, with both MBSR and MBCT as a major focus. All of these U.K.-based programs are taught on a part-time basis over 2 to 3 years to professionals, and provide coverage of the experiential and didactic elements of MBCT, along with its evidence base.

A more likely scenario, especially for instructors living in North America, is that you find yourself attending an MBCT clinical workshop, a silent mindfulness retreat for therapists, seeking supervision from a practicing MBCT instructor, or starting a peer supervision group. These are all useful experiences, but to help you chart how far along you are in the process, it may be useful to have a roadmap. We have therefore decided to list what we consider to be the normal minimal requirements for teaching MBCT for mood disorders (see Figure 21.1). Our intention is to help instructors situate their continuing professional education within a more modular progression of training experiences that can lead to MBCT adherence and competence. Our second motivation is to avoid the situation in which people with just a little experience of mindfulness meditation feel that, once they have read the book, they are competent to run MBCT classes (see Figure 21.1).

SUPPORTING OUR PATIENTS

We have developed an MBCT workbook[160] for patients to use as they work their way through the 8-week program (though it can also be used outside the program with or without a therapist). Along with describing the content in each session, patients are provided a rationale for the different exercises and helpful hints for their growing practice. It is an essential resource designed to function as a single source for the handouts, home practice sheets, calendars, poems, CDs, and other content covered during the 8 weeks.

For people who are interested in reading about how the practice of mindfulness can be broadened to deal with milder but more ubiquitous mental states, such as worry and unhappiness, *The Mindful Way through Depression*[76] can be very helpful. It features seven guided meditations narrated by Jon Kabat-Zinn and provides the reader with more extensive background to these practices than would typically be provided in an MBCT class. In the spirit of reinforcing an ongoing commitment to the

These are normal minimal requirements for teaching MBCT for mood disorders.

1. An ongoing commitment to a personal mindfulness practice through daily formal and informal practice.

2. A professional qualification in clinical practice and mental health training that includes the use of structured, evidence-based therapeutic approaches to treating affective disorders (e.g., CBT, interpersonal psychotherapy, behavioral activation).

3. Knowledge and experience of the populations to which the mindfulness-based approach will be delivered, including experience of teaching, therapeutic, or other care provision with groups and individuals.

4. Completion of an in-depth, rigorous, mindfulness-based teacher training program or supervised pathway with a minimum duration of 12 months. (A "supervised pathway" might include attending three 8-week courses, the first as participant, the second as trainee, and the third as co-teacher, as well as attending workshops on theoretical and practical aspects of teaching the core practices and curriculum.)

5. Ongoing adherence to the framework for ethical conduct as outlined within his or her profession.

6. Engagement in an ongoing peer supervision process with an experienced *mindfulness-based teacher(s)*, which should include receiving periodic feedback on teaching from an experienced, mindfulness-based teacher through video recordings, a supervisor sitting in on teaching sessions, or co-teaching including scheduled feedback sessions.

For the purposes of continuing professional development we recommend:

1. Participation in residential, teacher-led mindfulness meditation retreats.

2. Ongoing peer supervision with mindfulness-based *colleagues*, built and maintained as a means to share experiences and learn collaboratively.

3. Engagement in *further training* to develop skills and understanding in delivering mindfulness-based approaches, which includes keeping up to date with the current evidence base for mindfulness-based approaches.

FIGURE 21.1. Training guidelines for teaching mindfulness-based cognitive therapy.

principles and practices of MBCT, a number of centers give this book to patients at the last group session. *Mindfulness: A Practical Guide to Finding Peace in a Frantic World,* by Mark Williams and Danny Penman,[161] is another option for those who wish to taste shorter meditation practices to see whether this is something they wish to explore further through the full MBCT program. It includes meditations narrated by Mark Williams (see *www.franticworld.com* and *www.oxfordmindfulness.org*).

Using a similar format to *The Mindful Way through Depression*,[76] *The Mindful Way through Anxiety*[162] is meant for people who suffer from disturbing fears and anxiety and want to learn how the integration of traditional exposure techniques with mindfulness training can help them live more fully. As well, *The Mindful Path to Self-Compassion*[163] offers helpful guidance in addressing self-blame, judgment, and perfectionism through developing mindfulness and compassionate responses to difficulties.

Epilogue

We have come to the end of this edition. Our aim has been to tell the story of how our previous research and clinical work led us to realize the urgency of the fact that depression has emerged as a global problem and needs a new approach. We have described how we looked toward the mindfulness approach that Jon Kabat-Zinn developed at UMass, and how we needed then to return to psychological science to guide the development of MBCT. So here we have provided a tapestry—an interweaving of new understandings from research, together with clinical teaching about its implementation.

We hope that this book, written as a result of our own experience, can provide a map for you that will act as a guide and an encouragement as you make your own journey. If you wish to teach MBCT (or to deepen your teaching of mindfulness in any context), you'll find that you need to sustain your teaching by returning again and again to two essential foundations: the learning that comes from your own daily practice and the learning that comes from the approach's empirical grounding within psychological science.

From this point forward, we hope that your own understanding, practice, and personal engagement with the material allow you to guide those who come to you seeking help, so you will feel more able to show them how they, too, can draw on their own powerful inner resources to cultivate kind and self-compassionate courses of action. In time, those who participate in your classes, guided by your teaching, will appreciate the enormous power of this work: that in addition to enabling them to step out of ruminative thought loops or respond to warning signs, this practice can help them to expand their quality of life and experience, moment by moment, to find a wholly new way of living based neither in fear nor in brooding over the past, but in embracing the "full catastrophe" of daily life with more courage, compassion, and joy than they had ever imagined.

As we end this second edition, we pay tribute to the many participants we have been privileged to meet on this extraordinary journey—in our classes and in our research studies—who, whether they know it or not, have been our teachers and our guides, and whose experiences have helped shape the field. Through their courage, the way we understand depression and the way we offer help to those who suffer from it will never be the same again.

References

1. Lepine JP, Gastpar M, Mendlewicz J, Tylee A. Depression in the community: The first pan-European study DEPRES. *International Clinical Psychopharmacology* 1997; *12*:19–29.

2. Parikh SV, Wasylenki D, Goering P, Wong J. Mood disorders: Rural/urban differences in prevalence, health care utilization and disability in Ontario. *Journal of Affective Disorders* 1996; *38*:57–65.

3. Weissman MM, Bruce LM, Leaf PJ. Affective disorders. In Robins LN, Regier DA, eds. *Psychiatric disorders in America: The Epidemiologic Catchment Area study.* New York: Free Press, 1990:53–80.

4. Kessler RC, Berglund P, Demler O, Jin R, Koretz D, Merikangas KR, Rush AJ, Walters EE, Wang PS. The epidemiology of major depressive disorder: Results from the National Comorbidity Survey Replication (NCS-R). *Journal of the American Medical Association* 2003; *289*:3095–3105.

5. Hasin DS, Goodwin RD, Stinson FS, Grant BF. Epidemiology of major depressive disorder: Results from the National Epidemiologic Survey on Alcoholism and Related Conditions. *Archives of General Psychiatry* 2005; *62*:1097–1106.

6. Keller MB, Lavori PW, Mueller TI, Coryell W, Hirschfeld RMA, Shea MT. Time to recovery, chronicity and levels of psychopathology in major depression. *Archives of General Psychiatry* 1992; *49*:809–816.

7. Sargeant JK, Bruce ML, Florio LP, Weissman MM. Factors associated with 1-year outcome for major depression in the community. *Archives of General Psychiatry* 1990; *47*:519–526.

8. Boyd JH, Burke JD, Gruneberg E, Holzer CE III, Rae DS, George LK, Karno M, Stoltzman R, McEvoy L, Nestadt G. Exclusion criteria of DSM-III: A study of co-occurrence of hierarchy-free syndromes. *Archives of General Psychiatry* 1984; *41*:983–959.

9. National Institute for Health and Clinical Excellence. *Depression: The treatment and management of depression in adults.* NICE guidance, Clinical Guidelines CG90, 2009.

10. Wells KB, Sturm R, Sherbourne CD, Meredith LS. *Caring for depression*. Boston: Harvard University Press, 1996.

11. Broadhead WE, Blazer DG, George LK, Tse CK. Depression, disability days and days lost from work in a prospective epidemiological survey. *Journal of the American Medical Association* 1990; *264*:2524–2528.

12. Adler DA, McLaughlin TJ, Rogers WH, Chang H, Lapitsky L, Lerner D. Job performance deficits due to depression. *American Journal of Psychiatry* 2006; *163*:1569–1576.

13. Murray CL, Lopez AD. *The global burden of disease: A comprehensive assessment of mortality and disability from disease, injuries and risk factors in 1990 and projected to 2020*. Boston: Harvard University Press, 1998.

14. Nathan KI, Musselman DL, Schatzberg AF, Nemeroff CB. Biology of mood disorders. In Nemeroff CB, ed. *The American Psychiatric Press textbook of psychopharmacology*. Washington, DC: American Psychiatric Press, 1995:439–478.

15. Healy D. *The antidepressant era*. Cambridge, MA: Harvard University Press, 1997.

16. Fournier JC, DeRubeis RJ, Hollon SD, Dimidjian S, Amsterdam JD, Shelton RC, Fawcett J. Antidepressant drug effects and depression severity: A patient-level meta-analysis. *Journal of the American Medical Association* 2010; *303*:47–53.

17. Fava GA, Offidani E. The mechanisms of tolerance in antidepressant action. *Progress in Neuro-Psychopharmacology and Biological Psychiatry* 2011; *35*:1593–1602.

18. Lewinsohn PM, Antonuccio DO, Steinmetz JL, Teri L. *The Coping with Depression course: A psychoeducational intervention for unipolar depression*. Eugene, OR: Castalia Press, 1984.

19. Becker RE, Heimberg RG, Bellack AS. *Social skills training treatment for depression*. Elmsford, NY: Pergamon Press, 1987.

20. Beck AT, Rush AJ, Shaw BF, Emery G. *Cognitive therapy of depression*. New York: Guilford Press, 1979.

21. Klerman GL, Weissman MM, Rounsaville BJ, Chevron E. *Interpersonal psychotherapy of depression*. New York: Basic Books, 1984.

22. Hollon SD, Stewart M, Strunk, D. Enduring effects for cognitive behavior therapy in the treatment of depression and anxiety. *Annual Review of Psychology* 2006; *57*:285-315.

23. Keller MB, Lavori PW, Lewis CE, Klerman GL. Predictors of relapse in major depressive disorder. *Journal of the American Medical Association* 1983; *250*:3299–3304.

24. Kessler RC, Demler O, Frank RG, Olfson M, Pincus HA, Walters EE, Wang P, Wells KB, Zaslavsky AM. Prevalence and treatment of mental disorders, 1990 to 2003. *New England Journal of Medicine* 2005; *352*:2515–2523.

25. Judd LL. The clinical course of unipolar major depressive disorders. *Archives of General Psychiatry* 1997; *54*:989–991.

26. Kupfer DJ. Long-term treatment of depression. *Journal of Clinical Psychiatry* 1991; *52 Suppl*:28–34.

27. Coryell W, Endicott J, Keller MB. Outcome of patients with chronic affective

disorder: A five year follow up. *American Journal of Psychiatry* 1990; *147*:1627–1633.

28. American Psychiatric Association. *Diagnostic and statistical manual of mental disorders* (4th ed., text rev.). Washington, DC: American Psychiatric Publishing, 2000.

29. Glen AI, Johnson AL, Shepherd M. Continuation therapy with lithium and amitriptyline in unipolar depressive illness: A randomized, double blind, controlled trial. *Psychological Medicine* 1984; *14*:37–50.

30. Frank E, Prien RF, Jarrett RB, Keller MB, Kupfer DJ, Lavori PW, Rush AJ, Weissman MM. Conceptualization and rationale for consensus definitions of terms in major depressive disorder. *Archives of General Psychiatry* 1991; *48*:851–855.

31. Gelenberg A, Freeman M, Markowitz J, Rosenbaum J, Thase M, Trivedi M, Van Rhoads R. *Practice guideline for the assessment and treatment of major depressive disorder* (3rd ed.). Washington, DC: American Psychiatric Publishing, 2006.

32. Hollon SD, DeRubeis RJ, Shelton RC, Amsterdam JD, Salomon RM, O'Reardon JP, Lovett ML, Young PR, Haman KL, Freeman BB, Gallop R. Prevention of relapse following cognitive therapy vs medications in moderate to severe depression. *Archives of General Psychiatry* 2005; *62*:417–422.

33. Rush AJ, Trivedi MH, Wisniewski SR, Nierenberg AA, Stewart JW, Warden D, Niederehe G, Thase ME, Lavori PW, Lebowitz BD, McGrath PJ, Rosenbaum JF, Sackeim HA, Kupfer DJ, Luther J, Fava M. Acute and longer-term outcomes in depressed outpatients requiring one or several treatment steps: A STAR*D report. *American Journal of Psychiatry* 2006; *163*:1905–1917.

34. Post RM. Transduction of psychosocial stress into the neurobiology of recurrent affective disorder. *American Journal of Psychiatry* 1992; *149*:999–1010.

35. Lin EH, Von Korff M, Katon W, Bush T, Simon GE, Walker E, Robinson P. The role of the primary care physician in patients' adherence to antidepressant therapy. *Medical Care* 1995; *33*:67–74.

36. Lewis E, Marcus SC, Olfson M, Druss BG, Pincus HA. Patients' early discontinuation of antidepressant prescriptions. *Psychiatric Services* 2004; *55*:494.

37. Reuters/Health. Few patients satisfied with antidepressants, 1999. Available at *www.reuters.com.*

38. Frank E, Kupfer DJ, Perel JM, Cornes C, Jarrett DB, Mallinger AG, Thas ME, McEachran AB, Grochocinski VJ. Three year outcomes for maintenance therapies in recurrent depression. *Archives of General Psychiatry* 1990; *47*:1093–1099.

39. Blackburn IM, Eunson KM, Bishop S. A two-year naturalistic follow-up of depressed patients treated with cognitive therapy, pharmacotherapy, and a combination of both. *Journal of Affective Disorders* 1986; *10*:67–75.

40. Evans MD, Hollon SD, DeRubeis J, Piasecki JM, Grove WM, Tuason VB. Differential relapse following cognitive therapy and pharmacotherapy for depression. *Archives of General Psychiatry* 1992; *49*:802–808.

41. Shea MT, Elkin I, Imber S, Sotsky SM, Watkins JT, Collins JF, Pilkonis PA, Beckham E, Glass DR, Dolan RT, et al. Course of depressive symptoms over follow

up: Findings from the NIMH Treatment of Depression Collaborative Research Program. *Archives of General Psychiatry* 1992; *49*:782–787.

42. Simons A, Murphy G, Levine J, Wetzel R. Cognitive therapy and pharmacotherapy for depression: Sustained improvement over one year. *Archives of General Psychiatry* 1986; *43*:43–50.

43. Vittengl JR, Clark LA, Dunn TW, Jarrett RB. Reducing relapse and recurrence in unipolar depression: A comparative meta-analysis of cognitive-behavioral therapy's effects. *Journal of Consulting and Clinical Psychology* 2007; *75*:475–488.

44. Beck AT. *Cognitive therapy and the emotional disorders.* New York: International Universities Press, 1976.

45. Kovacs MB, Beck AT. Maladaptive cognitive structures in depression. *American Journal of Psychiatry* 1978; *135*:525–533.

46. Weissman M, Beck AT. *Development and validation of the Dysfunctional Attitude Scale.* Paper presented at the meeting of the Association for Advancement of Behavior Therapy, Chicago, 1978.

47. Ingram RE, Atchley RA, Segal ZV. *Vulnerability to depression: From cognitive neuroscience to prevention and treatment.* New York: Guilford Press, 2011.

48. Teasdale JD. Negative thinking in depression: Cause, effect or reciprocal relationship? *Advances in Behaviour Research and Therapy* 1983; *5*:3–25.

49. Teasdale JD. Cognitive vulnerability to persistent depression. *Cognition and Emotion* 1988; *2*:247–274.

50. Segal ZV, Ingram RE. Mood priming and construct activation in tests of cognitive vulnerability to unipolar depression. *Clinical Psychology Review* 1994; *14*:663–695.

51. Miranda J, Persons JB. Dysfunctional attitudes are mood state dependent. *Journal of Abnormal Psychology* 1988; *97*:76–79.

52. Miranda J, Persons JB, Byers C. Endorsement of dysfunctional beliefs depends on current mood state. *Journal of Abnormal Psychology* 1990; *99*:237–241.

53. Segal ZV, Gemar MC, Williams S. Differential cognitive response to a mood challenge following successful cognitive therapy or pharmacotherapy for unipolar depression. *Journal of Abnormal Psychology* 1999; *108*:3–10.

54. Segal ZV, Kennedy S, Gemar M, Hood K, Pedersen R, Buis T. Cognitive reactivity to sad mood provocation and the prediction of depressive relapse. *Archives of General Psychiatry* 2006; *63*:749–755.

55. Kendler KS, Thornton LM, Gardner CO. Stressful life events and previous episodes in the etiology of major depression in women: An evaluation of the "kindling" hypothesis. *American Journal of Psychiatry* 2000; *157*:1243–1251.

56. Segal ZV, Williams JMG, Teasdale JD, Gemar MC. A cognitive science perspective on kindling and episode sensitization in recurrent affective disorder. *Psychological Medicine* 1996; *26*:371–380.

57. Nolen-Hoeksema S, Morrow J. A prospective study of depression and posttraumatic stress symptoms after a natural disaster: The 1989 Loma Prieta earthquake. *Journal of Personality and Social Psychology* 1991; *61*:115–121.

58. Treynor W, Gonzalez R, Nolen-Hoeksema, S. Rumination reconsidered: A psychometric analysis. *Cognitive Therapy and Research* 2003; *27*:247–259.

59. Lyubomirsky S, Nolen-Hoeksema S. Effects of self-focused rumination on negative thinking and interpersonal problem solving. *Journal of Personality and Social Psychology* 1995; *69*:176–190.

60. Teasdale JD, Segal ZV, Williams JMG. How does cognitive therapy prevent relapse and why should attentional control (mindfulness) training help? *Behaviour Research and Therapy* 1995; *33*:225–239.

61. Barber JP, DeRubeis, R. On second thought: Where the action is in cognitive therapy. *Cognitive Therapy and Research* 1989; *13*:441–457.

62. Simons AD, Garfield S, Murphy G. The process of change in cognitive therapy and pharmacotherapy for depression. *Archives of General Psychiatry* 1984; *49*:45–51.

63. Ingram RE, Hollon SD. Cognitive therapy for depression from an information processing perspective. In Ingram RE, ed. *Information processing approaches to clinical psychology*. Orlando, FL: Academic Press, 1986:261–284.

64. Teasdale JD. The impact of experimental research on clinical practice. In Emmelkamp PMG, Everaerd WTAM, Kraaimmaat F, van Son MJM, eds. *Advances in theory and practice in behaviour therapy*. Amsterdam: Swets & Zeitlinger, 1988:1–18.

65. Linehan MM, Armstrong HE, Suarez A, Allmon D, Heard H. Cognitive-behavioral treatment of chronically parasuicidal borderline patients. *Archives of General Psychiatry* 1991; *48*:1060–1064.

66. Kabat-Zinn J. *Wherever you go, there you are: Mindfulness meditation in everyday life*. New York: Hyperion, 1994.

67. Kabat-Zinn J. *Full castastrophe living: Using the wisdom of your body and mind to face stress, pain, and illness*. New York: Dell, 1990.

68. Kabat-Zinn J, Lipworth L, Burney R, Sellers W. Four-year follow-up of a meditation-based program for self-regulation of chronic pain: Treatment outcomes and compliance. *Clinical Journal of Pain* 1986; *2*:159–173.

69. Kabat-Zinn J, Massion AO, Kristeller J, Peterson LG, Fletcher KE, Pbert L, Lenderking WR, Santorelli SF. Effectiveness of a meditation-based stress reduction program in the treatment of anxiety disorders. *American Journal of Psychiatry* 1992; *149*:936–943.

70. Miller J, Fletcher K, Kabat-Zinn J. Three year follow-up and clinical implications of a mindfulness-based stress reduction intervention in the treatment of anxiety disorders. *General Hospital Psychiatry* 1995; *17*:192–200.

71. McLean P, Hakstian A. Clinical depression: Relative efficacy of outpatient treatments. *Journal of Consulting and Clinical Psychology* 1979; *47*:818–836.

72. Öst L-G. Efficacy of the third wave of behavioral therapies: A systematic review and meta-analysis. *Behaviour Research and Therapy* 2008; *46*:296–321.

73. Watzlawick P, Fisch R, Weakland J. *Change: Principles of problem formation and problem resolution*. New York: Norton, 1974.

74. Linehan MM. *Cognitive-behavioral treatment of borderline personality disorder.* New York: Guilford Press, 1993.

75. Wegner D. Ironic processes of mental control. *Psychological Review* 1994; *101*:34–52.

76. Williams JMG, Teasdale JD, Segal ZV, Kabat-Zinn J. *The mindful way through depression: Freeing yourself from chronic unhappiness.* New York: Guilford Press, 2007.

77. Miller WR, Rose GS. Toward a theory of motivational interviewing. *American Psychologist* 2009; *64*:527–537.

78. Crane C, Williams JMG. Factors associated with attrition from mindfulness based cognitive therapy for suicidal depression. *Mindfulness* 2010; *1*:10–20.

79. Feldman C. *The Buddhist path to simplicity.* London: Thorsons, 2001.

80. Salzberg S. Mindfulness and loving kindness. *Contemporary Buddhism* 2011; *12*:177–182.

81. Feldman C, Kuyken W. Compassion in the landscape of suffering. *Contemporary Buddhism* 2011; *12*:143–155.

82. Kabat-Zinn J. *Coming to our senses.* New York: Hyperion, 2006.

83. Barnhofer T, Chittka T, Nightingale H, Visser C, Crane C. State effects of two forms of meditation on prefrontal EEG asymmetry in previously depressed individuals. *Mindfulness* 2010; *1*:21–27.

84. Germer CK. *The mindful path to self compassion: Freeing yourself from destructive thoughts and emotions.* New York: Guilford Press, 2009.

85. Friedman RS, Förster J. Implicit affective cues and attentional tuning: An integrative review. *Psychological Bulletin* 2010; *136*:875–893.

86. Hayes SC, Wilson KG, Gifford EV, Follette VM, Strosahl K. Experimental avoidance and behavioral disorders: A functional dimensional approach to diagnosis and treatment. *Journal of Consulting and Clinical Psychology* 1996; *64*:1152–1168.

87. Oliver M. *Dream work.* Boston: Grove/Atlantic, 1986.

88. Hollon SD, Kendall P. Cognitive self-statements in depression: Development of an Automatic Thoughts Questionnaire. *Cognitive Therapy and Research* 1980; *4*:383–395.

89. Goldstein J. *Insight meditation: The practice of freedom.* Boston: Shambhala, 1994.

90. Crane R. *Mindfulness-based cognitive therapy.* London: Routledge, 2009.

91. Kolb DA. *Experiential learning: Experience as a source of learning and development.* Englewood Cliffs, NJ: Prentice Hall, 1984.

92. Padesky C. *Socratic questioning: Changing minds or guiding discovery?* London: European Congress of Behavioural and Cognitive Therapies, 1993.

93. Santorelli S. *Heal thyself: Lessons on mindfulness in medicine.* New York: Bell Tower, 1999.

94. Barks C, Moyne J. *The essential Rumi.* San Francisco: Harper, 1997.

95. Rosenberg L. *Breath by breath.* Boston: Shambhala, 1998.

96. Fennell M. Depression. In Hawton K, Salkovskis P, Kirk J, Clark D, eds. *Cognitive*

behaviour therapy for psychiatric problems. Oxford, UK: Oxford University Press, 1989:169–234.

97. Mathew KL, Whitney HS, Kenny MA, Denson LA. The long-term effects of mindfulness-based cognitive therapy as a relapse prevention treatment for major depressive disorder. *Behavioural and Cognitive Psychotherapy* 2010; *38*:561–576.

98. Dobson KS, Hollon SD, Dimidjian S, Schmaling KB, Kohlenberg RJ, Gallop RJ, Rizvi SL, Gollan JK, Dunner DL, Jacobson NS. Randomized trial of behavioral activation, cognitive therapy, and antidepressant medication in the prevention of relapse and recurrence in major depression. *Journal of Consulting and Clinical Psychology* 2008; *76*(3):468–477.

99. Bennett-Levy J, Butler G, Fennell M, Hackmann A, Meuller M, Westbrook, D. *Oxford guide to behavioural experiments in cognitive therapy*. Oxford, UK: Oxford University Press, 2004.

100. Oliver M. *House of light*. Boston: Beacon Press, 1990.

101. Carmody J, Baer RA. Relationships between mindfulness practice and levels of mindfulness, medical and psychological symptoms and well-being in a mindfulness-based stress reduction program. *Journal of Behavioral Medicine* 2008; *31*:23–33.

102. Mausbach BT, Moore R, Roesch S, Cardenas V, Patterson TL. The relationship between homework compliance and therapy outcomes: An updated meta-analysis. *Cognitive Therapy and Research* 2010; *34*:429–438.

103. Teasdale JD, Segal ZV, Williams JMG, Ridgeway V, Soulsby J, Lau M. Prevention of relapse/recurrence in major depression by mindfulness-based cognitive therapy. *Journal of Consulting and Clinical Psychology* 2000; *68*:615–623.

104. Ma SH, Teasdale JD. Mindfulness-based cognitive therapy for depression: Replication and exploration of differential relapse prevention effects. *Journal of Consulting and Clinical Psychology* 2004; *72*:31–40.

105. Kendler KS, Thornton LM, Gardner CO. Stressful life events and previous episodes in the etiology of major depression in women: An evaluation of the "kindling" hypothesis. *American Journal of Psychiatry* 2000; *157*:1243–1251.

106. Bondolfi G, Jermann F, der Linden MV, Gex-Fabry M, Bizzini L, Rouget BW, Myers-Arrazola L, Gonzalez C, Segal Z, Aubry JM, Bertschy G. Depression relapse prophylaxis with mindfulness-based cognitive therapy: Replication and extension in the Swiss health care system. *Journal of Affective Disorders* 2010; *122*:224–231.

107. Godfrin KA, van Heeringen C. The effects of mindfulness-based cognitive therapy on recurrence of depressive episodes, mental health and quality of life: A randomized controlled study. *Behaviour Research and Therapy* 2010; *48*:738–746.

108. Kuyken W, Byford S, Taylor RS, Watkins E, Holden E, White K, Barrett B, Byng R, Evans A, Mullan E, Teasdale JD. Mindfulness-based cognitive therapy to prevent relapse in recurrent depression. *Journal of Consulting and Clinical Psychology* 2008; *76*:966–978.

109. Segal ZV, Bieling P, Young T, MacQueen G, Cooke R, Martin L, Bloch R,

Levitan RD. Antidepressant monotherapy vs sequential pharmacotherapy and mindfulness-based cognitive therapy, or placebo, for relapse prophylaxis in recurrent depression. *Archives of General Psychiatry* 2010; *67*:1256–1264.

110. Jarrett RB, Kraft D, Doyle J, Foster BM, Eaves GG, Silver PC. Preventing recurrent depression using cognitive therapy with and without a continuation phase. *Archives of General Psychiatry* 2001; *58*:381–388.

111. Piet J, Hougaard E. The effect of mindfulness-based cognitive therapy for prevention of relapse in recurrent major depressive disorder: A systematic review and meta-analysis. *Clinical Psychology Review* 2011; *31*:1032–1040.

112. Hofmann SG, Sawyer AT, Witt AA, Oh D. The effect of mindfulness-based therapy on anxiety and depression: A meta-analytic review. *Journal of Consulting and Clinical Psychology* 2010; *78*:169–183.

113. Semple R, Lee J. *Mindfulness-based cognitive therapy for anxious children.* Oakland, CA: New Harbinger, 2011.

114. Bogels S, Hoogstad B, van Dun L, de Schutter S, Restifo K. Mindfulness training for adolescents with externalizing disorders and their parents. *Behavioural and Cognitive Psychotherapy* 2008, *36*:193–209.

115. Bowen S, Chawla N, Marlatt GA. *Mindfulness-based relapse prevention for addictive behaviors: A clinician's guide.* New York: Guilford Press, 2011.

116. Dimidjian S, Goodman SH. Nonpharmacological interventions and prevention strategies for depression during pregnancy and the postpartum. *Clinical Obstetrics and Gynecology* 2009; *52*:498–515.

117. McManus F, Muse K, Surawy, C, Williams JMG. A randomized clinical trial of mindfulness-based cognitive therapy vs. unrestricted services for health anxiety. *Journal of Consulting and Clinical Psychology* in press.

118. Rimes K, Wingrove J. Mindfulness-based cognitive therapy for people with chronic fatigue syndrome still experiencing excessive fatigue after cognitive behaviour therapy: A pilot randomized study. *Clinical Psychology and Psychotherapy* in press.

119. Philippot P, Nef F, Clauw L, Romrée M, Segal Z. A randomized controlled trial of mindfulness-based cognitive therapy for treating tinnitus. *Clinical Psychology and Psychotherapy* in press.

120. Chadwick P, Hughes S, Russell D, Russell I, Dagnan D. Mindfulness groups for distressing voices and paranoia: A replication and randomized feasibility trial. *Behavioural and Cognitive Psychotherapy* 2009; *37*:403–412.

121. Britton WB, Haynes PL, Fridel KW, Bootzin RR. Polysomnographic and subjective profiles of sleep continuity before and after mindfulness-based cognitive therapy in partially remitted depression. *Psychosomatic Medicine* 2010; *72*:539–548.

122. Piet J, Hougaard E, Hecksher MS, Rosenberg NK. A randomized pilot study of mindfulness-based cognitive therapy and group cognitive-behavioral therapy for young adults with social phobia. *Scandinavian Journal of Psychology* 2010; *51*:403–410.

123. Craigie MA, Rees CS, Marsh A, Nathan P. Mindfulness-based cognitive therapy for generalized anxiety disorder: A preliminary evaluation. *Behavioural and Cognitive Psychotherapy* 2008; *36*:553–568.

124. Kim B, Lee S-H, Kim YW, Choi TK, Yook K, Suh SY, Cho SJ, Yook K-H. Effectiveness of a mindfulness-based cognitive therapy program as an adjunct to pharmacotherapy in patients with panic disorder. *Journal of Anxiety Disorders* 2010; *24*:590–595.

125. Shawyer F, Meadows GN, Judd F, Martin PR, Segal Z, Piterman L. The DARE study of relapse prevention in depression: Design for a phase 1/2 translational randomised controlled trial involving mindfulness-based cognitive therapy and supported self monitoring. *BMC Psychiatry* 2012; *12*:3.

126. Foley E, Baillie A, Huxter M, Price M, Sinclair E. Mindfulness-based cognitive therapy for individuals whose lives have been affected by cancer: A randomized controlled trial. *Journal of Consulting and Clinical Psychology* 2010; *78*:72–79.

127. Bartley T. *Mindfulness-based cognitive therapy for cancer.* Hoboken, NJ: Wiley-Blackwell, 2011.

128. Schroevers MJ, Brandsma R. Is learning mindfulness associated with improved affect after mindfulness-based cognitive therapy? *British Journal of Psychology* 2010; *101*:95–107.

129. Geschwind N, Peeters F, Drukker M, van Os J, Wichers M. Mindfulness training increases momentary positive emotions and reward experience in adults vulnerable to depression: A randomized controlled trial. *Journal of Consulting and Clinical Psychology* 2011; *79*:618–628.

130. Crane C, Winder R, Hargus E, Amarasinghe M, Barnhofer T. Effects of mindfulness-based cognitive therapy on specificity of life goals. *Cognitive Therapy and Research* 2012; *36*:182–189.

131. Arch J, Craske, M. Mechanisms of mindfulness: Emotion regulation following a focused breathing induction. *Behaviour Research and Therapy* 2006; *44*:1849–1858.

132. Kenny M, Williams M. Treatment-resistant depressed patients show a good response to mindfulness-based cognitive therapy. *Behaviour Research and Therapy* 2007; *45*:617–625.

133. Eisendrath SJ, Delucchi K, Bitner R, Fenimore P, Smit M, McLane M. Mindfulness-based cognitive therapy for treatment-resistant depression: A pilot study. *Psychotherapy and Psychosomatics* 2008; *77*:319–320.

134. Barnhofer T, Crane C, Hargus E, Amarasinghe M, Winder, R Williams JMG. Mindfulness-based cognitive therapy as a treatment for chronic depression: A preliminary study. *Behaviour Research and Therapy* 2009; *47*:366–373.

135. van Aalderen J, Donders A, Giommi F, Spinhoven P, Barendregt H, Speckens A. The efficacy of mindfulness-based cognitive therapy in recurrent depressed patients with and without a current depressive episode: A randomized controlled trial. *Psychological Medicine* 2011; *3*:1–13.

136. Williams JMG, Alatiq Y, Crane C, Barnhofer T, Fennell MJV, Duggan DS, Hepburn S, Goodwin GM. Mindfulness-based cognitive therapy (MBCT) in bipolar disorder: Preliminary evaluation of immediate effects on between-episode functioning. *Journal of Affective Disorders* 2008; *107*:275–279.

137. Stange P, Eisner LR, Hölzel B, Peckham A, Dougherty D, Rauch SL, Nierenberg A, Lazar S, Deckersbach T. Mindfulness-based cognitive therapy for bipolar disorder: Effects on cognitive functioning. *Journal of Psychiatric Practice* 2011; *17*:410–419.

138. Weber B, Jermann F, Gex-Fabry M, Nallet A, Bondolfi G, & Aubry JM. Mindfulness-based cognitive therapy for bipolar disorder: A feasibility trial. *European Psychiatry* 2010; *25*:334–337.

139. Miklowitz DJ, Alatiq Y, Goodwin GM, Geddes JR, Fennell MJV, Dimidjian S, Hauser M, Williams JMG. A pilot study of a mindfulness-based cognitive therapy for bipolar disorder. *International Journal of Cognitive Therapy* 2009; *4*:373–382.

140. Allen M, Bromley A, Kuyken W, Sonnenberg SJ. Participants' experiences of mindfulness-based cognitive therapy: "It changed me in just about every way possible." *Behavioural and Cognitive Psychotherapy* 2009; *37*:413–430.

141. Dimidjian S, Segal Z. The clinical science of mindfulness training: Patient outcomes and change mechanisms. *American Psychologist* in press.

142. Williams JMG, Teasdale J, Segal Z, Soulsby J. Mindfulness-based cognitive therapy reduces overgeneral autobiographical memory in formerly depressed patients. *Journal of Abnormal Psychology* 2000; *109*:150–155.

143. Hargus E, Crane C, Barnhofer T, Williams JM. Effects of mindfulness on meta-awareness and specificity of describing prodromal symptoms in suicidal depression. *Emotion* 2010; *10*:34–42.

144. Heeren A, Van Broeck N, Philippot P. The effects of mindfulness on executive processes and autobiographical memory specificity. *Behaviour Research and Therapy* 2010; *47*:403–409.

145. Kuyken W, Watkins E, Holden E, White K, Taylor RS, Byford S, Evans A, Radford S, Teasdale JD, Dalgleish T. How does mindfulness-based cognitive therapy work? *Behaviour Research and Therapy* 2010; *48*:1105–1112.

146. Baer RA, Smith GT, Allen KB. Assessment of mindfulness by self-report: The Kentucky Inventory of Mindfulness Skills. *Assessment* 2004, *11*:191–206.

147. Neff K. The development and validation of a scale to measure self-compassion. *Self and Identity* 2003; *2*:223–250.

148. Beiling P, Hawley L, Corcoran K, Bloch R, Levitan R, Young T, MacQueen G, Segal Z. Mediators of treatment efficacy in mindfulness-based cognitive therapy, antidepressant pharmacotherapy, or placebo for prevention of depressive relapse. *Journal of Consulting and Clinical Psychology* 2012; *80*:365–372.

149. Fresco DM, Moore MT, van Dulmen MH, Segal ZV, Ma SH, Teasdale JD, Williams JM. Initial psychometric properties of the Experiences Questionnaire: Validation of a self-report measure of decentering. *Behavior Therapy* 2007; *38*:234–246.

150. Leary MR, Tate EB, Adams CE, Allen AB, Hancock J. Self-compassion and reactions to unpleasant self-relevant events: The implications of treating oneself kindly. *Journal of Personality and Social Psychology* 2007; *92*:887–904.

151. Raes F, DeWulf D, Van Heeringen C, Williams JMG. Mindfulness and reduced cognitive reactivity to sad mood: Evidence from a correlational study and a non-randomized waiting list controlled study. *Behaviour Research and Therapy* 2009; *47*:623–627.

152. Davidson RJ, Kabat-Zinn J, Schumacher J, Rosenkranz M, Muller D, Santorelli SF, Urbanowski F, Harrington A, Bonus K, Sheridan JF. Alterations in brain and immune function produced by mindfulness meditation. *Psychosomatic Medicine* 2003; *65*:564–570.

153. Barnhofer T, Duggan D, Crane C, Hepburn S, Fennell MJ, Williams JM. Effects of meditation on frontal alpha-asymmetry in previously suicidal individuals. *NeuroReport* 2007; *18*:709–712.

154. Lazar SW, Kerr C, Wasserman RH, Gray JR, Greve D, Treadway MT, McGarvey M, Quinn BT, Dusek JA, Benson H, Rauch SL, Moore CI, Fischl B. Meditation experience is associated with increased cortical thickness. *NeuroReport* 2005; *16*:1893–1897.

155. Hölzel BK, Carmody J, Vangel M, Congleton C, Yerramsetti SM, Gard T, Lazar SW. Mindfulness practice leads to increases in regional brain gray matter density. *Psychiatry Research: Neuroimaging* 2011; *191*:36–42.

156. Farb NAS, Segal ZV, Mayberg H, Bean J, McKeon D, Fatima Z, Anderson AK. Attending to the present: Mindfulness meditation reveals distinct neural modes of self-reference. *Social Cognitive and Affective Neuroscience* 2007; *2*:313–322.

157. Watkins E, Teasdale JD. Rumination and overgeneral memory in depression: Effects of self-focus and analytic thinking. *Journal of Abnormal Psychology* 2001; *110*:353–357.

158. Farb NAS, Anderson AK, Mayberg H, Bean J, McKeon D, Segal ZV. Minding emotions: Mindfulness training alters the neural expression of sadness. *Emotion* 2010; *10*:25–33.

159. Goldstein J, Kornfeld J. *Seeking the heart of wisdom: The path of insight meditation.* Boston: Shambhala, 1987.

160. Teasdale JD, Williams JMG, Segal, ZV. *The mindfulness-based cognitive therapy workbook.* New York: Guilford Press. Manuscript in preparation.

161. Williams JMG, Penman D. *Mindfulness: A practical guide to finding peace in a frantic world.* London: Piatkus Books, 2011.

162. Orsillo SM, Roemer L. *The mindful way through anxiety: Break free from chronic worry and reclaim your life.* New York: Guilford Press, 2011.

163. Germer CK. *The mindful path to self-compassion: Freeing yourself from destructive thoughts and emotions.* New York: Guilford Press, 2009.

Index

List of Audio Files

Track	Title	Run Time
1	Welcome and Introduction	00:30
2	Raisin Exercise	09:13
3	Body Scan	37:47
4	10-Minute Sitting Meditation—Mindfulness of the Breath	11:20
5	Mindful Movement—Formal Practice	38:25
6	Stretch and Breath Meditation	40:41
7	Mindful Walking	32:24
8	3-Minute Breathing Space—Regular Version	04:08
9	3-Minute Breathing Space—Responsive Version	04:58
10	20-Minute Sitting Meditation	20:32
11	Sitting Meditation	36:46
12	Working with Difficulty Meditation	24:08
13	Bells at 5 Minutes, 10 Minutes, 15 Minutes, 20 Minutes, and 30 Minutes	30:32